Clinical Nutrition
in Athletic Training

Clinical Nutrition in Athletic Training

Editor

Mark Knoblauch, PhD, LAT, ATC, CSCS

Clinical Associate Professor

Clinical Coordinator, Second-Year MAT Students

Coordinator of Research

Department of Health and Human Performance

University of Houston

Houston, Texas

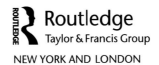

Routledge
Taylor & Francis Group

NEW YORK AND LONDON

First published 2023 by SLACK Incorporated

Published 2024 by Routledge
605 Third Avenue, New York, NY 10158

and by Routledge
4 Park Square, Milton Park, Abingdon, Oxon, OX14 4RN

Routledge is an imprint of the Taylor & Francis Group, an informa business

The *2020 Standards for Accreditation of Professional Athletic Training Programs* listed at the beginning of each chapter are cited from Commission on Accreditation of Athletic Training Education. *Standards and Procedures for Accreditation of Professional Programs in Athletic Training.* Author; 2022.

Library of Congress Control Number: 2022946474

Cover Artist: Lori Shields

ISBN: 9781630918040 (pbk)
ISBN: 9781003523079 (ebk)

DOI: 10.4324/9781003523079

Contents

Acknowledgments

Writing a textbook can be as difficult as it can be rewarding. Without the assistance of the team of writers involved in developing *Clinical Nutrition in Athletic Training,* this book would not exist. Therefore, my first and most directed "thank you" as editor goes out to each of the contributing authors who took time out of their schedules over the past year to develop the outstanding chapters in this book. While it is not always easy for a book production schedule to be adhered to, the authors involved in this project met each deadline without fail. It is because of their efforts that this book became a reality.

Because the process of writing can be a time-consuming ordeal, the families and loved ones of each contributing author also deserve a special thanks for being accepting of the time, effort, and sometimes even frustration involved with each author's desire to get their chapter "just right." Only once the book is in print is the time and effort spent writing finally realized, and those who supported each chapter author deserve to be recognized.

Personally, I want to thank every colleague of mine who offered support, encouragement, and guidance along the journey of moving this book from concept to completion. I also want to acknowledge my family for allowing me the time needed to write and organize this book.

Finally, I want to thank the publisher, SLACK Incorporated, for being accepting of my vision for this project and giving it the chance to come to fruition.

About the Editor

Mark Knoblauch, PhD, LAT, ATC, CSCS is a clinical associate professor and clinical coordinator of the Master of Athletic Training program at the University of Houston in Texas. He has been certified as an athletic trainer since 1996, and has worked clinically at both the university and junior college level. Mark received his PhD in Kinesiology from the University of Houston and completed a post-doctoral fellowship in Molecular Physiology and Biophysics from Baylor College of Medicine in Houston, Texas, where his research focus was on skeletal muscle damage and signaling mechanisms. He is a member of the National Athletic Trainers' Association (NATA), the National Strength and Conditioning Association, and the Southwest Athletic Trainers' Association (SWATA) and is a site visitor for the Commission on Accreditation of Athletic Training Education. As a professional he has been involved with several committees for the NATA and SWATA, and has written several books in the areas of diet, fitness, and vestibular disorders, as well as served as editor of the book *Professional Writing in Kinesiology and Sports Medicine.*

Contributing Authors

Melissa Brown, PhD, RD, CSSD, LD (Chapter 10)
Department of Nutrition and Public Health
University of Saint Joseph
West Hartford, Connecticut

Melanie Clark, MS, RD, CSSD, LD (Chapter 5)
Sports Dietitian
Sun Devil Athletics
Arizona State University
Tempe, Arizona

Kyla Cross, MS, MPH, RD, LD (Chapters 5 and 8)
Sport Dietitian for the Columbus Crew
Columbus, Ohio

Jon P. Gray, EdD (Chapter 12)
Instructional Professor
Department of Health and Human Performance
University of Houston
Houston, Texas

Layci Harrison, PhD, LAT, ATC (Chapter 7)
Clinical Assistant Professor
Master of Athletic Training Program
Department of Health and Human Performance
University of Houston
Houston, Texas

Christina Curry King, MS, RD, CSSD, LD (Chapter 6)
Sports Dietitian
Memorial Hermann
Rockets Sports Medicine Institute
Houston, Texas

Tara LaRowe, PhD, RDN, CSSD, CD (Chapter 11)
Assistant Teaching Professor
Department of Nutritional Sciences
University of Wisconsin—Madison
Madison, Wisconsin

Tracey Ledoux, PhD, RD (Chapter 12)
Department of Health and Human Performance
University of Houston
Houston, Texas

Tabbetha D. Lopez, PhD, RD, LD (Chapter 12)
Assistant Professor and Dietetic Internship Director
Sam Houston State University
Huntsville, Texas

Mindy A. Patterson, PhD, RDN (Chapter 2)
Associate Professor, Nutrition and Food Sciences
Co-Director, Institute for Women's Health
Institute of Health Sciences
Texas Woman's University
Houston, Texas

Andrea Rudser-Rusin, MA, ATC, RD, CSSD (Chapter 1)
SportWise Nutrition & Consulting, LLC
Adjunct Faculty
DePaul University
Chicago, Illinois

Brett Singer, MS, RD, CSSD, LD (Chapters 5 and 8)
Memorial Hermann
Rockets Sports Medicine Institute
Houston, Texas

Sarah Snyder, MS, RD, CSSD, LD, CSCS (Chapter 4)
Director of Nutrition
Baltimore Ravens
Baltimore, Maryland

E. Joanna Soles, DHSc, ATC, LAT (Chapter 13)
University of the Incarnate Word
Associate Professor/Clinical Education Coordinator
Department of Athletic Training
San Antonio, Texas

Cathy Tillery, MS, RD, CSSD, LD (Chapter 9)
Woodstock, Georgia

Mandy Tyler, MEd, RD, CSSD, LD, LAT (Chapter 13)
Sports Dietitian Consultant
Bulverde, Texas

Penny Wilson, PhD, RDN (Chapter 15)
Eating For Performance
Vail, Colorado

Preface

Nutrition is a key component of an individual's overall health and wellness. Among active individuals, the role of nutrition is often enhanced due to the body's need for fuel in response to an increased activity level, as well as to ensure an adequate supply of nutrients to allow the body to properly recover from the physical stresses imposed by physical activity. In addition to fueling and recovery concerns, the importance of proper nutrition within the context of physical activity also warrants an understanding of those ancillary aspects of nutrition, such as eating disorders and weight management, as well as the wide variety of available diets that can serve to provide a strong foundation for engaging in productive physical activity.

Athletic trainers, who often work closely with physically active individuals in a variety of settings, can utilize many of the underlying principles of clinical nutrition to enhance patient care. For those athletic trainers working in an athletic setting, there is no doubt that nutrition—when coupled with factors such as proper workout plans and adequate recovery—can be a vital component of a quality sports performance plan. Separately, for those athletic trainers employed in nontraditional settings involving patients or clients who often have individualized goals, such as running a 5K or simply improving their health, nutrition can play a key role in their overall success. Bone and heart health, fatigue, blood pressure, endurance, and a wealth of other conditions can often be influenced by nutrition, and it is vital that athletic trainers understand the role and the importance of nutrition in overall health.

Clinical Nutrition in Athletic Training is written for students as well as practicing athletic trainers in order to strengthen their understanding of many of the clinical-based aspects of nutrition. To accomplish this, the book pulls together an assembly of experienced athletic trainers and dietitians to cover the most relevant topics that athletic trainers can use to improve patient care for physically active individuals. The book opens with an introduction to the role that nutrition can play in physical activity, followed by an overview of macronutrients and micronutrients. The various energy systems are then reviewed, after which hydration principles as well as the role of supplements in nutrition is discussed. Next, nutrition's role in weight management and injury recovery is outlined, followed by an overview of how nutrition and physical activity are linked. Then, pathologies associated with nutrition are discussed, followed by a chapter discussing the various eating disorders as well as how proper nutrition can be maintained while traveling. Lastly, food package labels are discussed before closing with details on how athletic trainers can conduct an effective nutrition counseling session. Collectively, these chapters are intended to provide the athletic trainer with essential information in clinical nutrition that can improve their athlete's, patient's, or client's ability to achieve their fitness and activity goals.

The influence of nutrition in areas of health and wellness cannot be overstated. This book was written to address the influence that nutrition can have in helping athletic trainers relay the most relevant information that can, in turn, improve patient care. The content of the book is focused toward clinical nutrition; therefore, detailed chemical processes and intricate physiological events are largely avoided in most chapters, instead focusing mainly on the clinical application of various nutrition concepts. And while the principles of nutrition are themselves quite science-based, the tone of the book is focused on presenting these principles in a clear and understandable fashion. In the end, we hope that you find the book to be engaging as well as beneficial to your own education and practice.

Chapter 1

The Basis for Nutrition

Andrea Rudser-Rusin, MA, ATC, RD, CSSD

Commission on Accreditation of Athletic Training Education *2020 Standards*

CAATE has established the *2020 Standards for Accreditation of Professional Athletic Training Programs* at the master's level to meet the learning needs of the athletic trainer and the skills that they are expected to perform. These include nutrition-related knowledge and skills in the Patient-Centered Care Core Competencies.[1] This chapter addresses the following *2020 Standards for Accreditation of Professional Athletic Training Programs*:

- Standard 55: Students must gain foundational knowledge in statistics, research design, epidemiology, pathophysiology, biomechanics and pathomechanics, exercise physiology, nutrition, human anatomy, pharmacology, public health, and health care delivery and payor systems.

- Standard 56: Advocate for the health needs of clients, patients, communities, and populations.

- Standard 58: Incorporate patient education and self-care programs to engage patients and their families and friends to participate in their care and recovery.

- Standard 59: Communicate effectively and appropriately with clients/patients, family members, coaches, administrators, other health care professionals, consumers, payors, policy makers, and others.

- Standard 61: Practice in collaboration with other health care and wellness professionals.

- Standard 69: Develop a care plan for each patient. The care plan includes (but is not limited to) the following:
  - Assessment of the patient on an ongoing basis and adjustment of care accordingly
  - Collection, analysis, and use of patient-reported and clinician-rated outcome measures to improve patient care
  - Consideration of the patient's goals and level of function in treatment decisions
  - Discharge of the patient when goals are met, or the patient is no longer making progress
  - Referral when warranted
- Standard 73: Select and incorporate interventions (for pre-op patients, post-op patients, and patients with nonsurgical conditions) that align with the care plan. Interventions include (but are not limited to) the following:
  - Home care management
  - Cardiovascular training

Knoblauch M, ed. *Clinical Nutrition in Athletic Training* (pp 1-12).
© 2023 Taylor & Francis Group.

- Standard 79: Develop and implement strategies to mitigate the risk for long-term health conditions across the lifespan. These include (but are not limited to) the following conditions:
  - Cardiovascular disease
  - Diabetes
  - Obesity
  - Osteoarthritis
- Standard 81: Plan and implement a comprehensive preparticipation examination process to affect health outcomes.

Therefore, familiarity with the tools/resources available and how to use these tools, understanding the relationship of lifestyle factors to chronic disease, and the role of proper fueling on performance and injury prevention and recovery are within the scope. Combined, understanding these concepts is essential for a professional working under the umbrella of "sports medicine."

Learning Objectives

After reviewing this chapter, readers will be able to:

- Explain the history, development, and relationships of the *Healthy People* initiative, the *Dietary Guidelines for Americans, Physical Activity Guidelines for Americans*, and MyPlate.
- Apply the basic tools available for building a healthy diet, including applying the *Dietary Guidelines, 2020-2025* at all life stages, as well as using MyPlate and all its new resources.
- Explain the *Physical Activity Guidelines* and identify the additional health benefits of regular physical activity beyond the more familiar cardiovascular fitness benefits.
- Describe the SportWise Fueling Plate and its application for fueling activity and recovery, as well as meeting micronutrient needs.
- Define energy balance (ie, when a positive or negative energy balance may be seen) and why RED-S can be detrimental to an individual's health and performance.
- Identify areas of nutrition needing further research relative to injury management and understand the current limitations to studying acute injuries.
- Differentiate the roles that the registered dietitian/nutritionist, registered dietitian/nutritionist with the CSSD credential, and the nutritionist can have when working with newly active, active, and high-level persons.

Introduction: Nutrition and the Athletic Trainer

The study of nutrition and its role in health, disease management, and prevention has grown significantly since the turn of the 21st century. The combined efforts of various government agencies have made it their mission to encourage people to take control of their health by establishing nutrition and physical activity guidelines and tools that are more actionable and user friendly. On the other end of the spectrum, sport and exercise nutrition has also grown by leaps and bounds. Colleges and universities, professional sports, military and tactical groups, and commercial sporting and training organizations nationwide are adding registered dietitians to their staff to educate athletes on how to properly fuel their bodies to optimize performance and reduce the risk of injury. All the while, the athletic trainer is in the trenches working with the patient/athlete on a daily basis. In these cases, the athletic trainer may be the first medical professional that the patient encounters with perceived knowledge of nutrition who might be able to help them on their journey back to health or achieve their performance goals. While not a nutrition expert, working within the scope of practice as an athletic trainer still requires a thorough understanding of the concepts of nutrition. In fact, the CAATE *Standards* for accreditation of professional athletic training programs include nutrition-related objectives.[1] Those *Standards* have been delineated at the beginning of this chapter.

Sidebar 1-1

Chronic diseases, such as heart disease, cancer and diabetes, are responsible for 7 out of every 10 deaths among Americans each year, and account for 75% of the nation's health spending. Many of the risk factors that contribute to the development of these diseases are preventable.[3]

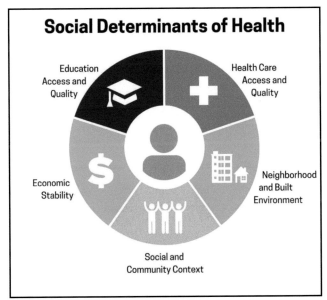

Figure 1-1. Social determinants of health (SDOH) consider environments that affect people's health, functioning, and quality-of-life outcomes and risks. The 5 domains of the SDOH include Education Access and Quality, Health Care Access and Quality, Neighborhood and Built Environment, Social and Community Context, and Economic Stability. (Reproduced from US Department of Health and Human Services, Office of Disease Prevention and Health Promotion. *Healthy People 2030*. Retrieved July 15, 2022 from https://health.gov/healthypeople/priority-areas/social-determinants-health.)

"Let Food Be Thy Medicine, and Medicine Be Thy Food" —Hippocrates

In 2014, the World Health Organization (WHO) attributed more than two-thirds of deaths worldwide to chronic diseases: cancer, cardiovascular disease, chronic respiratory disease, and diabetes. Well-established evidence shows that the incidence of these diseases share modifiable risk factors—alcohol consumption, cigarette smoking, body mass index (BMI), unhealthy diet, and physical inactivity—that account for more than two-thirds of these diseases.[2] It was reported that regardless of sex, there was a positive, dose-response relationship for BMI >25 and risk of first chronic disease;

Sidebar 1-2

This is a summary of the *Health Care Access and Quality Objectives*, with the goal of increasing access to comprehensive, high-quality health care services[5]:

- Reduce the proportion of people who cannot get medical care and prescription medicines when they need them.

- Increase the proportion of people with a usual primary care provider (PCP), and the ability of PCP and behavioral health professionals to provide more high-quality care to patients who need it.

- Increase the proportion of adults whose health care providers involve them in decisions as much as they want, and decrease the proportion of adults who report poor communication with their health care providers.

- Increase in the proportion of adults whose health care providers verify their understanding, and those with limited English proficiency report their providers explain things clearly.

whereas, there is an inverse response when investigating the daily consumption of fruits and vegetables and levels of physical activity and first chronic disease. Multimorbidity (having 2 or more and 3 or more chronic diseases from a list of 9) places a significant strain on the health care system, as individuals with multimorbidity have complex care needs and greater health expenditures.[2]

Chronic diseases, such as heart disease, cancer, and diabetes, are responsible for 7 out of every 10 deaths among Americans each year and account for 75% of the nation's health spending (Sidebar 1-1).[3] Later chapters will further explore the association of diet and chronic diseases.

Since the initial publication in 1979, every 10 years the federal government publishes a national public health agenda with science-based objectives to "increase the quality and years of healthy life" and "eliminate health disparities."[4] And so began the *Healthy People* initiative. Now in its fifth iteration, *Healthy People 2030* aims to improve health and well-being over the next decade for people of all ages—infants, children and adolescents, adults and older adults, and general population. Shifting slightly from previous versions to now focus on health equity, it does so by also prioritizing social determinants of health (SDOH) and improving outcomes related to health literacy (Sidebar 1-2). These are priority areas an athletic trainer will encounter almost daily (Figure 1-1).[5,6]

Figure 1-2. *Dietary Guidelines for Americans, 2020-2025.* (Reproduced with permission from US Department of Agriculture and US Department of Health and Human Services. *Dietary Guidelines for Americans, 2020-2025.* 9th ed. December 2020. Available at DietaryGuidelines.gov.)

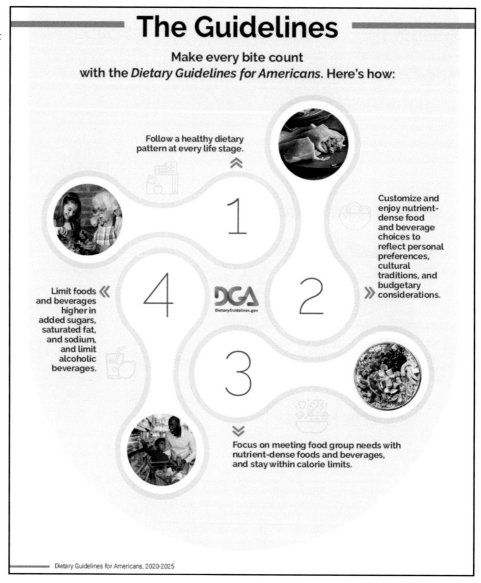

Guides to Building a Healthy Diet and Lifestyle

Every 5 years the US Department of Health and Human Services and the US Department of Agriculture (USDA) jointly publish the *Dietary Guidelines for Americans.*

Each edition of the *Dietary Guidelines* reflects the current body of nutrition science, helps health professionals and policymakers guide Americans to make healthy food and beverage choices, and serves as the science-based foundation for vital nutrition policies and programs across the United States.[4]

The *Dietary Guidelines, 2020-2025* supports messages presented in *Healthy People 2030,* encouraging healthy eating at all stages of the lifespan, to promote health, and reduce the risk of all-cause morbidity and mortality of persons of all ages.[7] See Figure 1-2 for the 4 guidelines for creating healthy, adaptable eating plans.

The *Dietary Guidelines, 2015-2020* emphasized making smart choices from all food groups, choosing nutrient-dense foods, and balancing intake with physical activity to maintain weight.[8] Building upon those recommendations, the *Dietary Guidelines, 2020-2025* reinforces that "healthy eating is key to a healthy life." It is with the current *Dietary Guidelines* that we see, for the first time, recommendations are provided for each life stage, from birth through older adulthood (Sidebar 1-3).[7]

Keeping in mind the themes throughout the *Dietary Guidelines*—"Make Every Bite Count" and "Small Changes Matter"—a health practitioner may guide the conversation with a patient as they seek to improve and maintain health by applying the 3 key, guiding principles[7]:

Sidebar 1-3

The ninth edition of the *Dietary Guidelines* is the first to provide guidance for healthy dietary patterns by life stage (including women who are pregnant or lactating) to meet nutrient needs, promote health, and help prevent chronic disease.[7]

- **Birth through 23 months:** Lowers the risk of overweight/obesity, type 1 diabetes, iron deficiency, peanut allergy, and asthma.

- **Children and adolescents:** Lowers adiposity and total and low-density lipoprotein (LDL) cholesterol.

- **Women who are pregnant or lactating:** Supports favorable cognitive development in the child and folate status in women during pregnancy and lactation.

- **Adults, including older adults:** Lowers the risk of all-cause mortality, cardiovascular disease and mortality, obesity, type 2 diabetes, and certain cancers. Supports lifestyle to lower total and LDL cholesterol, blood pressure, BMI, waist circumference, and body fat—of which all are risk factors to the aforementioned diseases. Supports favorable bone health, contributing to lower risk of hip fracture.

1. Meet nutritional needs primarily from nutrient-dense foods and beverages
2. Choose a variety of options from each food group
3. Pay attention to portion size

The *Dietary Guidelines* can be applied to persons of all ages, sizes, and activity level (including athletes).

The relationship between diet and physical activity contributes to achieving and maintaining a healthy body weight and reducing the risk for developing high blood pressure, high cholesterol, diabetes, heart disease, stroke, and cancer,[4] to name a few. In fact, 4 of the top 10 leading causes of death are related to poor diet and insufficient physical activity. Only 1 in 4 adults and 1 in 5 adolescents in the United States meet physical activity guidelines for aerobic and muscle-strengthening activities. Unfortunately, 26% of men and 19% of women, and only 20% of adolescents, report achieving sufficient activity.[9] As such, *Physical Activity Guidelines for Americans* has been written to help promote health and reduce the risk of chronic disease. *Physical Activity Guidelines* (Figure 1-3) is issued by the US Department of Health and Human Services.

The *Physical Activity Guidelines, Second Edition,* cites that being physically active is one of the most important actions that people of all ages can take to improve their health and includes recommendations for preschool (ages 3 to 5) through adulthood.[10] In fact, being physically active was identified as one of the Leading Health Indicators of the *Healthy People 2020 Midcourse Review* (Figure 1-4). At the time of writing the *Healthy People 2030* report, Americans were still at the baseline for general physical activity objectives. Children and adolescents received a "getting worse" status for objectives (3) relating to increasing proportion of children and/or adolescents participating in aerobic and muscle strengthening activities and participation in sport. It is the newly active, or those exercising to improve their health, with whom the *Dietary Guidelines* and *Physical Activity Guidelines* will be best for the athletic trainer to use to begin conversations of lifestyle changes.

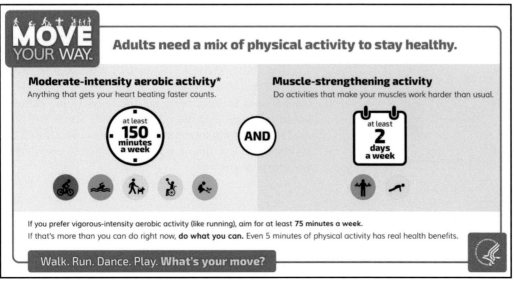

Figure 1-3. *Physical Activity Guidelines for Americans.* (Reproduced with permission from Office of Disease Prevention and Health Promotion, https://health.gov/paguidelines/second-edition/.)

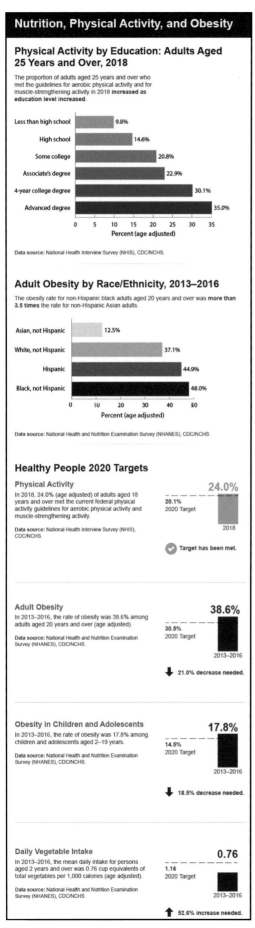

Nutrition, Physical Activity, and Obesity

Physical Activity by Education: Adults Aged 25 Years and Over, 2018

The proportion of adults aged 25 years and over who met the guidelines for aerobic physical activity and for muscle-strengthening activity in 2018 **increased as education level increased.**

Education	Percent
Less than high school	9.8%
High school	14.6%
Some college	20.8%
Associate's degree	22.9%
4-year college degree	30.1%
Advanced degree	35.0%

Percent (age adjusted)

Data source: National Health Interview Survey (NHIS), CDC/NCHS.

Adult Obesity by Race/Ethnicity, 2013–2016

The obesity rate for non-Hispanic black adults aged 20 years and over was **more than 3.5 times** the rate for non-Hispanic Asian adults.

Race/Ethnicity	Percent
Asian, not Hispanic	12.5%
White, not Hispanic	37.1%
Hispanic	44.9%
Black, not Hispanic	48.0%

Percent (age adjusted)

Data source: National Health and Nutrition Examination Survey (NHANES), CDC/NCHS.

Healthy People 2020 Targets

Physical Activity — **24.0%**
In 2018, 24.0% (age adjusted) of adults aged 18 years and over met the current federal physical activity guidelines for aerobic physical activity and muscle-strengthening activity. 20.1% 2020 Target. 2018. Target has been met.

Data source: National Health Interview Survey (NHIS), CDC/NCHS.

Adult Obesity — **38.6%**
In 2013–2016, the rate of obesity was 38.6% among adults aged 20 years and over (age adjusted). 30.5% 2020 Target. 2013–2016. 21.0% decrease needed.

Data source: National Health and Nutrition Examination Survey (NHANES), CDC/NCHS.

Obesity in Children and Adolescents — **17.8%**
In 2013–2016, the rate of obesity was 17.8% among children and adolescents aged 2–19 years. 14.5% 2020 Target. 2013–2016. 18.5% decrease needed.

Data source: National Health and Nutrition Examination Survey (NHANES), CDC/NCHS.

Daily Vegetable Intake — **0.76**
In 2013–2016, the mean daily intake for persons aged 2 years and over was 0.76 cup equivalents of total vegetables per 1,000 calories (age adjusted). 1.16 2020 Target. 2013–2016. 52.6% increase needed.

Data source: National Health and Nutrition Examination Survey (NHANES), CDC/NCHS.

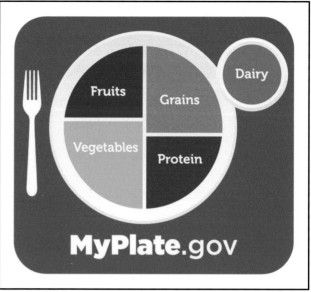

Figure 1-5. MyPlate. (Reproduced with permission from www.myplate.gov.)

Putting It Into Practice

The nutrition facts label is a tool plentiful of information, but very misunderstood. Chapter 14 will take a more in-depth look at the new, overhauled label. In the meantime, the key understanding should be that the changes made to the new label are reflective of the most recent scientific findings of the relationship of individual nutrients and health of Americans—think *Healthy People* and *Dietary Guidelines*. It is the role of the athletic trainer, again often the first point of contact for persons on a journey to health and wellness, to know the meaning of items listed on the label and why. Most importantly, while we as people eat food, nutrients do matter. It is the nutrition facts label that can empower the patient/athlete to make wise food choices for improved quality of life, better performance, and efficient recovery, based on the individual nutrients of that particular food item and the needs of the individual. See Chapters 2 and 3 for a more in-depth understanding of the role each nutrient (macronutrients and micronutrients, respectively) plays in health and performance, and see Chapter 14 to better understand the power of using the nutrition facts label to build a healthy diet.

The USDA MyPlate (Figure 1-5) is a visual representation of the advice contained in the *Dietary Guidelines*. It was released in 2011 replacing the Food Guide Pyramid (or Eating Right Pyramid or MyPyramid), which had been used in a variety of formats for nearly 2 decades. The USDA MyPlate is a tool that is readily accessible to everyone at www.myplate.gov.[11]

Figure 1-4. Leading health indicators: nutrition, physical activity, and obesity. (Reproduced with permission from the US Department of Health and Human Services, Office of Disease Prevention and Health Promotion. https://www.healthypeople.gov/2020/leading-health-indicators/infographic/nutrition-physical-activity-and-obesity-5?width=618&height=100%25&date=Sep-2019.)

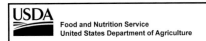

USDA Food and Nutrition Service
United States Department of Agriculture

MyPlate.gov

Start *simple* with **MyPlate** Plan

The benefits of healthy eating add up over time, bite by bite. Small changes matter. Start Simple with MyPlate.

A healthy eating routine is important at every stage of life and can have positive effects that add up over time. It's important to eat a variety of fruits, vegetables, grains, protein foods, and dairy or fortified soy alternatives. When deciding what to eat or drink, choose options that are full of nutrients. Make every bite count.

Food Group Amounts for 1,800 Calories a Day for Ages 14+ Years

Fruits	Vegetables	Grains	Protein	Dairy
1½ cups	**2½ cups**	**6 ounces**	**5 ounces**	**3 cups**
Focus on whole fruits	Vary your veggies	Make half your grains whole grains	Vary your protein routine	Move to low-fat or fat-free dairy milk or yogurt (or lactose-free dairy or fortified soy versions)
Focus on whole fruits that are fresh, frozen, canned, or dried.	Choose a variety of colorful fresh, frozen, and canned vegetables—make sure to include dark green, red, and orange choices.	Find whole-grain foods by reading the Nutrition Facts label and ingredients list.	Mix up your protein foods to include seafood; beans, peas, and lentils; unsalted nuts and seeds; soy products; eggs; and lean meats and poultry.	Look for ways to include dairy or fortified soy alternatives at meals and snacks throughout the day.

Limit — Choose foods and beverages with less added sugars, saturated fat, and sodium. Limit:
- Added sugars to **<45 grams** a day.
- Saturated fat to **<20 grams** a day.
- Sodium to **<2,300 milligrams** a day.

Activity — Be active your way:
Children 6 to 17 years old should move **60 minutes** every day. Adults should be physically active at least **2½ hours** per week.

Figure 1-6. Sample USDA MyPlate Plan, based on a 50-year-old, 5′5″ female weighing 135 pounds. She is currently not meeting the physical activity recommendation of at least 150 minutes of moderate-intensity physical activity per week. (Reproduced with permission from https://myplate-prod. azureedge.us/sites/default/files/2021-08/2020MyPlatePlan_1800cals_Age14%2B.pdf.)

While the USDA MyPlate has certain limitations, it is not meant to be a one size fits all; it is a starting point for improved health. The MyPlate Plan shows food group targets (what and how much to eat) within your calorie allowance. It is an interactive tool that is customized, with results based on the user's individual age, sex, height, weight, and physical activity level. The MyPlate Plan in Figure 1-6 is a sample of the individualized report that one receives when they use the Plate Planner tool. Also added with the most recent version of MyPlate is a QR code for using the Shop Simple tool to assist in shopping healthy and budget-wise in your area, the Start Simple with MyPlate App, and MyPlate on Alexa. All of these tools are available to everyone for free at https://www. myplate.gov/resources/tools.

Making appropriate food choices requires consumers to have some nutrition knowledge and understanding of how to use the tools available. It is with the guidance of the learned athletic trainer that the patient can begin putting the Key Recommendations of the *Dietary Guidelines* and the *Physical Activity Guidelines* into practice by using the MyPlate resources.

Finding a Balance

Nutritional balance is easier to illustrate to the client when tools such as the *Dietary Guidelines'* Key Recommendations, the nutrition facts label, and MyPlate, are available as guides for the athletic trainer's use. However, nutrition balance can easily be disrupted, and energy imbalance is often a result. Energy balance represents the individual meeting the fueling needs by the food and beverages they consume, relative to the energy expended through activities of daily living, exercise, and metabolism (Figure 1-7).[11] There is a clear link between "energy balance" and "health and performance."

When the energy intake exceeds the energy output, a positive energy balance occurs that will result in weight gain. Sometimes, positive energy balance is intentional, as in situations where one seeks to gain body mass. Most often this is done in hopes of increasing lean body mass, but gaining both muscle and fat occurs in most cases. In cases where a positive energy balance is not intentional and unhealthy patterns of adipose tissue are accumulated, one's health suffers. In fact, in America approximately 1 in 3 adults (34.0%) and 1 in 6

Figure 1-7. This teeter-totter–like image demonstrates the factors that contribute to one's energy (caloric) balance. (arka38/Shutterstock.com.)

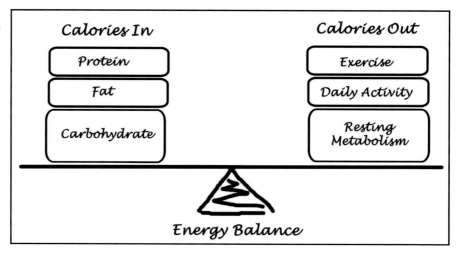

children and adolescents (16.2%) are obese (see Figure 1-4).[3] This is discussed further in Chapters 7 and 11.

When the energy intake falls short of the demands of energy expenditure, a negative energy balance occurs and weight loss will result. Negative energy balance may be intentional, with the end goal being to change body composition. When one's goal is to lower body fat for performance, improve their power to weight ratio, or for aesthetic purposes, they walk a delicate line and health can suffer. When the energy deficit is too great, low energy availability (LEA), can occur. In situations of LEA, physiological mechanisms (think regulatory hormones) reduce the amount of energy used for cellular maintenance, thermoregulation, growth, bone development, and reproduction. Extremely low energy intakes may impair performance and increase risk of nutritional deficiencies and illness, ultimately resulting in a clustering of physiological decrements described as Relative Energy Deficit in Sport (RED-S). The International Olympic Committee's interdisciplinary expert group defines RED-S as,

> compromised physiological function including, but not limited to, metabolic rate, menstrual function, bone health, immunity, protein synthesis, and cardiovascular health. The cause of this syndrome is energy deficiency relative to the balance between energy intake and energy expenditure required for health and activities of daily living, growth, and sporting activities.[12]

Because an athletic trainer will encounter a range of athletes from weekend warriors to the full-time professional, identifying imbalances can be difficult to identify. Familiarizing oneself with the RED-S model will better arm the athletic trainer to identify LEA in women and active men. Chapters 7, 11, and 12 will explore these topics in further depth. The goal of the RED-S model is to identify those at risk early, to prevent health complications and to allow early treatment to restore the normal function to the body.[13]

Performance Nutrition

Athletes can help themselves by eating well-balanced diets and avoid overconsuming or the opposite end of the spectrum, LEA. After all, *food is fuel*. Success in athletic activities that demand the ability to generate power, show great endurance, or demonstrate focus requires adequate fuel. It is well known that carbohydrates are the major fuel for muscle activity in high-intensity exercise (see Chapter 2 for more on macronutrient guidelines). When the stored carbohydrate (muscle glycogen) is depleted, the ability to generate power and intensity is lessened. It is during this submaximal exercise that fat begins to contribute a greater portion to the fuel utilized to power the activity. Perhaps one of the greatest areas where the self-coached (or the coach who fails to keep up with current literature) makes the most common mistake is in performance-fueling decisions—high carbohydrate, low carbohydrate, high fat, high protein, liquid fuel, train fasted ... the list goes on. What is best for the athlete from a performance standpoint? The correct answer is, "It depends." Chapter 10 will explore the energy requirements specific to different types of activity and the corresponding macronutrient recommendations. The SportWise Fueling Plate (Figure 1-8) from SportWise Nutrition & Consulting, LLC[14] is a tool the athletic trainer, coach, or parent can rely on to fuel the athlete properly, according to the energy needs of the day.

Use of the SportWise Fueling Plate can be an effective tool and successfully executed if there is an understanding of the demands of exercise. After all, no 2 days are alike for an athlete. Chapter 4 will offer a refresher of the energy systems and the role nutrition plays, in relation to performance.

Bear in mind that the body of knowledge of sport and exercise nutrition is meager when comparing to other bodies of research related to exercise physiology and performance ergogenics. However, this is an exciting time for nutrition in sports. More value is being placed on diet periodization,

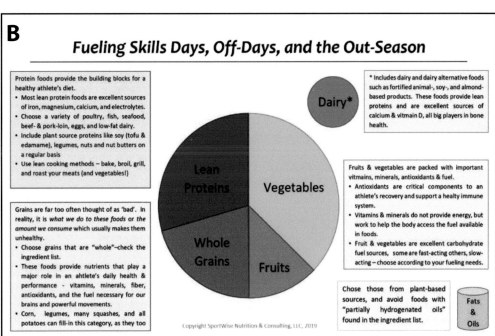

Figure 1-8. (A) SportWise Fueling Plate eating plan ideal for an athlete at a meal where they have (or will) partake in a moderate- or high-intensity workout; or on a day when 2-a-day workouts are on the schedule and the fuel tank needs to be full for the next workout. (B) SportWise Fueling Plate for those meals/days where activity is light, but balanced nutrition is still essential. (Reproduced with permission from www.SportWiseNutrition.com.)

not only from the perspective of the annual training cycle but also in the microcycles within the competitive seasons. What is known at this time in sport science is that to improve health, perform at the highest level possible, and support the demands of training, balanced nutrition is essential. Areas where further research is merited is nutrition specific to injury recovery.

Nutrition in Injury Prevention and Return to Sport

Exploring the influence of nutrition on injury prevention and injury recovery is a challenging one. At this time we do not have a solid grasp on the specific application of nutrients in injured athletes, especially in the acutely injured state (eg, we cannot go around breaking legs for the sake of satisfying our curiosity). Therefore, our *(n)* is limited to the human studies relative to that which is available in the animal model. Where we have made significant ground is in the area

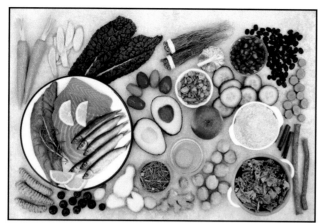

Figure 1-9. A well-balanced diet, which includes a variety of colorful fruits and vegetables, roots, seeds, nuts, and food rich in omega-3 fatty acids, can provide invaluable nutrients and phytochemicals essential to maintaining health and remaining in recovery. (marilyn barbone/Shutterstock.com.)

of concussion and head injury research, but questions still remain to be answered.[15] What we do know from studying chronic disease and starvation is that adequate and balanced nutrition is essential. Figure 1-9 shows food representative of food groups providing nutrients and phytochemicals that are invaluable to maintaining or returning the athlete to health. The Nutrition for Injury Recovery and Nutrition-Influenced Disorders chapters (Chapters 8 and 11, respectively) will take a more in-depth look into the role that one's diet can have on one's return to the playing field.

Working With Nutrition Professionals

This chapter has served as an introduction to the relationship that nutrition plays in health and performance (injury management included), and to emphasize the need for the athletic trainer to have a thorough understanding of these relationships. While the CAATE *Standards* include nutrition-related knowledge and skills, working within the scope of practice as an athletic trainer may still require a referral to a nutrition professional. Therefore, a thorough understanding of the value each allied health practitioner can contribute to the sports medicine team is essential. It is this team that makes the whole greater than the sum of all parts. From a nutrition and fueling standpoint, in the United States, the athletic trainer will come upon both nutritionists and registered dietitian nutritionists (RDN).[16] The titles are not interchangeable, yet "nutritionist" can be inclusive of both (Sidebar 1-4). The title "nutritionist" is not as regulated as "dietitian," and tends to have a broader, more general meaning. The title of "nutritionist" is also not generally protected, meaning that it can be used by anyone. Nutritionists often do not have any professional training and, therefore, should be neither diagnosing nor treating any diseases. One of the major differences is that a dietitian can help the patient/client

---

Sidebar 1-4

Every Registered Dietitian Is a Nutritionist, but Not Every Nutritionist Is a Registered Dietitian.

"The 'RD' and 'RDN' credential can only be used by practitioners who are currently authorized by the Commission on Dietetic Registration of the Academy of Nutrition and Dietetics."[16]

---

develop nutrition-related intervention plans for the management of their health problems and diseases. While nutritionists can certainly offer support in these areas, most of their work deals with food behavior. RDNs are food and nutrition experts who have completed a minimum of a bachelor's degree at an accredited college/university, completed an accredited supervised practice program, and passed a national examination.[17] As with any medical professional, RDNs must complete continuing professional educational requirements to maintain their RDN credential. Some states have licensure/registration standards these professionals must also meet.

RDNs who have specialized experience in sports dietetics, and have met minimum requirements, may sit for an advanced certification exam. Passing of the exam demonstrates that the RDN is CSSD (Board-Certified as a Specialist in Sports Dietetics) and has successfully demonstrated they have specific knowledge, skills, and expertise for competency in sports dietetics practice.[18] Specialty certification differentiates sports dietitians from those who are less qualified to provide sports nutrition services.

Conclusion

The *Standards* established by the CAATE include nutrition-related knowledge and skills in the *Patient-Centered Care Core Competencies*.[1] Without understanding of basic concepts related to health and performance, the athletic trainer is poorly equipped in their role as a health care provider. The information included in this introductory chapter has provided tools for the athletic trainer's "toolbox" to be well-equipped. Familiarity with the "tools" introduced in this chapter (*Healthy People, Dietary Guidelines, Physical Activity Guidelines,* USDA MyPlate, and SportWise Fueling Plate) and the background to their development allows the athletic trainer to begin the conversations of balanced nutrition and performance fueling more easily.

In the forthcoming chapters, the reader will dive deeper into the topics introduced in this introductory chapter. Application of the basic concepts and their relationship to health, disease, performance, and recovery will be explored in further depth. Knowledge of the consequences of nutrition imbalance, be it overnutrition or LEA, will enable the athletic trainer to sit in the forefront, to advocate **for** the patient and **to** the community of the importance of nutrition programming, and to ensure access to the appropriate professionals of the multidisciplinary team.

Case Studies

Case Study 1

You are in a clinic working with Alice, a 45-year-old female, 2 months status post ACL repair. You compliment her on her noticeable, significant weight loss. During your conversation Alice explains she began eating a vegetarian diet. She reports she has lost 40 pounds in the past 4 months and now her BMI is 32. She continues to explain that her dietary changes were motivated by her surgeon telling her she has some arthritis in her knee and needs to lose weight, lowering her BMI to under 30 (it was 38 at that time). "Just 2 more points to go!" she proclaims. She goes on to explain she is enjoying the diet while still including eggs and dairy, is eating 3 meals a day, and snacks on Melba toast, cherry tomatoes, and cottage cheese. Alice speaks with excitement of her progress. She chuckles a bit when telling, "despite always feeling cold, I crave chewing on ice, even more since going vegetarian and my recent weight loss." Alice's tone then changes and she appears disheartened when she tells of getting winded easily during workouts and just doesn't have the "oomph" for daily chores; "I thought it was going to get easier as I got more fit and had less weight to carry around."

1. Based on the information gained during this conversation, what nutrients may be of concern?
2. What may be contributing to Alice's cold intolerance and fatigue with activity?
3. Can Alice meet all her nutrient needs while following a lacto-ovo vegetarian diet?

Case Study 2

A collegiate men's volleyball player visited his athletic trainer, hoping to receive some guidance as to how he could improve his body composition, "you know, lose the fluff," he states. He goes on to say that it is his junior year, his chance to step up and be a team leader. In doing so, he feels he needs to clean up his diet, be healthy, and really needs to perform at his best—be explosive in his performance and quick on his feet. Having been told by his mom to "cut the carbs, because they make you fat," he has eliminated grain-based food. As the session continued, he reported that he has cut out all the grains, likes to eat fruits and vegetables, and will eat any kind of meat. Seemingly disappointed, the athlete goes on to tell, "by mid-week I'm not feeling strong and explosive throughout the workouts and am making mistakes I would not normally make."

1. With all the media touting "low carb" and the role carbohydrates are playing in the obesity epidemic, what should the athletic trainer tell the athlete?
2. Does this athlete's diet need a complete overhaul?
3. What tool might the athletic trainer introduce to the athlete to get him started in achieving better balance in his diet?
4. How could choosing a low carbohydrate diet put this athlete at risk for injury?

Case Study 3

A female runner is training for a 10K race, one she has completed several years in a row. This year she is training harder than in years past. Despite her new job being high pressure and working 10-hour days to keep up, she is still hoping to PR and break 50 minutes. She is complaining that she just does not seem to be able to hit the run paces she was able to run earlier in the summer. She is a bit confused because a few weeks back she began "eating clean." Upon the advice of her sister, who is a holistic nutritionist, she has even been trying to follow a plant-based diet. She will include dairy-based ice cream, "because I can't give up everything."

1. How might you help this athlete understand the fueling demands of an athlete?
2. Is she at risk for injury or illness? If so, what?
3. What advice could you give this athlete to help her fuel throughout the busy days, to be ready for her next training session?

References

1. Commission on Accreditation of Athletic Training Education. *Standards for Accreditation of Professional Athletic Training Programs at the Master's Level (2020 Standards).* Accessed December 15, 2019. https://caate.net/Portals/0/Documents/Standards%20and%20Procedures%20for%20Accreditation%20of%20Professional%20Programs.pdf
2. Ng R, Sutradhar R, Yao Z, Wodchis WP, Rosella LC. Smoking, drinking, diet and physical activity—modifiable lifestyle risk factors and their associations with age to first chronic disease. *Int J Epidemiol.* 2020;49(1):113-130. doi:10.1093/ije/dyz078
3. Office of Disease Prevention and Health Promotion. *Healthy People 2020.* Accessed September 9, 2019. https://www.healthypeople.gov/2020/
4. US Department of Health and Human Services, Office of Disease Prevention and Health Promotion. Healthy People 2020 [Internet]. *Leading Health Indicators: Nutrition, Physical Activity, and Obesity.* Accessed April 23, 2020. https://www.healthypeople.gov/2020/leading-health-indicators/infographic/nutrition-physical-activity-and-obesity-5?width=618&height=100%25&date=Sep-2019
5. US Department of Health and Human Services, Office of Disease Prevention and Health Promotion. *Healthy People 2030* [Internet]. Accessed July 14, 2022. https://health.gov/healthypeople

6. US Department of Health and Human Services, Office of Disease Prevention and Health Promotion. *Healthy People 2030.* Retrieved July 15, 2022 fromhttps://health.gov/healthypeople/priority-areas/social-determinants-health

7. US Department of Agriculture and US Department of Health and Human Services. *Dietary Guidelines for Americans, 2020-2025.* 9th ed. Accessed July, 17, 2022. https://DietaryGuidelines.gov

8. US Department of Health and Human Services and US Department of Agriculture. *2015–2020 Dietary Guidelines for Americans.* 8th ed. Accessed September 15, 2019. https://health.gov/our-work/nutrition-physical-activity/dietary-guidelines/previous-dietary-guidelines/2015

9. Office of Disease Prevention and Health Promotion. *Healthy People 2020.* Accessed April 23, 2020. https://www.healthypeople.gov/2020

10. US Department of Health and Human Services. *Physical Activity Guidelines for Americans.* 2nd ed. 2018. Accessed September 15, 2019. https://health.gov/our-work/nutrition-physical-activity/physical-activity-guidelines/current-guidelines

11. US Department of Agriculture—Center for Nutrition Policy & Promotion. *MyPlate.* Accessed July 15, 2022. https://www.myplate.gov/

12. Mountjoy M, Sundgot-Borgen J, Burke L, et al. The IOC consensus statement: beyond the female athlete triad—Relative Energy Deficiency in Sport (RED-S). *Br J Sports Med.* 2014;48:491-497. doi:10.1136/bjsports-2014-093502

13. Statuta SM, Asif IM, Drezner JA. Relative Energy Deficiency in Sport (RED-S). *Br J Sports Med.* 2017;51:1570-1571. doi.org/10.1136/bjsports-2017-097700

14. Rudser-Rusin A. SportWise Nutrition & Consulting, LLC. www.sportwisenutrition.com

15. Tipton K. Review article: nutrition support or exercise-induced injuries. *Sports Med.* 2015;45(suppl1):S93-S104. doi:10.1007/s40279-015-0398-4

16. Academy of Nutrition and Dietetics. *What is a Registered Dietitian Nutritionist?* Accessed July 15, 2022. https://www.eatrightpro.org/about-us/what-is-an-rdn-and-dtr/what-is-a-registered-dietitian-nutritionist

17. Academy of Nutrition and Dietetics. *Standards of Practice.* Accessed July 15, 2022. https://www.eatrightpro.org/practice/quality-management/standards-of-practice/

18. Sports and Human Performance Nutritionists, a dietetic practice group of the Academy of Nutrition and Dietetics. *The Board Certified Specialist in Sports Dietetics (CSSD) is the Premier Professional Sports Nutrition Credential in the US* Accessed July 15, 2022. https://www.shpndpg.org/professional-resources/cssd

Chapter 2

Macronutrients

Mindy A. Patterson, PhD, RDN

Commission on Accreditation of Athletic Training Education *2020 Standards*

This chapter addresses the following *2020 Standards for Accreditation of Professional Athletic Training Programs*:

- Standard 62: Provide athletic training services in a manner that uses evidence to inform practice.
- Standard 83: Educate and make recommendations to clients/patients on fluids and nutrients to ingest prior to activity, during activity, and during recovery for a variety of activities and environmental conditions.

Overview of Macronutrients

Adequate dietary intake is necessary for optimizing nutritional status and influencing physical performance. Poor dietary intake patterns have been linked to suboptimal training; inadequate strength, flexibility, and stamina; attenuated muscle growth and development; and injury and ineffective recovery.[1] Thus, the role of the athletic trainer to educate physically active individuals on proper nutrition cannot be undermined so that performance can be maximized.

Nutrition is the science that links the nutrients from the foods and beverages we consume to how those nutrients impact overall health. When nutrients are consumed, they must be digested, absorbed, utilized, metabolized, and excreted. The nutrients must go through each process efficiently to maximize its utilization so health and performance can be optimized. Six nutrients have been classified: carbohydrates, protein, fat, vitamins, minerals, and water. The nutrients that provide energy, or kilocalories (also known as calories), include carbohydrates, protein, and lipids (also known as fat). These nutrients are macronutrients because they are needed in large amounts (eg, grams). Vitamins and minerals are classified as micronutrients because they are needed in small amounts (eg, micrograms).

Macronutrients contain carbon and are therefore considered organic compounds. Once consumed, macronutrients are broken down into smaller components, such as glucose from carbohydrates, peptides or amino acids from proteins, or fatty acids (FA) from lipids. These smaller compounds are absorbed across the small intestine and

Knoblauch M, ed. *Clinical Nutrition in Athletic Training* (pp 13-24).
© 2023 Taylor & Francis Group.

Learning Objectives

After reviewing this chapter, readers will be able to:

- Know the types of macronutrients and their main functions.
- Define "calorie" and how it is measured.
- Understand how energy from macronutrients can be used for other cellular processes.
- Define and classify different types of carbohydrates.
- Know the structural components of carbohydrates and their main functions.
- Understand how carbohydrates and fiber are digested, absorbed, and utilized in the body.
- Know the dietary requirements for carbohydrates in healthy individuals and athletes.
- Compare and contrast different types of fibers, and the types that active individuals should avoid prior to exercise.
- Know the basic structure, functions, classifications, and food sources of lipids.
- Identify the fat-soluble vitamins and their primary functions.
- Understand how lipids and cholesterol are digested, absorbed, and utilized.
- Know the requirements and recommendations for dietary lipids, essential fatty acids, and cholesterol.
- Know the basic functions and properties of proteins and amino acids.
- Understand how amino acids are classified and why some are essential.
- Understand how proteins and amino acids are digested and absorbed.
- Identify high-quality protein sources and how quality is measured.
- Know the dietary recommendations for both healthy and exercising individuals.

transported to primarily the liver and peripheral tissues. The fate of the smaller compounds depend on the energy needs of the host. If the host needs energy, glucose and FA will be broken down further to produce energy (eg, adenosine triphosphate or ATP), a process known as catabolism. If energy is abundant, the smaller compounds are used to build new molecules such as glycogen, proteins, or triacylglycerol (TAG), which is known as anabolism.

During the catabolism of macronutrients, chemical bonds are broken to produce energy and heat (Sidebar 2-1). Glycolysis is the catabolic process for glucose, while beta-oxidation is the process that breaks down FAs. Protein catabolism does not directly generate energy per se, but instead provides certain amino acids that can form new glucose and can generate energy. The energy from glucose and FA catabolism can be housed in the highly energetic compound ATP, which provides energy when a phosphate bond is broken. The ATP generated from catabolism can either be directly produced within the cell (ie, substrate level phosphorylation) or captured in cofactors, such as NADH and $FADH_2$, that ultimately donate electrons to oxygen to produce ATP (ie, oxidative phosphorylation). Oxygen must be present for ATP to be produced by oxidative phosphorylation. However, ATP produced by substrate level phosphorylation can occur without oxygen, or anaerobic, conditions. The energy generated from ATP or cofactors is used to fuel other processes in the cell, such as muscle contraction, and building new proteins and other large molecules.

Sidebar 2-1

Breaking a chemical bond releases heat and forms compounds that store energy and serve as energy sources for other reactions. Such compounds include ATP, which provides energy when a phosphate bond is broken, or cofactors that ultimately donate electrons to oxygen to produce ATP. The energy is needed for exertion, building new compounds (anabolism), transporting molecules across membranes, and transferring genetic information.

The energy capacity of a macronutrient can be described by the term "kilocalorie," even though the term "calorie" is used (Sidebar 2-2). A calorie is the amount of energy (heat) required to increase the temperature of 1 g of water by 1 °C. The amount of energy in food is quantified as a kilocalorie because it provides enough energy (heat) to increase 1 kg of water by 1 °C. Carbohydrates provide 4 kcal/g, protein provides 4 kcal/g, and lipids provide 9 kcal/g. The macronutrients that contain more kcal per gram, such as lipids, generate more ATP than macronutrients providing less kcal/g, such as carbohydrates.

Each macronutrient has several important roles in the body. For example, the glucose from carbohydrates can undergo glycolysis to produce energy for all tissues and cells or be stored as glycogen for future energy utilization. Some tissues prefer glucose as an energy source, such as the brain, while some cells can only use glucose as an energy substrate, such as the red blood cells. Without glucose, the amount of energy available to perform an exercise in active individuals is reduced, which could lead to ineffective performance. In contrast to carbohydrates, protein provides the amino acids necessary for protein synthesis and repair, maintains tissue structure and function (including bone), and generates the enzymes necessary for metabolism. Low or inadequate protein intake in active individuals can lead to reduced muscle mass and performance, attenuated tissue repair following exercise, and insufficient metabolic processes. The final macronutrient, lipids, is the primary storage form of energy in the body. Lipids also maintain cell membrane structure, conduct molecular signaling and regulation, produce cofactors (eg, ubiquinone in the electron transport chain and vitamin K in the formation of blood clots) and hormones (eg, testosterone and cortisol), and have antioxidant capabilities (eg, vitamin E). In active individuals, lipids serve as an energy source during endurance exercise when glycogen is depleted and helps to support bone and tissue structure.

Carbohydrates

Carbohydrates are a class of compounds containing carbon, oxygen, and hydrogen with the formula $C(H_2O)$. Carbohydrates can be divided into "available" or "unavailable." Available carbohydrates are hydrolyzed (ie, broken down in the presence of water) by digestive enzymes to ultimately produce glucose for the body. An example would include fully digestible starches and simple sugars. Unavailable carbohydrates do not ultimately produce glucose and do not directly provide energy to the host. Unavailable carbohydrates include fibers that are not broken down in the small intestine because their bonds are not recognized or accessible to digestive enzymes. Because unavailable carbohydrates are not digested in the small intestine, they enter the large intestine intact. Carbohydrates can also be categorized by the time it takes for them to be digested and absorbed. Simple carbohydrates are digested and absorbed quickly and raise blood glucose levels rapidly. Complex carbohydrates are digested and absorbed slowly, producing a slower rise in blood glucose compared to simple carbohydrates.

Classification

Carbohydrates can be classified according to the type and number of sugar units, or monomers, and how the monomers are linked together. For example, monosaccharides include 1 monomer, disaccharides have 2 monomers, oligosaccharides have a few (3 to 12) monomers, and polysaccharides have many monomers linked together. The type of link, or bond, between the sugar units is important because enzymes are specific to the type of bond they hydrolyze.

Monosaccharides are named according to the number of carbons within the monomer and whether either an aldehyde or ketone is present. An aldehyde has a carbon-oxygen double bond linked to a hydrogen and is located at the end of the molecule. Ketones have the carbon-oxygen double bond between 2 functional groups and is located in the middle of the molecule. For example, a 6-carbon monosaccharide with an aldehyde is an "aldohexose." A 5-carbon monosaccharide with a ketone is a "ketopentose." The nutritionally relevant monosaccharides are glucose, galactose, and fructose. They are nutritionally relevant because they are the products of carbohydrate digestion that are absorbed and utilized in the body. Monosaccharides are found in fruit, milk, honey, and other simple carbohydrates.

A disaccharide is formed when 2 monosaccharides are joined together via a glycosidic bond, which is a covalent bond that links 2 sugar monomers together. The disaccharides are maltose (glucose + glucose), lactose (glucose + galactose), and sucrose (glucose + fructose). Disaccharides are found in table sugar, honey, fruit and fruit juice, sugary drinks, and milk. In fact, many sports drinks include sucrose to assist in hydration after intense exercise. Disaccharides are also known as simple carbohydrates.

Oligosaccharides typically include 3 to 12 monomers and are not hydrolyzed by digestive enzymes in the small intestine; therefore, they are considered a dietary fiber. However, many oligosaccharides are fermented by gut microbes in the large intestine to produce short chain fatty acids (SCFAs; eg, acetate, propionate, and butyrate) that can elicit additional roles in the body. For example, butyrate can be used as a fuel source by the intestinal cells to assist in maintaining gut health. Propionate can be used as a substrate to generate new glucose. Acetate can be absorbed and used by the peripheral tissues as an energy source. Examples of oligosaccharides include fructooligosaccharides found in onions, asparagus, and wheat and inulin that occurs naturally in garlic, leeks, and onions.

Polysaccharides contain many monomers linked in a linear and/or branched fashion and are classified as complex carbohydrates. Homopolysaccharides consist of only 1 type of monosaccharide, while heteropolysaccharides contain at least 2 different types of monosaccharides. The most common homopolysaccharide is starch, which is stored as granules in plants. Starch contains glucose linked via both alpha 1,4 linear bonds and alpha 1,6 branch points. The linear linkages are called "amylose," while the sections with the branch points are called "amylopectin." About 20% to 25% of starch consists of amylose, while the remainder is comprised of amylopectin. Interestingly, plants with higher amounts of amylopectin—or branch points—are digested more rapidly than plants with higher amylose concentrations. This is because more branch points create more locations for enzymes to access for rapid glucose hydrolysis. Starch is found in potatoes, corn, peas, beans, and grain products (Figure 2-1).

Consuming complex carbohydrates is ideal for maximizing glycogen stores prior to exercise as well as during recovery. However, some types of complex carbohydrates contain slowly digestible starch that can take anywhere from 20 to 100 minutes to fully digest, and may not be ideal as a rapid energy source during exercise. Simple carbohydrates provide the muscle a rapid source of energy via glucose to sustain exercise. Immediately before and during exercise—especially during endurance events—simple carbohydrates require little digestion and are rapidly absorbed. For this reason, many sports beverages and foods that are used immediately before and during endurance events primarily contain simple carbohydrates.

Digestion and Absorption

Carbohydrate digestion occurs within the mouth, stomach, and small intestine. Digestion of starch begins in the mouth where salivary amylase hydrolyzes alpha 1,4 bonds. The products, oligosaccharides and maltose, enter the stomach where little digestion occurs due to the low pH environment. The low pH of the stomach denatures salivary amylase, which in turn renders it inactive. As the food products move to the duodenum, pancreatic amylase is released from the pancreas to further cleave alpha 1,4 bonds and produces maltose, maltotriose, and "limit dextrins." Limit dextrins are a smaller starch molecule with both alpha 1,4 and alpha 1,6 bonds intact. As the partially digested food products move further down the duodenum, pancreatic amylase and isomaltase—located on the luminal side of the gastrointestinal tract—hydrolyze the limit dextrins to ultimately produce maltose. The luminal (facing the inside of the small intestine tract) enzymes maltase, sucrase, and lactase cleave the disaccharides maltose, sucrose, and lactose, respectively. These enzymes are found within the brush border of the small intestinal cell, also known as an "enterocyte." The end products of starch and carbohydrate digestion include the monosaccharides glucose, galactose, and fructose. All 3 are absorbed across the enterocyte via transporters. The transporters are located within the plasma membrane of the enterocytes to facilitate complete absorption of the monosaccharides. Once absorbed, the monosaccharides travel via the portal blood to the liver. In the liver, galactose and fructose are chemically processed, ultimately producing glucose. Carbohydrates that are not digested in the small intestine (eg, fiber) enter the large intestine where some are fermented by the gut microbiota to produce methane, hydrogen, and SCFAs.

Factors that influence the digestion and absorption of carbohydrates include the presence of other nutrients in the food matrix that impact transit time (eg, fat, fiber), osmolality, malabsorption (lack of intact gut mucosal lining, lack of effective transporter expression), ineffective pancreatic enzyme release due to surgery or genetic condition (eg, cystic fibrosis), and impaired luminal enzyme expression. All of these factors must be considered in athletes and active individuals. For example, high osmolarity foods and beverages are concentrated with solutes and can promote the influx of water into the gastrointestinal tract to neutralize solute concentration. Excessive water in the gastrointestinal tract can cause stomach pain, discomfort, and distress, all of which are problematic during exercise. Another example of factors that impact the digestion and absorption of carbohydrates is the malabsorption of the disaccharide lactose found in dairy products. Lactase is a luminal enzyme located on the brush border of enterocytes and cleaves lactose to form galactose and glucose during digestion. Some ethnic groups, older adults, and individuals with certain genetic conditions have minimal lactase expression. Failure to break down lactose in the small intestine allows it to enter the large intestine, causing an osmotic effect. In addition, gut microbes rapidly feed on lactose to produce gas, which can cause abdominal bloating, pain, and diarrhea. Athletes and active individuals with minimal lactase expression may need to consume lactose-free dairy to minimize gastrointestinal distress during exercise.

Requirements and Recommendations

Both complex and simple carbohydrates are found in abundance in the food supply. Complex carbohydrates are found in starchy foods. The starchy foods include grains (bread, cereal, rice, pasta) and vegetables such as potatoes and corn. Food sources rich in mono- and disaccharides include simple carbohydrates. Sources of simple carbohydrates include dairy (milk, yogurt), fruit (apples, bananas, grapes), snack foods (cake, candy, cookies, crackers), and sugary drinks (soda, sports drinks).

The Acceptable Macronutrient Distribution Range (AMDR) for carbohydrates in healthy adults is 45% to 65% of total calories.[1] For example, if 2500 kcal are consumed daily by active individuals, between 1125 kcal (281 g) and 1625 kcal (406 g) should come from carbohydrates. Many active individuals who engage in moderate exercise for the purposes of maintaining health do not need different carbohydrate recommendations than the AMDR. However, athletes and active individuals training for a competitive event (eg, marathon, triathlon) may need to follow different carbohydrate recommendations as their carbohydrate needs may be higher.

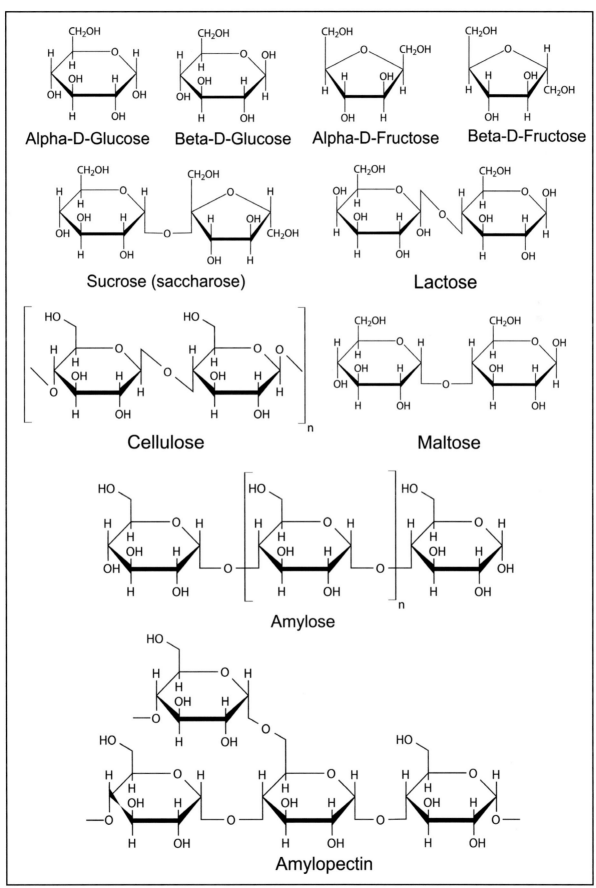

Figure 2-1. Molecular structures. (chromatos/Shutterstock.com.)

Table 2-1

Carbohydrate Recommendations for Athletes and Active Individuals

ACTIVITY LEVEL	CARBOHYDRATE INTAKE PER DAY
Light (low intensity)	3 to 5 g/kg body weight
Moderate (~1 hour/day)	5 to 7 g/kg body weight
High (endurance, ~1 to 3 hour/day)	6 to 10 g/kg body weight
Very High (extreme, >4 to 5 hour/day)	8 to 12 g/kg body weight

Adapted from Thomas DT, Erdman KA, Burke LM. American College of Sports Medicine joint position statement. Nutrition and athletic performance. *Med Sci Sports Exerc.* 2016;48(3):543-568. doi:10.1249/MSS.0000000000000852

Carbohydrates and Exercise

Carbohydrates are the recommended fuel source for athletes for several reasons. Glucose is versatile in that it can produce energy under both aerobic and anaerobic conditions.[2] For example, compared to lipids, glucose yields more ATP from oxygen.[3] Glycogen stores can be maximized by consuming appropriate amounts of carbohydrate and limiting physical activity. With continued intake of carbohydrates (especially simple carbohydrates) during prolonged or intermittent high-intensity exercise, glucose becomes readily available to effectively fuel the muscle cell to sustain performance.[2]

While recommendations should be individualized to the athlete's preference and tolerance, general recommendations have been established. The American College of Sports Medicine and Academy of Nutrition and Dietetics[2] have specific carbohydrate recommendations for athletes based on exercise intensity and duration, which are based on body weight, and can be found in Table 2-1.

Pre-event carbohydrate intake should include 1 to 4 g/kg of body weight about 1 to 4 hours prior to exercise. Additional carbohydrate is not needed if the duration of exercise is less than 30 minutes. However, for endurance and intermittent, high-intensity exercise lasting 1 to 2 hours, then 30 g per of carbohydrate/hour are recommended. In some instances, endurance exercise lasting more than 2 to 3 hours, up to 60 to 90 g carbohydrate can be consumed per hour. For athletes with gastrointestinal discomfort during exercise, low-fiber, low glycemic index carbohydrates may be necessary. In addition, because glucose and fructose are absorbed into the enterocyte using different transporters, using foods rich in these monosaccharides may benefit the athlete due to rapid utilization for energy production.

Dietary Fiber

The US Food and Drug Administration has not officially adopted a definition for fiber; however, the definition from the Institute of Medicine (IOM) is most commonly used in the United States. The IOM defines dietary fiber as "nondigestible carbohydrates and lignin that are intrinsic and intact in plants as well as components of plant cell walls that are resistant to hydrolysis by human enzymes."[1] The IOM also considers isolated fibers that have shown physiological benefits in humans to be functional fibers. Thus, the sum of dietary and functional fibers equal total dietary fiber.

Types of fiber include cellulose, hemicellulose, pectins, gums, mucilages, and lignin. Each fiber has distinct physiological properties that can include viscosity (ability to hold water) and fermentability (ability to be fermented in the large intestine by gut microbes to produce metabolites such as SCFAs). However, the nutrition facts label still classifies dietary fiber as being soluble or insoluble, but these terms do not translate into physiological function. Additional properties include gel-forming fibers, such as gels, mucilages, and some hemicelluloses, while others may be structural in nature. Gel-forming fibers dissolve in water to form a viscous gel that can bind to nutrients (including cholesterol) in the gastrointestinal tract to reduce utilization. They also slow gastric emptying to promote fullness and satiety. Structural fibers are typically nonviscous and are poorly fermentable, thus they contribute to stool bulk.

Other fibers include inulin, fructans, and resistant starch. Inulin and fructans including fructooligosaccharides are highly, and often rapidly, fermentable. Inulin is found in chicory root and is often used as an added fiber in commercial food products. The characteristics of these fibers may not be ideal for athletes, especially if consumed before an event. The rapid fermentation can cause gastrointestinal distress, gas, cramping, and bloating. In contrast, resistant starches are found in starchy foods, such as just-ripe bananas, legumes, potatoes that have been cooked then chilled, stir-fried rice, and some types of breads, grains, and cereals.[4] There are 5 types of resistant starches, and types 2 and 3 are fermented but are tolerated more than rapidly fermentable fibers.[5]

The energy contribution from dietary fibers come from SCFAs produced from microbial fermentation in the large intestine. The SCFAs are absorbed and utilized systemically to contribute approximately 10% of host energy.

Although fiber is not an essential nutrient, the health benefits of consuming adequate fiber have allowed for an adequate intake to be established. The current daily recommendations for fiber include 25 g for women and 38 g for men, or 14 g per 1000 kcal.[1] On average, US adults consume ~15 g of fiber daily, which is considered inadequate. Consuming a mix of fibers in appropriate amounts can promote gastrointestinal health, assist with weight and glucose control, and reduce the risk of certain cancers and cardiovascular disease.[6]

Athletes and active individuals who experience gastrointestinal distress during a competitive event may need to reduce the amount of fiber consumed 1 to 2 days prior to the event. Some rapidly fermented fibers can release methane and other gasses that can contribute to gastrointestinal discomfort and bloating, which would interfere with the ability to exercise. Therefore, active individuals should use a "trial and error" approach when ingesting fiber prior to exercise in an effort to minimize gastrointestinal distress.

Lipids

Lipids are primarily hydrophobic compounds that contain carbon, hydrogen, and oxygen.

Some lipids have hydrophilic areas that attract aqueous solutions. The structure of lipids depicts their function and physical properties. Lipids have several functions, including providing an energy source (9 kcal/g), promoting energy storage, generating signaling molecules such as eicosanoids that have many biological functions, and assisting with cell membrane fluidity and function. The fat-soluble vitamins (A, D, E, and K) are considered lipids.

Vitamins A and D also function as hormones that bind to DNA within cells to up- or downregulate the production of enzymes. Vitamin E is a key antioxidant, and vitamin K is involved in blood coagulation and the binding of calcium in bone. In addition to the fat-soluble vitamins, lipids also include FAs, TAG, phospholipids, and sterols. Linoleic acid (omega-6) and alpha-linolenic (omega-3) acid are the only lipids considered essential because humans do not have the appropriate enzymes to form these FAs in the body.

Classification

FAs are the simplest lipid structure that can vary in carbon length and degree of saturation. Saturated fatty acids (SFAs) have carbons that are "saturated" with hydrogen and the carbons are linked via single bonds. SFAs are linear and are able to pack tightly against one another. Due to the linear structure, SFAs are solid at room temperature. Unsaturated

fatty acids (UFAs) contain one or more double bonds. The double bond imposes a "kink" in the FA structure that decreases the ability of the UFAs to pack together tightly; therefore, UFAs exist in fluid form at room temperature. If the UFA has one double bond, it is a monounsaturated fatty acid (MUFA). When the FA contains more than one double bond, it is a polyunsaturated fatty acid (PUFA). The location of the hydrogens around the double bond classifies the UFA as being either "*cis*" or "*trans*." The UFA has a *cis* configuration if the hydrogens are on the same side of the double bond, and the *trans* configuration has hydrogens on the opposite sides of the double bond. Almost all naturally occurring UFAs are in the *cis* configuration except minor amounts produced in ruminant animals and some plants. The majority of *trans* FAs are incorporated into processed foods and oils to increase the shelf life due to the stability of the *trans* FA at higher temperatures for a long period of time. However, *trans* FA no longer have "Generally Recognized as Safe" status from the US Food and Drug Administration, meaning they are no longer safe for human consumption and cannot be added to foods (Sidebar 2-3). *Trans FAs* have been linked to cardiovascular disease and other conditions.[7]

Approximately 95% of dietary lipids consumed are in the form of TAG, which contains a 3-carbon glycerol backbone with FAs attached to each carbon via an ester linkage. The FAs in TAG can differ in carbon length and saturation. Phospholipids, cholesterol, and free FAs make up the remaining 5% of dietary lipids (Figure 2-2).

Digestion and Absorption

Lipid digestion is an efficient process where approximately 95% of all lipids ingested are utilized. Due to the nonpolar, hydrophobic properties of lipids, they must be emulsified before they are absorbed. Prior to emulsification, the lipids must be broken down by enzymes into simpler compounds. The digestion process of lipids begins in the stomach where one FA is cleaved from TAG by a lipase released from the stomach's chief cells. The products resulting from stomach lipid digestion are glycerol with 2 FAs, or diacylglycerol. Undigested TAG, diacylglycerol, and free FAs travel from the stomach to the duodenum, or upper part of the small intestine, where the majority of lipid digestion occurs.

Figure 2-2. Triglycerides and fatty acids. (Alila Medical Media/Shutterstock.com.)

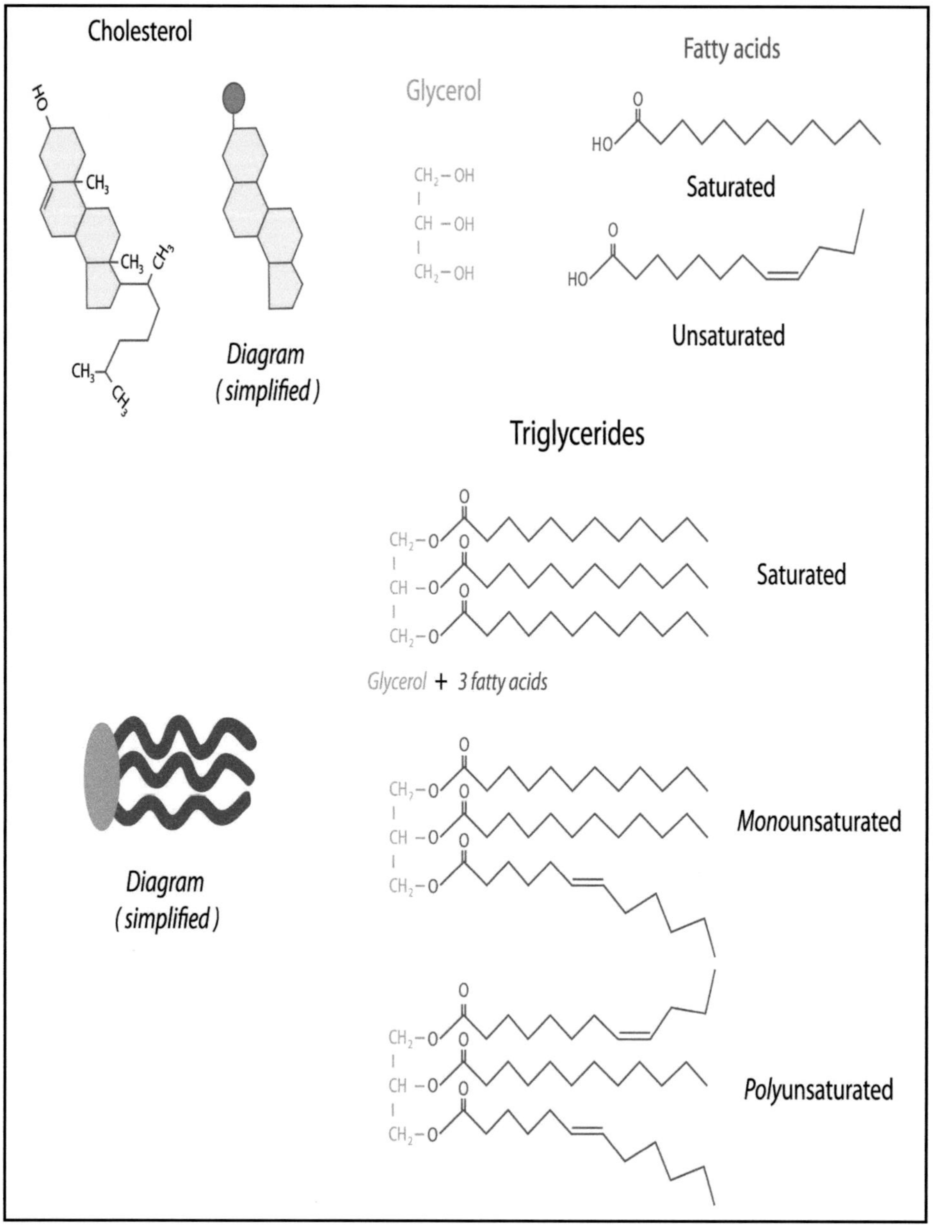

As lipids enter the duodenum, enzymes are secreted from the pancreas to continue breaking down the lipids. In addition to pancreatic enzymes, bile acids must enter the small intestine to facilitate lipid emulsification. Bile acids are released from the gallbladder via the bile acid duct, which is triggered by the hormone cholecystokinin. Cholecystokinin is secreted from the I cells of the small intestine, which is released by the presence of the lipids in the duodenum. This hormone functions to stimulate gallbladder contraction and release bile acids. The bile acids act as detergent to emulsify the lipids and promote micelle formation. Micelles are aggregates that include a nonpolar (water-fearing) core and polar (water-loving) shell. Micelles allow the aqueous layer lining of the absorptive cells (enterocytes) in the small intestine to interact with the nonpolar lipids in the micelles. Without this interaction, the lipids would not be absorbed (Sidebar

Sidebar 2-4

Athletes or active individuals without a gallbladder may have a hard time digesting lipids. In some cases, a lower fat diet is recommended for these individuals.

2-4), with the exception of small chain FAs (~<12 carbons in length) that can be directly absorbed across the enterocyte for entry into the portal circulation.

Within the micelle, additional lipases continue to break down lipids and form the final products of lipid digestion: glycerol, FAs, monoacylglycerol (glycerol + 1 FA), phosphatidic acid from phospholipase, and cholesterol. These products, along with fat-soluble vitamins, are now incorporated into the micelle and are ready to be absorbed into the enterocyte.

As the micelle encounters the aqueous layer that lines the small intestine, the contents of the micelle are absorbed across the enterocyte. Bile acids, however, are not absorbed with the micelle contents. Instead, bile acids travel to the distal ileum where they are reabsorbed via a process known as "enterohepatic circulation."

Through a series of complex processes within the enterocyte, TAG, phospholipids, and cholesterol are reformed and packaged into chylomicrons. Chylomicrons are a lipoprotein that carries exogenous, or dietary, lipids to the tissues (Sidebar 2-5). From the enterocyte, chylomicrons enter the lymph and ultimately the blood via the thoracic duct. Once in the blood, chylomicrons deliver primarily FAs from TAG to the muscle (for energy production) or adipose tissue (for storage). The glycerol backbone of TAG is not taken up by the tissues and instead travels back to the liver for utilization. As the lipids are removed from the chylomicron, they become smaller in size to become a chylomicron remnant. The chylomicron remnants are ultimately absorbed by the liver.

Lipoproteins are the proteins that transport lipids to and from the tissues in the body. They are necessary because lipids are nonpolar and would not be effectively transported in the blood, which is a polar solution. Lipoproteins are classified according to size, density (mass per amount of volume), and the type of lipids they deliver to the tissues. Chylomicrons are largest, least dense, and carry dietary TAG to the tissues. Additional lipoproteins in order of largest to smallest size include very low–density lipoproteins (VLDLs), low-density lipoproteins (LDLs), and high-density lipoproteins (HDLs). VLDLs are formed in the liver and function to deliver endogenous TAG to the tissues. As VLDLs release FAs from TAG to enter the tissues (primarily muscle and adipose), they become smaller to eventually become LDLs. LDLs are rich in cholesterol and are absorbed by peripheral tissues and the endothelial cells that line the interior of blood vessels. The function of LDL is to deliver cholesterol to the cells. HDL is a dense, protein-rich lipoprotein formed in the liver and is involved in reverse-cholesterol transport. Reverse-cholesterol transport is a process that transports cholesterol from the peripheral tissues to HDLs where the cholesterol is returned to the liver.

Requirements and Recommendations

The AMDR for lipids is 20% to 35% of energy for adults, but 25% to 35% of energy for men and women between 14 and 18 years of age.[1] The recommendation for linoleic acid is 17 g and 12 g daily and the alpha-linolenic acid requirements include 1.6 g and 1.1 g daily for adult men and women from 19 to 50 years of age, respectively. In addition, no more than 10% of energy should come from saturated fat

Sidebar 2-5

A lipoprotein is a molecule that is made of lipids and proteins. They function to transport lipids and cholesterol, both exogenous (from the diet) and endogenous (made in the body), to and from the tissues.

and no *trans FA* should be consumed. The American Heart Association recommends SFA to be replaced with MUFA and PUFA.[8] Dietary cholesterol has been shown to have no influence on blood cholesterol concentrations; therefore, cholesterol recommendations are no longer applicable. Instead of cholesterol, SFA have been linked to dyslipidemia that may lead to the development of cardiovascular disease.

Dietary sources of lipids include animal products, seafood, nut and seed oils, and processed foods. Saturated FA sources include beef, poultry with skin, lamb, pork, dairy (butter, cheese, full- and reduced-fat yogurt and milk), and oils made from palm and coconut. Sources of PUFA include soybean, corn, and sunflower oils as well as some nuts (walnuts) and seeds (flaxseed). Monounsaturated FA can be found in olive and canola oil, avocados, and nuts and seeds. *Trans fats* are found in processed foods and can be identified by the term "partially hydrogenated oil" in the ingredient list. However, *trans FA* should no longer be added to processed foods because they are no longer considered safe. Linoleic acid can be found in plant oils (ie, sunflower, corn, peanut) but cold-water fish, canola, and soybean oils are good sources of alpha-linolenic acid.

Essential fatty acids (EFA; linoleic and alpha-linolenic) are important because they can synthesize signaling molecules such as eicosanoids, an umbrella term that includes leukotrienes, thromboxanes, and prostaglandins. The EFA can be incorporated into cell membranes where a signal or trauma to the cell can stimulate the release of the EFA into the cytosol. Here, enzymes can convert the EFA to an eicosanoid that can act in either a paracrine or autocrine fashion. Typically, linoleic acid can form eicosanoids that are pro-inflammatory in nature and promote vasoconstriction. Alpha-linolenic acid forms eicosanoids that promote anti-inflammatory reactions and can cause vasodilation. In addition, alpha-linolenic acid can be elongated and desaturated to form docosahexaenoic acid (DHA) and eicosapentaenoic acid (EPA) that have additional functions that assist with neuroprotection. However, the conversion of alpha-linolenic acid to DHA and EPA is inefficient; therefore, dietary sources of these FAs should be recommended. Cold-water fatty fish (eg, salmon and tuna), fortified eggs, and some algal sources contain DHA and EPA.

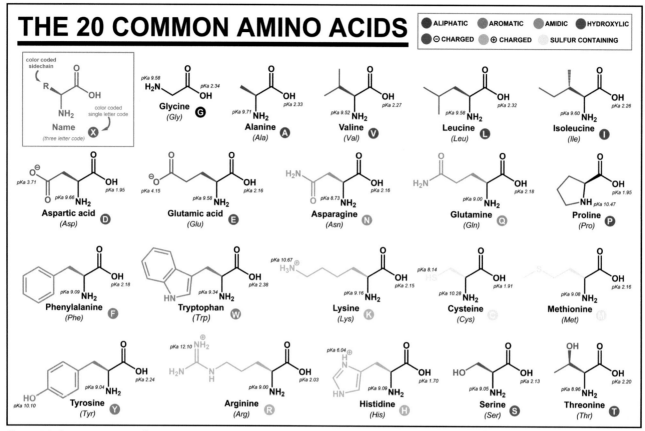

Figure 2-3. Common amino acids. (Cristian Victor Rete/Shutterstock.com.)

Lipids and Exercise

Lipids are an important fuel source for both active individuals and athletes, especially those engaged in moderately intense exercise activities. Intramuscular and adipose stores provide a source of free FAs to be oxidized for ATP production during activity, especially when glucose availability is limited. Increasing dietary lipid intake in conjunction with reduced carbohydrate intake does not appear to improve performance when compared to normal recommended carbohydrate and lipid intake for athletes.[1]

Protein

Protein is an important macronutrient that has structural and regulatory roles. Protein is a structural component of bone, muscle, and tissues and regulates cellular growth and repair. The regulatory roles of protein function as enzymes, hormones, transport proteins, neurotransmitters, and antibodies. Protein also plays a role in the maintenance of fluid balance and assists in regulating the pH of fluids. Protein can also provide energy as a minor function.

Proteins are made of amino acids (AAs) linked together via peptide bonds. AAs can be either nonessential (dispensable) or essential (indispensable). The nonessential AAs can be made in the body, while essential AAs are not. Essential AAs must be consumed in the diet in recommended amounts to meet the needs of the individual. Of the 20 total AAs, 11 are nonessential and include alanine, arginine, aspartic acid, asparagine, cysteine, glutamic acid, glutamine, glycine, proline, serine, and tyrosine. The essential AAs are isoleucine, leucine, lysine, methionine, phenylalanine, threonine, tryptophan, valine, and histidine (children only). Some AAs are considered conditionally essential, where they must be supplied in the diet under special circumstances, such as inborn errors of metabolism. Two conditionally essential AAs are cysteine (which is formed from methionine) and tyrosine (which is formed from phenylalanine; Figure 2-3).

Classification

All AAs have an amino group, carboxylic group, hydrogen, and functional group surrounding the central carbon atom. The properties of AAs are based on the size, charge, and type of functional (or "R") group. For example, isoleucine, leucine, and valine are known as branched-chain AAs (BCAAs) because of their functional group (Figure 2-4). Due to their functional group, the BCAAs are preferentially metabolized by the muscle instead of the liver, as in the other AAs. Other AAs have special functions, such as tryptophan and tyrosine, that can form key neurotransmitters.

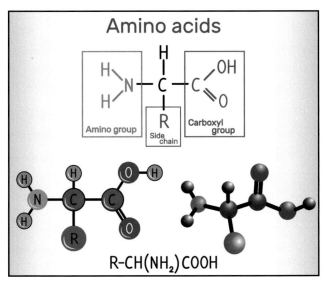

Figure 2-4. Branched-chain amino acids. (Bacsica/Shutterstock.com.)

Tryptophan can form melatonin and serotonin, while tyrosine can produce 2 catecholamines: epinephrine and norepinephrine. Thyroid hormones are also made from tyrosine. Furthermore, some AA can undergo post-translational modification to assist with the formation of collagen, which is found in bone, muscle, and tendons.

Proteins have 4 main structures based on complexity: primary, secondary, tertiary, and quaternary. The primary structure of a protein involves the AA linked via peptide bonds in a linear manner to form a polypeptide chain. The secondary structures include beta-pleated sheets (a least 2 or more polypeptide sheets lined together laterally) and alpha-helices (the polypeptide "winds up" to form a helix). These secondary structures are found in fibrous proteins, such as collagen and keratin. The 3-dimensional arrangement of proteins is the tertiary structure. The tertiary structure is important for protein function (eg, enzymes) and signaling. Quaternary structures exist when polypeptides interact with each other to form a subunit. An example is hemoglobin, which is itself made of 4 subunits. Proteins are not functional until they become a tertiary or quaternary structure.

Digestion and Absorption

Protein digestion begins in the stomach where the acidic environment serves to denature the protein. Once denatured, pepsins (enzymes) are released into the stomach to break down proteins into larger peptides and AAs. From here, the peptides enter the small intestine where trypsinogen is released from the pancreas. Trypsinogen is a zymogen, meaning it must be "activated" before it can become fully functional. Enterokinase, another enzyme housed on the enterocyte membrane, converts trypsinogen (the zymogen) to trypsin (the active form). Active trypsin can activate other enzymes that begin to break down peptides into smaller

components. The final products of protein digestion include free AAs and small peptides.

The majority of AAs and peptide absorption occurs in the jejunum portion of the intestine. Transporters absorb the AAs and peptides across the enterocyte based on their shape and chemical properties. Free AAs are absorbed via active transport (ie, requires energy) across the small intestine lumen and have different fates once inside the enterocyte. The AAs can be used for the synthesis of new proteins, be oxidized to produce energy, be converted to other AAs or metabolites, or pass through unaltered. Some AAs are preferentially absorbed more than others. The BCAAs are absorbed faster than methionine, followed by essential AAs, then the nonessential AAs. Small peptides are transported more efficiently than AAs into the enterocyte. A common transporter, Pept1, uses energy to absorb the small peptides (Sidebar 2-6).

Requirements and Recommendations

Good sources of protein include meat, poultry, pork, fish and shellfish, dairy, eggs, beans and legumes, nuts and seeds, and grains. Protein quality is important to consider when assessing adequate protein intake and needs. Foods that contain all 9 essential AAs in adequate amounts to meet growth and development and are digested effectively are considered high quality. If just one essential AA is limiting, or lower than recommendations, whole-body protein synthesis becomes inadequate. Animal proteins and soy protein isolate contain all 9 essential AAs. However, some foods have components that inhibit the digestion and absorption of proteins and AAs. These components include phytates, trypsin inhibitors, isoflavones, or fiber and can diminish the protein quality of a protein-rich food.[9]

The Protein Digestibility Corrected Amino Acid Score (PDCAAS) is a common method to assess protein quality. The animal proteins milk, whey, egg, and plant protein soy isolate have a PDCAAS of 1.0.[10] However, this method does not consider the true bioavailability of the AAs. Thus, the Digestible Indispensable Amino Acid Score (DIAAS) is more accurate because it reflects ileal digestibility. The DIAAS is important because it measures digestibility at the end of the small intestine to capture the peptides and AAs that have not been absorbed. Most animal proteins (eg, whey) have a higher DIAAS than plant proteins (eg, soy) because plant proteins often have limiting amounts of isoleucine, lysine, methionine, threonine, and tryptophan.[11,12]

The AMDR for protein for adults is 10% to 35% of energy, or 56 g for men and 46 g for women.[1] The recommended dietary allowance for adults is 0.8 g/kg body weight.

Protein and Exercise

Some populations including athletes and older adults may benefit from higher amounts of dietary protein. To sustain appropriate protein status, 1.2 to 2.0 g/kg of protein depending on type of exercise (ie, endurance or resistance training) is recommended for most athletes and older adults.[1] The upper limit of protein intake may also be recommended for athletes undergoing energy restriction or recovery from an injury.[13]

In addition to protein amount, the timing of intake of protein must also be considered in athletes to maximize muscle protein synthesis (MPS). Some studies have shown that consuming protein with ~10 g of an essential AA within 1 to 2 hours post-exercise improves MPS[14] or ~15 to 30 g protein for most active individuals and athletes. Leucine (700 to 3000 mg) consumed acutely with other high-quality protein sources has also been shown to upregulate MPS.[13]

Conclusion

Active individuals and athletes must consume adequate amounts of all macronutrients for optimal performance and recovery. Carbohydrates provide energy in the form of glucose to the muscle as a sustained energy source. Lipids provide energy stores to be used during exercise, especially endurance activities. Protein is necessary for structural components of the body, including muscle and maintains metabolic processes, during exercise. Inappropriate intake of macronutrients can attenuate performance, cause injury, and hinder recovery.

Discussion Questions

1. How can performance be maintained when athletes or active individuals reduce the intake of all macronutrients for the purposes of reducing calories and ultimately body weight?

2. How can vegan athletes ensure they consume adequate protein and essential amino acids to sustain or improve performance?

References

1. Institute of Medicine. *Dietary Reference Intakes for Energy, Carbohydrate, Fiber, Fat, Fatty Acids, Cholesterol, Protein, and Amino Acids.* National Academies Press; 2015.

2. Thomas DT, Erdman KA, Burke LM. Nutrition and athletic performance. *Med Sci Sports Exerc.* 2016;48(3):543-568. doi:10.1249/MSS.0000000000000852

3. Spriet LL. Recent advances in sports nutrition. *Sports Med.* 2014;44(1):S3-S4. doi:10.1007/s40279-014-0170-1

4. Patterson MA, Maiya M, Stewart ML. Resistant starch intakes in the United States: a narrative review. *J Acad Nutr Diet.* 2020;120:222-236.

5. Shen D, Bai H, Li Z, Yu Y, Zhang H, Chen L. Positive effects of resistant starch supplementation on bowel function in healthy adults: a systematic review and meta-analysis of randomized controlled trials. *Int J Food Sci Nutr.* 2017;68(2):149-157. doi:10.1080/09637486.2016.1226275

6. Dahl WJ, Stewart ML. Position of the Academy of Nutrition and Dietetics: health implications of dietary fiber. *J Acad Nutr Diet.* 2015;115(11):1861-1870. doi:10.1016/j.jand.2015.09.003

7. Stender S, Dyerberg J. Influence of trans fatty acids on health. *Ann Nutr Metab.* 2004;48(2):61-66.

8. Sacks FM, Lichtenstein AH, Wu JHY, et al. Dietary fats and cardiovascular disease: a presidential advisory from the American Heart Association. *Circulation.* 2017;136(3):e1-e23. doi:10.1161/CIR.0000000000000510

9. Food and Agriculture Organization of the United Nations. *Dietary Protein Quality Evaluation in Human Nutrition: Report of an FAO Expert Consultation.* 2013.

10. Schaafsma G. The protein digestibility-corrected amino acid score. *J Nutr.* 2000; 130(7):1865S-1867S. doi:10.1093/jn/130.7.1865S

11. Mathai JK, Liu Y, Stein HH. Values for digestible indispensable amino acid scores (DIAAS) for some dairy and plant proteins may better describe protein quality than values calculated using the concept for protein digestibility-corrected amino acid scores (PDCAAS). *Br J Nutr.* 2017;117(4):490-499. doi:10.1017/S0007114517000125

12. Rogerson D. Vegan diets: practical advice for athletes and exercisers. *J Int Soc Sports Nutr.* 2017;14:36. doi:10.1186/s12970-017-0192-9

13. Jager R, Kerksick CM, Campbell BI, et al. International Society of Sports Nutrition Position Stand: protein and exercise. *J Int Soc Sports Nutr.* 2017;14(20). doi:10.1186/s12970-017-0177-8

14. Gorissen SHM, Crombag JJR, Senden JMG, et al. Protein content and amino acid composition of commercially available plant-based protein isolates. *Amino Acids.* 2018;50(12):1685-1695. doi:10.1007/s00726-018-2640-5

Chapter 3

Micronutrients

Mark Knoblauch, PhD, LAT, ATC, CSCS

Commission on Accreditation of Athletic Training Education *2020 Standards*

This chapter addresses the following *2020 Standards for Accreditation of Professional Athletic Training Programs*:

- Standard 55: Students must gain foundational knowledge in statistics, research design, epidemiology, pathophysiology, biomechanics and pathomechanics, exercise physiology, nutrition, human anatomy, pharmacology, public health, and health care delivery and payor systems.
- Standard 83: Educate and make recommendations to clients/patients on fluids and nutrients to ingest prior to activity, during activity, and during recovery for a variety of activities and environmental conditions.

Learning Objectives

After reviewing this chapter, readers will be able to:

- Identify the various micronutrients as well as differentiate between vitamins and minerals.
- Understand the function of micronutrients within the body.
- Identify the recommended intakes for the major micronutrients.
- Recognize deficiencies that can result from inadequate intake of micronutrients.

Knoblauch M, ed. *Clinical Nutrition
in Athletic Training* (pp 25-40).
© 2023 Taylor & Francis Group.

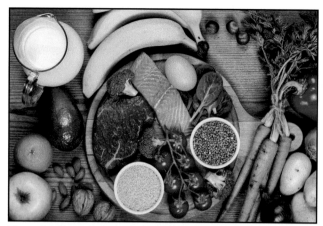

Figure 3-1. For active individuals, the importance of a balanced diet is critical to ensure an adequate intake of micronutrients. (Evan Lorne/Shutterstock.com.)

Introduction

For most active individuals, macronutrients such as carbohydrates and proteins are typically emphasized in the diet due to the critical roles that these nutrients play in energy supply as well as in tissue growth and repair, both of which are essential for maintaining a healthy and active lifestyle. Without an adequate intake of macronutrients, an individual cannot expect to perform at their best; therefore, it is understandable that most individuals tend to prioritize carbohydrates, fats, and proteins when planning out their diet. While macronutrients are certainly relevant for active individuals, micronutrients also play a significant role in normal body function as well as in maintenance of overall health. Enzyme function, hormone production, and even gene expression are among the many body processes that require the assistance of one or more of the various micronutrients. Without an adequate dietary intake of micronutrients, these body processes can become impaired to the point that complications ranging from relatively minor inconveniences (eg, skin rash), to significant impairment, or even death can occur. Fortunately, healthy individuals who consume a Western-based diet are unlikely to experience micronutrient deficiency, and in those rare situations when a deficiency does occur, it can often be quickly remedied through a simple dietary modification (Figure 3-1).

In most cases, an athletic trainer's involvement with micronutrients will likely arise through a deficiency experienced by an athlete, patient, or client—even if only temporarily (eg, "electrolyte imbalance"), such as what could occur in response to strenuous activity. Often, these individuals will make note of some sort of performance impairment such as fatigue or lack of endurance, or they may complain of symptoms related to a structural or systemic issue such as bone loss or perhaps excessively low blood pressure. When overt conditions such as disease or injury are not the underlying cause of such issues, a simple micronutrient deficiency may be to blame. Given the extensive involvement

that micronutrients play in the body's normal physiological function as well as what symptoms can occur in response to a deficiency, it is important for athletic trainers to be able to understand these roles specific to how micronutrients are involved in an individual's health and wellness.

Based on the number of micronutrients that exist, as well as the wide-ranging involvement that micronutrients have in metabolism, a full chapter could easily be written on each micronutrient specific to aspects such as its molecular structure or its involvement in cell signaling or gene transcription pathways. For the clinical athletic trainer, however, the most relevant micronutrient information is typically tied to broader topics such as a particular micronutrient's general influence on cell structure or metabolism, as well as nutrition-specific aspects such as dietary sources or complications that can result from a particular micronutrient deficiency. In understanding these clinical-based components of micronutrients, athletic trainers can better recognize how specific micronutrients factor into maximizing one's performance. Therefore, this chapter is designed to orient athletic trainers to the role that the more common macronutrients play in overall health and wellness. For those micronutrients covered, aspects including each micronutrient's function within the body, as well as primary dietary sources, will be discussed. In addition, complications that patients can experience as a result of micronutrient deficiencies will be outlined.

What Are Micronutrients?

At its simplest, a micronutrient is any dietary substance that the body requires in relatively small quantities. Several micronutrients such as magnesium and zinc have daily intake levels of less than 1 g per day while others, such as some vitamins, have recommended intake levels of less than 1 mg per day. These relatively small micronutrient recommendations differ considerably from the much higher intake recommendations for macronutrients which, in the case of carbohydrates, can easily exceed 100 g per day—or even several hundred grams per day among elite or highly competitive athletes.

Though the recommended intake levels for micronutrients are quite low, it is important to recognize that micronutrients are essential in nature such that they are not synthesized within the body. Therefore, an adequate supply of micronutrients must be obtained from the diet. Without sufficient intake, many of the body's metabolic processes will not function normally and the individual will likely develop some degree of ailment. For example, every grade school student has probably heard the story of how sailors adrift at sea for months at a time without access to fruits and vegetables developed scurvy in response to an inadequate supply of vitamin C. Scurvy, however, is far from the only micronutrient deficiency that can occur. For example, iodine deficiency is known to negatively influence thyroid hormone production,[1]

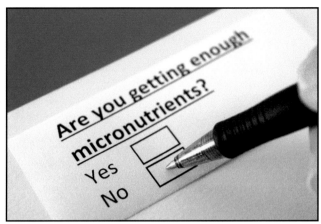

Figure 3-2. While most individuals obtain adequate micronutrients from their diet, those on special diets or who do not eat a balanced diet may be lacking consumption of key micronutrients. (Yeexin Richelle/Shutterstock.com.)

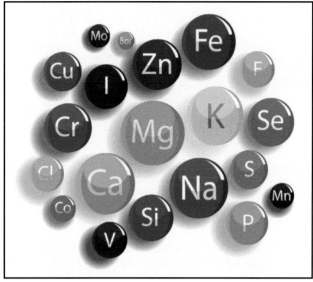

Figure 3-3. Not all micronutrients are alike—the wide range of physiological uses of the various minerals and vitamins warrants different intake levels for each. (Sadovnikova Olga/Shutterstock.com.)

and a deficiency in vitamin A has been shown to cause severe vision problems.[2] For most individuals living in the United States, however, disorders resulting from micronutrient deficiency are relatively uncommon thanks in large part to an ample food supply as well as focused research that has outlined the body's requirement for micronutrients (Figure 3-2).

The relative rarity of micronutrient deficiencies in developed countries is due in large part to targeted research that has identified the importance of micronutrients in maintaining proper health. As far back as the early 1900s, the nutritional significance of micronutrients was recognized as rats soon died after being fed a diet containing no macronutrients while rats fed an unpurified diet survived.[3] Over time, it was revealed that purified diets lacked an array of nutritional components that were essential for normal health. This in turn led to intense study into what we now know as micronutrients, and the resulting research has allowed for the identification of many disorders or diseases that are linked to specific micronutrients.

There are generally 2 groups of micronutrients—minerals and vitamins—that can be further separated into 4 categories: macrominerals, microminerals, fat-soluble vitamins, and water-soluble vitamins. Macrominerals such as calcium or sodium consist of a specific set of minerals that are required at a level that exceeds 100 mg per day, while microminerals, or "trace" minerals, such as zinc or copper are required in amounts of less than 100 mg per day.[4] Separately, fat-soluble vitamins are those that, when consumed in excess amounts, can be stored within the body. Water-soluble vitamins cannot be stored; therefore, any unneeded water-soluble vitamin is quickly excreted (Figure 3-3).

Although more than 30 different vitamins and minerals are needed for normal body function, several micronutrients have multiple roles within the body. Sodium, for example, is involved in signal transmission (eg, depolarization) as well as in fluid regulation. Similarly, calcium is essential for both bone formation as well as cellular signaling processes. The variety of roles that micronutrients play highlights the need for a thorough understanding by athletic trainers of not only the individual micronutrients that are significantly involved with physical activity but also their primary function(s) within the body. The remainder of this chapter will focus on outlining the major micronutrients that our body requires in order to maintain its metabolic activity. The most common macrominerals will be discussed first, followed by microminerals, fat-soluble vitamins, and water-soluble vitamins.

Minerals

Macrominerals

Calcium

Within the human body, calcium is the fifth-most abundant substance after oxygen, carbon, hydrogen, and nitrogen and is the most abundant mineral. Calcium is the primary mineral contained within bone,[5] and this high bone content allows it to serve as the body's primary storage site for calcium. Not surprisingly, more than 99% of the body's calcium is contained within the skeletal system, while another 1% resides in the teeth and soft tissues. A trivial yet critical 0.1% exists within various body tissues where it is used in cellular signaling events such as those required for skeletal muscle contraction.

As a mineral, calcium is probably best known for its involvement in the regulation of bone mass, though it is also involved with the production of other substances within the body such as parathyroid hormone, vitamin D, and estrogen. Calcium serves to "mineralize" bone, thereby providing structure and serving to strengthen bone tissue (Figure

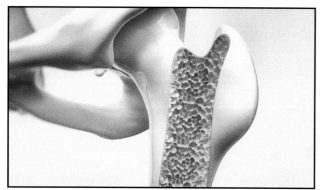

Figure 3-4. Calcium, along with other nutrients such as vitamin D, is crucial for maintenance of healthy bones. (Crevis/Shutterstock.com.)

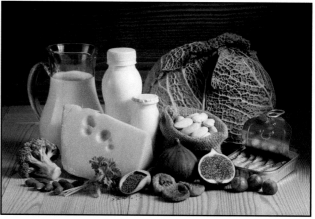

Figure 3-5. Foods rich in calcium include dairy products like milk or cheese, as well as several kinds of vegetables. (Evan Lorne/Shutterstock.com.)

3-4). Therefore, calcium is highly involved in the regulation of bone mass, as bone deposition requires an uptake of calcium from within the plasma, while bone resorption releases calcium from bone tissue. This in turn relegates bone tissue as a sort of reservoir for maintaining proper blood calcium levels to the point that bone strength may be sacrificed in order to maintain adequate calcium concentrations within the blood.[6] For otherwise healthy individuals, the calcium stored within bone tissue allows for maintenance of normal blood calcium levels when adequate calcium is not obtained through the diet. An understanding of how the body can sacrifice bone integrity in order to maintain blood calcium levels highlights the importance of maintaining an adequate intake of calcium within the diet so as to prevent the need for calcium resorption from bone.

Age-associated bone loss is well known, and calcium's involvement in bone loss over time has been the topic of much research. However, calcium is not likely the only factor involved in age-associated bone loss, as hip fracture rates have been shown to occur more frequently in developed countries where calcium intake is high than in developing countries where calcium intake is low.[7] This evidence suggests that fracture rates do not occur due to low calcium levels alone and may be influenced to some degree by factors such as protein intake, vitamin D status, or both. Still, if left unchecked, bone loss can have a significant impact on quality of life and can have a high financial cost in the event of bone injuries such as a hip fracture. However, when meeting or exceeding 800 mg/day of calcium intake, age-related bone loss can be counteracted. Such evidence emphasizes the point that athletic trainers should work to help ensure that all patients—particularly older individuals known to be at risk for bone loss—are consuming adequate calcium.

In addition to providing strength to the skeleton, calcium is a primary signaling molecule for the initiation of several cellular events. For example, myofibers utilize several physiologic events in order to elevate cytosolic calcium to more than 100 times the resting levels for the initiation of contraction.[8] At rest, calcium is stored within the sarcoplasmic reticulum (SR). In response to a neural signal from the brain, contraction initiates upon the release of calcium from the SR into the internal myofiber environment. This flood of calcium triggers a cascade of events that results in a shortening of the sarcomere. Immediately after calcium floods the myofiber interior, enzymes known as sarcoplasmic/endoplasmic reticulum calcium ATPase molecules start shuttling the released calcium back into the SR, diminishing the amount of free calcium within the internal myofiber environment and terminating the sarcomere's contraction.

Even small fluctuations in blood calcium can have significant consequences. For example, low blood calcium (ie, "hypocalcemia") can trigger seizures as well as muscle spasm, while high blood calcium levels ("hypercalcemia") can cause thirst, mental confusion, and fatigue.[9] With the exclusion of slightly higher (~1300 mg/day) calcium recommendations for older children and teenagers, kids and adults are generally recommended to take in around 1000 mg of calcium per day.[10]

Calcium Source

Some of the highest sources of dietary calcium include milk and milk products such as cheese, yogurt, and sour cream. Nuts, whole grain foods, and certain vegetables such as broccoli can also serve as significant sources of calcium (Figure 3-5). While spinach is often touted for its calcium content, the bioavailability of that calcium is relatively low.[11] When food-based calcium sources are inadequate, calcium-based supplements (600 to 1000 mg) can be used effectively to make up for dietary deficiencies. Still, the absorption of dietary calcium is relatively poor, as only around one-fourth to one-third of dietary calcium is absorbed.[3] This absorption rate is influenced by several factors, which can include age, dietary calcium content, or vitamin D status. Because of these absorption factors, recommended calcium intake has been the subject of debate.

Calcium Deficiency

Calcium deficiency is usually not the result of a lack of intake; rather, deficiency is often due to other factors such as vitamin D deficiency, decreased estrogen, or inadequate activity from the adrenal or parathyroid gland.[3] The most common indicators of calcium deficiency include poorly calcified bones in children, inadequate bone growth in children, and porous bone structure in adults.

Phosphorus

Phosphorus trails only calcium in terms of abundance within the body, and the human body contains on average around 750 g of phosphorus. While almost all cells require phosphorus, bones maintain around 85% of the total phosphorus content of the body.[3] In actuality, the body contains very little free phosphorus; instead, phosphorus exists predominantly as phosphate,[3] a molecule formed from a phosphorus atom surrounded by 4 oxygen atoms. While in its free form, phosphate is commonly referred to as "inorganic phosphate," or "Pi."

As a micronutrient, phosphorus is typically discussed alongside calcium given that the 2 elements are essential for the formation of bone, particularly when the calcium-to-phosphorus ratio is between 1 to 2:1.[12] Specifically, phosphorus supplies the anion required for the formation of hydroxyapatite that is necessary for bone mineralization.[13] Besides its role in bone formation, phosphorus also serves as a primary component of the phospholipid bilayer of cell membranes. Phosphorus combines with a lipid molecule to form a phospholipid that, when organized into the lipid bilayer, forms a barrier around individual cells that allows for regulated entry and exit of cellular materials (Figure 3-6). Physical activity, whether it be strenuous weightlifting or a light jog, can cause microdamage that involves disruption of cell membranes. Whereas phosphorus is a key constituent of these damaged membranes, an adequate intake of phosphorus can help ensure proper repair of activity-induced cell membrane damage.

Phosphorus also has several additional functions involving individual cellular processes. For example, phosphorus is involved in the production of DNA and is an essential component of the phosphorylation process that adds a phosphoryl group to a molecule. Phosphorus is involved in many enzymatic chemical processes, such as what occurs in the breakdown of glucose to pyruvate. Furthermore, phosphorus is a key element in many anabolic and catabolic processes and is highly involved in energy production within the body. This is because the phosphate groups of the ATP molecule are held together by bonds that, when broken, can release approximately twice the energy of normal bonds.[3]

Phosphate Sources

Phosphate can be found within many foods that are consumed in a normal diet. Meats, yogurt, and even soft drinks can be a significant source of phosphorus. Cola drinks

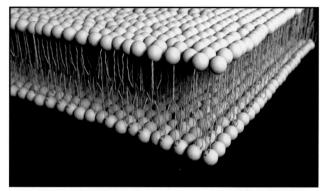

Figure 3-6. Phosphorus is a vital component of the lipid bilayer that is critical for healthy cell membranes. (raydingoz/Shutterstock.com.)

contain on average 44 to 62 mg of phosphorus, while diet colas contain 27 to 39 mg of phosphorus.[14] Men, on average, intake around 1.5 g of phosphate per day, while women consume on average 1.0 g,[3] both of which are much higher than the National Academies of Sciences, Engineering, and Medicine's (NASEM) recommendation of 700 mg per day. Adolescents, with their substantial bone growth, are recommended to consume at least 1250 mg per day.[15]

Phosphate Deficiency

Due to the wide variety of foods that most individuals in the United States consume, phosphate deficiency is unlikely. However, adults who consume a significant amount of aluminum-oxide antacids or eat a low-phosphate diet can experience phosphate-related symptoms such as muscle weakness, impaired growth, or bone pain. Hypophosphatemia can occur in up to 28% of patients with severe trauma, hyperventilation,[16] or other respiratory problems,[17] as well as in patients with infectious disease.[18] Furthermore, one study found that women who consumed more than 3 servings of cola per day exhibited lower bone mineral density in their hip than those who consumed less than 1 serving of cola per day.[19]

Sodium

Of all nutrients, sodium is likely the most overconsumed macronutrient within the average American diet. Sodium is typically consumed in one of its many compound forms such as sodium chloride (ie, table salt), sodium bicarbonate, or sodium phosphate. The vast majority (~75%) of sodium within the body is contained within the mineral makeup of bones,[3] while the remainder is largely held within the extracellular fluid where it exists as the primary extracellular electrolyte (Figure 3-7).

Within the body, sodium serves in 2 primary processes—fluid regulation and cellular signaling. To exert its effects on these beneficial physiological processes, sodium levels within the body must be maintained within a relatively small range. Normally, the body attempts to maintain a specific sodium concentration in the blood (ie, 135 to 145 mEq/L), and this range is maintained predominantly through a balance between sodium intake from the diet and excretion through

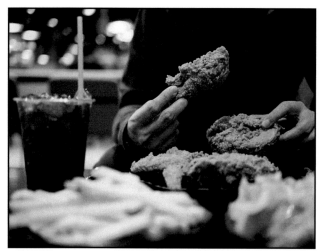

Figure 3-7. The high levels of sodium found in most processed or prepared foods contributes significantly to the excessive sodium that many Americans consume. (Boontoom Sae-Kor/ Shutterstock.com.)

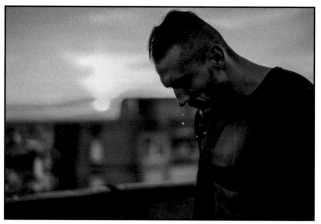

Figure 3-8. As an active individual sweats, small amount of minerals such as sodium are removed from the body. (Vladimir Borovic/ Shutterstock.com.)

urine and sweat. Fluctuations in total body fluid can alter the body's sodium concentration. Such fluctuations can occur through events such as fluid intake or significant sweat loss, each of which can require adjustments by the body to maintain an appropriate sodium concentration.

When the body's sodium concentration increases, such as in response to consumption of a high-sodium meal, antidiuretic hormone (ADH) is released that then triggers an increase in water resorption within the kidneys.[20] This resorption helps to dilute the existing sodium concentration in the body in an attempt to maintain a healthy level. Conversely, when the body's sodium concentration becomes low—as may occur after physical activity in hot weather—aldosterone is released within the body that then initiates a cascade of events, which ultimately leads to a retention of sodium from the filtrate and subsequent return of that retained sodium to the circulation. Through this careful balance of sodium resorption and excretion, adequate osmotic pressures can be maintained within the blood, extracellular space, and individual cells.

For the clinical athletic trainer, fluid regulation in response to sodium levels can be a major factor in the health of their athletes, patients, and clients. Athletes are known to engage in lengthy bouts of strenuous physical activity that can result in fluid loss as well as a loss of sodium that is contained within sweat (Figure 3-8). Patients or clients may engage in outdoor activity such as running or even mowing their yard on a hot day. In either case, the loss of sweat and sodium is not particularly problematic if the fluids are replenished. However, significant sweat loss followed by consumption of large amounts of water can be problematic if the amount of water is excessive (Sidebar 3-1). Conversely, consumption of a high sodium meal or even drinks such as tomato juice serve to increase the body's sodium concentration. To counter the sudden increase in sodium, the body may retain fluid in an attempt to lower the sodium concentration; however, this

Sidebar 3-1

Sodium regulation becomes particularly problematic when sodium and fluid is lost from the body (via urine or sweat) and only the fluid is replaced, such as in consuming a high amount of water. In such a case, the consumed water further dilutes the available sodium within the extracellular space, triggering low-sodium levels (ie, hyponatremia, or blood sodium levels <135 mEq/L) by throwing off the normal osmolarity of the body in an extensive process that can, in some cases, be fatal. Even a small amount of sodium consumed with water can alleviate this consequence; therefore, it is important for active individuals to understand the need to include an appropriate amount of sodium in their hydration plan.

in turn increases the body's fluid levels. When the retention of fluid becomes chronic in nature as a result of an ongoing high intake of sodium, it can be quite problematic, as it can result in conditions such as hypertension.

Besides fluid retention, sodium's second major function within the body is specific to cell signaling. One of the primary signaling events that sodium is involved with is specific to membrane depolarization that occurs through interaction with the sodium-potassium ATPase enzyme, also commonly known as the sodium-potassium pump. This pump capitalizes on the sodium ion's overall positive charge to create an electrochemical gradient that generates the depolarization/ repolarization mechanism essential for nerve transmission, muscle contraction, and other cellular signaling events. Based in part upon its role in membrane depolarization, it has traditionally been thought that sodium-related complications contribute to electrolyte-related conditions such as

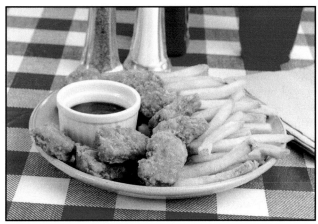

Figure 3-9. Sodium found within prepared foods is the primary source of sodium for many Americans, while sodium added via a salt shaker contributes a relatively small amount of additional sodium. (MSPhotographic/Shutterstock.com.)

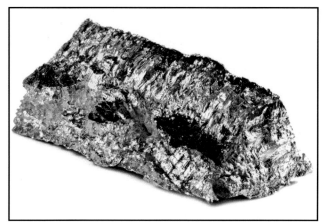

Figure 3-10. Magnesium in its raw form. (Bjoern Wylezich/Shutterstock.com.)

exercise-induced muscle cramping; however, evidence for a direct link between sodium intake and cramping remains to be clearly determined.[21]

Sodium Sources

Individuals often think of sodium as the compound sodium chloride, or "table salt." Although sodium is indeed a component of table salt, the terms should not be used interchangeably. Table salt is a compound comprised of 40% sodium and 60% chloride, and given the ubiquity of sodium chloride within prepared food items as well as in its use as a seasoning, it is not surprisingly a primary source of sodium consumption. Many food products contain a natural amount of sodium; however, the vast majority of dietary sodium intake occurs as a result of added sodium chloride from either its addition to processed or canned foods or from the salt shaker at the dinner table. Canned vegetables, meat products, and condiments often have a relatively high sodium level due to sodium's ability to act as an effective (and inexpensive) preservative. Furthermore, many food items often contain a relatively high sodium level due to the addition of salt for seasoning purposes, such as packaged foods that include seasoning packets, nuts, or potato chips (Figure 3-9).

Sodium Intake

Given the widespread nature of sodium in foods, it can be quite easy for athletes, patients, or clients to consume an excess amount of sodium. As such, sodium deficiency is quite rare. The average sodium intake for most individuals in the United States is around 3500 mg/day.[22] This high intake continues to occur despite the NASEM's adequate intake recommendation of 1500 mg/day for adults[23] and the US Food and Drug Administration's recommended limit of 2300 mg/day.[24] Both of these recommended intake levels are much higher than the body's minimum requirement of 200 to 500 mg/day to maintain physiological function,[25] though this minimal level should not generally be used as a dietary goal.

Rather, sodium intake should be adjusted based on factors such as activity level, as individuals engaged in endurance or vigorous exercise may need to replace sodium to a higher degree than nonactive individuals.

Magnesium

Magnesium is a grayish-white metal that is involved in more than 300 events within the body, particularly those events requiring enzymatic action[26] (Figure 3-10). The body contains on average 21 to 28 g of magnesium, with well over half of this amount contained within the skeleton[27] while the remaining magnesium exists largely within the intracellular environment.[26] A very small (~1%) amount of the body's total magnesium exists within the blood, where normal serum levels are found from 0.7 to 1.10 mmol/L.[28] Total magnesium levels within the body, like most all nutrients, are inherent to the net balance that exists between absorption of magnesium from the diet and that amount excreted from the kidneys and, to a small degree, sweat.

A primary role for magnesium is related to its involvement in energy production pathways including glycolysis and glucose homeostasis, where it serves as a cofactor in phosphorylation reactions that are required for ATP production. Similarly, magnesium has been shown to be involved in lipid metabolism and protein synthesis.[26] Specific to cell signaling, magnesium helps regulate the activity of ion channels such as the sodium-potassium pump required for nerve transmission, and is intricately involved in the process of muscle contraction. Magnesium helps regulate bone formation and also has a structural function within individual cells where it serves to stabilize mammalian cell membranes. Based on these wide-ranging actions, individuals involved in physical activity are well-served to maintain proper magnesium levels.

Generally, humans need approximately 300 to 400 mg of magnesium per day, though this amount can vary depending on factors such as activity level, gender, and age.[29] Available magnesium can be recirculated into the intestine via bile, which serves as a mechanism for regulating the body's

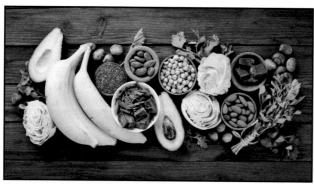

Figure 3-11. Plants, seeds, and nuts are excellent sources of magnesium. (YARUNIV Studio/Shutterstock.com.)

magnesium levels.[3] Regulation of magnesium levels is also facilitated within the kidney, as urine removes approximately 100 mg of magnesium per day from an adult who consumes around 300 mg/day. Therefore, both the intestinal and renal system are effective at maintaining adequate magnesium levels.

Magnesium Sources

Magnesium can be obtained through a wide variety of sources, yet primarily comes from plants. Vegetables, nuts, and meats are considered excellent sources of magnesium, and milk and other dairy-based products are relatively poor sources (Figure 3-11). When evaluating magnesium sources, it is important to note that processed foods lose much of their magnesium content. For example, grains that are processed prior to packaging can lose up to 80% of their magnesium content. This is particularly important in that only around 50% of dietary magnesium is absorbed[30] and is complicated by factors such as a high calcium that can adversely affect magnesium absorption. Furthermore, drugs such as digoxin or certain loop diuretics can alter magnesium levels within the body.[31]

Magnesium Deficiency

Though magnesium deficiency is relatively uncommon, symptoms resulting from a magnesium deficiency can range from rather mild—such as muscle spasm or twitching, nausea, or vomiting—to the more serious events of personality changes, convulsions, and/or coma.[3] It is important to note that magnesium deficiency is rarely related to dietary involvement alone; rather, any deficiency is more likely to occur in response to an existing comorbidity such as kidney disease, endocrine disorders, or alcoholism.[32] Also, individuals experiencing sustained bouts of diarrhea can be susceptible to short-term magnesium deficiency, and those individuals taking a thiazide diuretic are at risk for magnesium deficiency due to diuretics inhibiting the ability of the kidney to return magnesium from the filtrate to the body.[32] Athletic trainers should also note that any athlete, patient, or client exhibiting a magnesium deficiency should be evaluated for hypocalcemia, as magnesium plays a role in the parathyroid hormone—the calcium regulatory pathway that

is important for bone resorption.[33] Several pathologies have been suggested to be caused by alterations in magnesium levels, but the true influence magnesium has on these pathologies is debatable given that, as mentioned earlier, calcium can interfere with magnesium measures.[34] Because of the widespread range of foods that contain magnesium, individuals who consume a variety of foods are unlikely to reach a state of magnesium deficiency. Still, diseases such as high blood pressure, sickle cell anemia, and insulin resistance are suggested to be linked to magnesium abnormalities.[26] The true influence of magnesium on many of these diseases, however, is questionable given that alterations in magnesium homeostasis can be difficult to determine in a lab.[35]

Potassium

Potassium is a soft, waxy, silver-white colored element that is the predominant intracellular electrolyte. Potassium has multiple roles within the body including its involvement with membrane depolarization, where potassium's concentration inside or outside of the cell is regulated via the sodium-potassium ATPase enzyme in order to distribute the depolarization signal across the cell membrane. Potassium, like sodium, is a major contributor to the regulation of fluid levels within the body. Potassium also serves as a co-factor for enzymes, is involved in the metabolism of carbohydrates, and plays a role in the secretion of insulin.

Blood levels of potassium are closely maintained within a physiologic range as a result of the kidneys increasing or decreasing the amount of potassium that is removed from the filtrate. It has been shown that the pH level of urine can influence potassium secretion, as a higher acidity in the filtrate can increase the amount of potassium that is retained while a more alkaline urine can cause an increase in the excretion of potassium.[36] These blood levels of potassium can be influenced by physical activity, though sweat excretion of potassium is relatively minimal, at only around 5 mmol/L.[36] However, sustained exercise that induces a high sweat rate can lead to hypokalemia if potassium levels are not adequately replaced. In addition to excretion via urine and sweat, potassium can be excreted in small amounts in the feces. Therefore, in cases of severe diarrhea lasting a day or more, low potassium levels can develop.[3] Furthermore, patients on thiazide drugs (as well as loop diuretics) should be informed of the possibility of those drugs inducing a low potassium level.

Potassium intake recommendations vary across several countries. For example, Mexico and the United Kingdom recommend 90 mmol/day, while the United States and other countries recommend 120 mmol per day—both of which are higher than the 2002 Joint World Health Organization/Food and Agriculture Organization (WHO/FAO) of the United Nations Expert Consultation recommendation of 70 to 80 mmol/day.[37] Interestingly, no country's average population intake of potassium meets the 120 mmol/day recommendation that exists in the United States.[38] Failure to meet the recommended intake of potassium can have effects on aspects

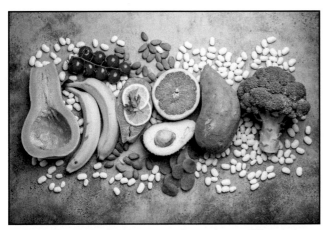

Figure 3-12. Potatoes, fish, bananas, and several types of fruits and vegetables are excellent sources of potassium. (Elena Eryomenko/Shutterstock.com.)

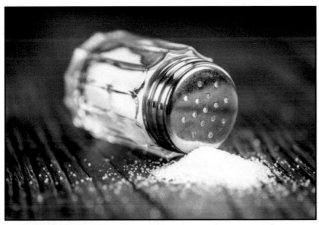

Figure 3-13. Along with sodium, table salt contributes a significant amount of chloride to an individual's diet. (HandmadePictures/Shutterstock.com.)

such as blood pressure and disease risk, as research has shown that increasing one's potassium intake correlates to favorable events such as a decrease in blood pressure and can also reduce one's risk of stroke.[39] Specific to RDA, NASEM in 2019 updated their Dietary Reference Intake such that 14- to 18-year-old individuals should obtain 3000 and 2300 mg per day respectively, while adult men and women aged 19 to 50 should seek to consume 3400 and 2600 mg of potassium per day, respectively.

Potassium Sources and Deficiency

Potassium is contained within almost all naturally occurring foods and has a high absorption rate of approximately 90% (Figure 3-12). Primary sources of potassium include orange juice, fish, potatoes, and bananas. Because potassium is found across a variety of foods, only those foods that are highly refined (pure sugars, oils, certain fats, etc.) are

Sidebar 3-2

Potassium has long been suspected to be involved in exercise-induced muscle cramping (EAMC), with sufferers often instructed to "eat a banana" to offset the sometimes debilitating cramps. However, more recent evidence has led away from potassium or other electrolyte as a potential cause of EAMC. Rather, current theories suggest EAMC is due more to a neurological excitability source.[67]

reported as lacking in potassium.[3] Potassium deficiencies are relatively mild but include muscle weakness, general malaise, and fatigue (Sidebar 3-2).

Chloride

The human body contains approximately 115 g of chloride on average which in turn makes up around 0.15% of the body's weight.[40] Chloride plays a role in several functions including preservation of the body's osmotic pressure and maintaining an acid-base balance such as required for stomach acid, and chloride is involved in the process of muscle contraction.[41] Within the body's tissue, intracellular chloride levels differ by cell type. For example, myofibers have a relatively low intracellular chloride content at 2 to 4 mEq/L while red blood cells have a much higher intracellular chloride content of 70 mEq/L.[42]

Chloride Sources and Deficiency

The source of most dietary chloride comes from salt (ie, sodium chloride) consumed within the diet (Figure 3-13).[41] Chloride from the diet is absorbed within the small intestine, in amounts that range from 7.8 to 11.8 g/day for men to 5.8 to 7.8 g/day for women in the United States.[43] Once in the body, chloride concentrations are largely regulated via a balance that is created between absorption within the intestinal tract and excretion by the kidney.[41] Approximately 99% of the chloride filtered within the kidneys is reabsorbed, ultimately resulting in approximately 180 mmol of chloride being excreted per day.

Disorders associated with high or low levels of chloride are relatively rare, given its presence within salt. However, abnormal chloride intake can have a direct effect on bicarbonate. For example, hypochloremia (or low levels of chlorine) will cause an increase in the reabsorption of bicarbonate that in turn triggers metabolic alkalosis.[40] Conversely, hyperchloremia often occurs in response to an intestinal or kidney-associated loss of bicarbonate (such as through diarrhea) that can generate an increase in chloride.

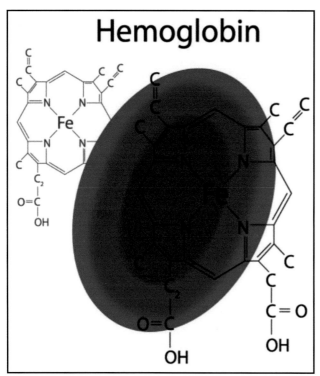

Figure 3-14. Iron (Fe) is a major component of hemoglobin, the oxygen-carrying component of the red blood cell. (yaruna/Shutterstock.com.)

Microminerals

Iron

Iron is the most plentiful metal in the body.[44] The total iron content in the body is around 4 g in men and 2.6 g in women, approximately 65% of which is contained within hemoglobin.[3] Iron is also quite abundant in the brain and liver. Iron is involved in several processes, including significant roles in regulating gene expression, synthesis of DNA and RNA, protein synthesis, enzyme activity, and transport of oxygen (Figure 3-14).[44]

Metabolism of iron is tied in with copper metabolism and may also involve other metals.[44] However, inflammation can affect iron homeostasis, as it has been shown that pro-inflammatory cytokines can alter iron homeostasis.[45] Furthermore, individuals with iron overload (ie, an excess of iron in the body) are at increased susceptibility to infection, particularly when compared against those with iron deficiency.[46] In older individuals, iron tends to accumulate and is associated with altered iron homeostasis, which is likely to contribute to general age-related deterioration.[47]

Iron is absorbed from the small intestine. Interestingly, the predominant method of "excretion" of iron from the body occurs not through the kidneys or intestines but rather as a result of the shedding of skin that accounts for 1 to 2 mg of iron loss per day.[48] Turnover and subsequent reuse of iron from red blood cells accounts for approximately 90% of iron recycling, with the additional 10% being obtained from the diet.[49]

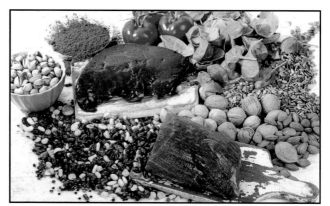

Figure 3-15. Sources of iron in the diet include meats, liver, and nuts, among various other foods. (Tatjana Baibakova/Shutterstock.com.)

Iron Sources and Deficiency

The RDA for men and post-menopausal women is 8 mg/day and for women is 18 mg/day. Significant sources of dietary iron include meats, nuts, liver, chickpeas, and fortified cereals (Figure 3-15). Failing to obtain an adequate intake of iron can influence fatigue, mood, and the ability to perform tasks.[50] And despite iron's abundance within foods, iron deficiency has been called the most common deficiency in the world, resulting in affected individuals being unable to produce enough hemoglobin to supply the body's need.[51] Similarly, iron deficiency is the most common cause for anemia, a condition particularly relevant to active individuals as it results from an inadequate number of red blood cells in the body and results in a diminished capacity for supplying oxygen to working muscles. Within athletic individuals, iron deficiency has been reported to exist at 3% to 11% in men and 15% to 35% in women.[52] The higher iron deficiency rate in women is largely due to menstruation, which results in an increased iron loss from the body.

Chromium

As a trace element, chromium is utilized by the body in its trivalent form as compared to its available hexavalent form that is actually toxic to the body and is a byproduct of pollution.[53] Chromium's role within the body includes aiding in enzyme activity and serving as a co-factor for insulin production,[54] and it is involved in carbohydrate metabolism as well as fatty acid and cholesterol synthesis.[51]

Adequate intake values for chromium have been suggested at 35 mg/day for men and 25 mg/day for women, both of which are less than a prior recommended intake of 50 to 200 mg/day.[55] Though quite common in foods, only very small amounts of chromium are typically found in dietary sources. The best sources for chromium include egg yolks, whole grains, bran cereals, and nuts.[56]

Zinc

Zinc has a role of serving as a cofactor for more than 70 different enzymatic reactions.[3] Though zinc was not originally recognized as an essential nutrient, it was later found to be absent or deficient in conditions that included stunted growth, anemia, enlarged liver and spleen, and mental lethargy.[3] Zinc serves several functions, including gene regulation and cell membrane stability, and is involved in protein synthesis as well as insulin production. Existing in a wide variety of food sources, zinc can be found in red meat, cheese, and plants, though plant sources are often rich in phytate which reduces the absorption of available zinc (Figure 3-16). Interestingly, zinc supplementation has been shown to decrease the level of high-density lipoprotein "C," thereby increasing the risk of cardiovascular disease in some individuals.[57] Deficiencies resulting from inadequate zinc intake, though relatively rare in developed societies, include skin lesions, growth retardation, impaired immunological function, and contribute to night blindness that is often associated with vitamin A deficiency.

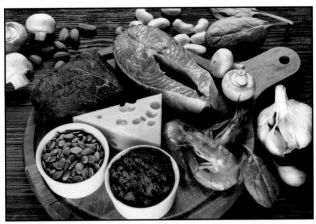

Figure 3-16. Meats and cheeses are excellent sources of zinc, along with several plant sources. (Evan Lorne/Shutterstock.com.)

Vitamins

The study of vitamins has been ongoing for more than a century when their discovery in rice bran was first thought to be the essential link to the disease of beriberi. As research continued over the first half of the 20th century, it became evident that vitamins had different roles and were even handled differently within the body (ie, fat-soluble versus water-soluble). Ongoing research has allowed understanding of the extensive role that vitamins play in metabolism and the association that vitamins have with many deficiency-based diseases.

Without an adequate supply of vitamins, body functions such as enzyme-mediated reactions cannot occur. This in turn can lead to issues such as muscle weakness, cardiac conditions, depression, and dry skin, among many other deficiency-related conditions that can affect almost all body tissues. Understanding the role that vitamins play in clinical nutrition is essential for maintaining proper body function. Therefore, this section will provide a general overview of several of the vitamins that can play a significant role in physical activity.

Water-Soluble Vitamins

B Vitamins

Eight B vitamins exist, and are often collectively referred to as b-complex vitamins. Included in the B vitamin group are thiamine (B_1), riboflavin (B_2), niacin (B_3), pantothenic acid (B_5), pyridoxine (B_6), biotin (B_7), folate (B_9), and cobalamin (B_{12}). The inconsistent numbering inherent to the B-complex vitamins results from prior numerical assignment being made to substances that were later classified as something other than a vitamin. The B-complex vitamins serve vital roles in acting predominantly as enzyme cofactors. Riboflavin, for example, is involved in the metabolism of flavin mononucleotide and flavin adenine dinucleotide.[58] Biotin plays a role in synthesis of the protein keratin that is essential for proper hair and nail growth, while folate plays a role in amino acid and nucleotide metabolism.[58]

B vitamins are significantly involved in carbohydrate and fat metabolism, and as such their intake is critical for active individuals.[58] The aforementioned biotin, for example, is produced within the gut yet plays important roles in gluconeogenesis, the synthesis of fatty acids, and the breakdown of amino acids, all processes that are highly relevant in fueling as well as tissue repair in active individuals. Similarly, pantothenic acid (ie, vitamin B_5) is involved in the metabolism of carbohydrates, fats, and proteins, all of which play a key role in an individual's ability to perform physical activity. A breakdown of the function, sources, and main deficiencies of B vitamins in humans is outlined in Table 3-1.

Given the array of B vitamins, food sources for this vitamin group are quite widespread (Figure 3-17). So much so, that for most individuals who consume a balanced diet, B-complex vitamin deficiency is rare. However, individuals who engage in vegetarian-type diets (eg, vegan) should ensure that they receive adequate intake of vitamins such as niacin or B_{12} that are found predominantly in animal products such as fish or liver but can also be found in nuts. For those who engage in higher physical activity levels (eg, athletes), adequate intake of B vitamins is essential due to the role that these vitamins play in macronutrient metabolism.[58]

Vitamin C

Vitamin C, or ascorbic acid, is a water-soluble vitamin that has an extensive array of functions within the body. One of its main roles is in the synthesis of collagen, as collagen cannot be formed without vitamin C.[57] Vitamin C is associated with hormone production as it assists in the conversion of dopamine to noradrenaline, and is also involved in amino acid metabolism.[58] In addition, vitamin C has been recognized for its significant anti-inflammatory effects.[58]

Table 3-1

Summary of Vitamin B Function, Dietary Source, and Symptoms Associated With Deficiency

B VITAMIN	NAME	MAIN FUNCTIONS	DIETARY SOURCES	DEFICIENCY SYMPTOMS
1	Thiamin	Carbohydrate metabolism	Wheat products Enriched flour and cereals	Beriberi Wernicke-Korsakoff syndrome
2	Riboflavin	Breakdown of fats, proteins, and carbohydrates	Milk and milk products Liver	Cracking of the lips Throat or mouth edema
3	Niacin	Oxidative phosphorylation	Liver Yeast Peanuts	Pellagra
5	Pantothenic acid	Red blood cell and hormone production	Meats Grains	Unknown
6	Pyridoxine	Amino acid metabolism	Meats Whole grains Vegetables	Weakness Insomnia Dermatitis
7	Biotin	Coenzyme for carboxylase enzymes	Vast sources	Unknown
9	Folate/folic acid	DNA synthesis	Leafy vegetables Bananas	Impaired cell division Anemia
12	Cobalamin	Red blood cell production Nerve health	Liver Shellfish Eggs	Certain neuropathies

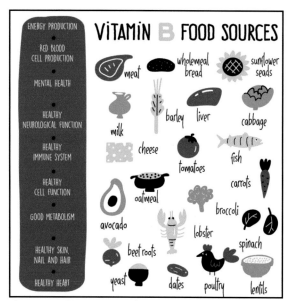

Figure 3-17. Dietary sources for vitamin B are extensive and include items that range from grains to vegetables to meat and fish. (Ekaterina Kapranova/Shutterstock.com.)

Normally, the body contains from 1500 to 2500 mg of vitamin C. Because of its water-soluble characteristic, any additional storage of vitamin C is not possible. Despite an inability to store vitamin C, a healthy diet should be expected to provide ample amounts necessary for metabolism. Sources of vitamin C predominantly include plant-based foods like potatoes or fruits, and it is often found in these foods at a much higher rate than other vitamins (Figure 3-18).[59] It is also noteworthy to point out that the cooking process destroys vitamin C; therefore, fresh fruits and vegetables are preferred as sources of vitamin C. When consumed at around 500 mg per day, such as might occur via supplementation, plasma levels of vitamin C do not increase. This is due in part to an increased urine excretion of vitamin C at these higher levels.[57]

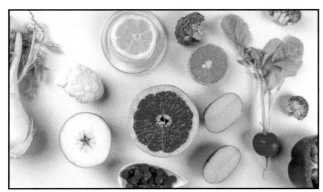

Figure 3-18. Fruits and vegetables such as potatoes are excellent sources of vitamin C. (DIVA.photo/Shutterstock.com.)

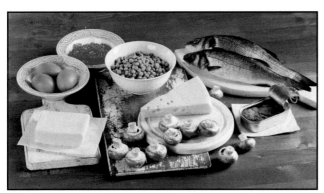

Figure 3-20. Quality vitamin D sources include fish as well as dairy products and mushrooms. (Tatjana Baibakova/Shutterstock.com.)

Fat-Soluble Vitamins

Four fat-soluble vitamins exist within the body—vitamins A, D, E, and K. Of these, vitamin D may be the most unique as it requires sunlight for synthesis before being further processed by the liver and kidneys, while the other fat-soluble vitamins are largely obtained through the diet.[58] Unlike water-soluble vitamins that generally cannot be stored within the body (vitamin B_{12} is found in very small amounts in the liver), fat-soluble vitamins can be stored within adipose tissue. Because of this ability for fat-soluble vitamins to be stored, medical conditions related to excess intake of fat-soluble vitamins are more common than with their water-soluble counterparts. Unlike water-soluble vitamins, however, fat-soluble vitamins are not involved in energy metabolism.[60] Rather, they are utilized for other functions such as serving as antioxidants and playing a role in the formation of bone.

Vitamin A

Vitamin A includes retinol as well as the carotenoids such as β–carotene. Retinol is critical for normal vision, and an early indicator of vitamin A deficiency is reduced visibility in low light settings, commonly known as "night blindness." Vitamin A is also involved in reproduction, cell

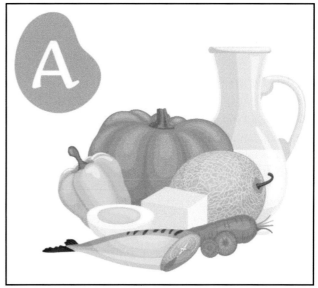

Figure 3-19. Meat-based products such as liver or eggs are good sources of vitamin A, along with some fruits and vegetables. (Ansty/Shutterstock.com.)

differentiation, and synthesis of certain glycoproteins, and also influences bone remodeling during growth.

Vitamin A has a high absorption rate, as up to 90% of consumed vitamin A ends up being absorbed within the intestine. Animal-based foods such as liver, egg yolk, and milk are good sources of vitamin A, and some foods such as margarine are often fortified with vitamin A.[57] Some vegetables as well as certain fruits such as pumpkins are also a good source of vitamin A (Figure 3-19). Recommended intake of vitamin A is age-dependent, with adult men and women second only to pregnant or lactating individuals. When failing to consume adequate vitamin A for extended periods, one of the most common deficiency-related complications is dry eye.

Vitamin D

Unlike other vitamins, vitamin D is not solely obtained from the diet but is rather a product of sunlight (ie, ultraviolet irradiation) affecting 7-dehydrocholesterol within the skin. The byproduct of this reaction, previtamin D_3 is then chemically processed through several steps to ultimately synthesize vitamin D. The amount of vitamin D synthesized by this process has been shown to be decreased among individuals with higher amounts of melanin within the skin as well as in older individuals.[57] As a result of vitamin D's metabolism requiring sunlight, vitamin D deficiency occurs in up to half of the world's population,[61] and among men in the United States, serum levels were found to have slightly decreased over a recent 20-year period due to suspected causes such as decreased milk consumption and increased use of sunscreen.[62]

Sources of vitamin D include mushrooms and meat products such as red meat, eggs, or liver (Figure 3-20). In the United States, certain food items such as milk, margarine, and certain cereals are often fortified with vitamin D.[63] Deficiencies related to inadequate vitamin D intake are often associated with bone health such as osteomalacia. However, certain medical conditions such as psoriasis, heart disease, and even obesity have been linked to vitamin D status,[57] though more research is needed to establish a definitive link with vitamin D.

Vitamin E

Vitamin E functions as a primary antioxidant within the body, and this antioxidant property appears to help prevent oxidation of the lipid bilayer, a negative consequence of physical activity.[64] However, a true physiological purpose for vitamin E has yet to be outlined. Still, premature infants are often given vitamin E, and certain childhood genetic disorders have been shown to exhibit very low plasma vitamin E levels. Sources of vitamin E include nuts, many vegetables and fruits, and vegetable oils. Vitamin E deficiency is rare in humans, resulting in little scientific evidence to support available dietary intake recommendations.[57]

Vitamin K

Vitamin K does not appear to have a well-understood role in overall health, though its main influence appears to be associated with blood and clotting. Clotting factors such as prothrombin are assembled in part through vitamin K's involvement as a cofactor,[57] and vitamin K does appear to influence the time required for blood to clot.[65] Similarly, deficiencies in vitamin K are generally tied to bleeding and coagulation, and certain anti-coagulant drugs such as warfarin operate by inhibiting vitamin K epoxide reductase, which is responsible for vitamin K recycling in the liver.[66] Sources of vitamin K within the diet largely include edible dark green leaves such as kale, spinach, and certain herbs such as mint and parsley.

Conclusion

As micronutrients, vitamins and minerals serve highly specific functions that facilitate events within the body required for normal metabolic activity. Without an adequate supply of micronutrients from the diet, these metabolic events can become compromised, eventually manifesting as some form of medical impairment. Fortunately, most individuals in the United States have little risk of micronutrient deficiency due to the ample availability and quantity of micronutrients within the diet. While most deficiencies are indeed rare, physical activity, as well as some medical conditions, can increase the risk for deficiency. This in turn increases the presence of symptoms associated with those deficiencies. For athletic trainers it is important to understand the physiological role of several of the more common micronutrients, as physical activity can be negatively affected when micronutrient levels within the body are influenced by factors such as inadequate intake or increased excretion. Maintaining proper micronutrient levels through careful monitoring of an athlete's, patient's, or client's intake of nutrients such as sodium, potassium, calcium, and vitamins can help contribute toward maximizing an individual's performance capabilities.

Discussion Questions

1. A client reports to you that they have just been feeling "off" since embarking on their recent vegetarian diet that began 2 months ago. They did not properly research the diet requirements, but decided to suddenly stop eating meat, fish, eggs, and milk. Outside of any macronutrient issues, how might micronutrients be involved in their concern of feeling "off" since switching to this new vegetarian diet?

2. A newly active individual purchased a treadmill and went from no real running ability to being able over the past 5 months to easily run 4 miles per day. Because she wants to try running longer distances, and because she feels that these longer distances will be too boring on the treadmill, she wants to begin running outdoors. Given that she has been running indoors in a climate-controlled environment, how might her micronutrient excretion change now given that she will be running in humid, 80 °F to 90 °F conditions each day?

References

1. Matovinovic J. Endemic goiter and cretinism at the dawn of the third millennium. *Annu Rev Nutr.* 1983;3(1):341-412. doi:10.1146/annurev.nu.03.070183.002013

2. Wolf G. A history of vitamin A and retinoids. *FASEB J.* 1996;10(9):1102-1107. doi:10.1096/fasebj.10.9.8801174

3. Berdanier C. *Advanced Nutrition: Micronutrients.* CRC Press; 1988.

4. Frassinetti S, et al. The role of zinc in life: a review. *J Environ Pathol Toxicol Oncol.* 2006;25(3). doi:10.1615/jenvironpatholtoxicoloncol.v25.i3.40

5. Epstein S. The problem of low levels of vitamin D and osteoporosis: use of combination therapy with alendronic acid and colecalciferol (vitamin D3). *Drugs Aging.* 2006;23(8):617-625. doi:10.2165/00002512-200623080-00001

6. Plowman SA, Smith DL. *Exercise Physiology for Health Fitness and Performance.* Lippincott, Williams & Wilkins; 2013.

7. World Health Organization, Food and Agricultural Organization of the United Nations. *Vitamin and Mineral Requirements in Human Nutrition.* World Health Organization; 2004.

8. Berchtold MW, Brinkmeier H, Muntener M. Calcium ion in skeletal muscle: its crucial role for muscle function, plasticity, and disease. *Physiol Rev.* 2000;80(3):1215-1265. doi:10.1152/physrev.2000.80.3.1215

9. Lambert H, Hakim O, Lanham-New SA. Major minerals: calcium and magnesium. *Essentials of Human Nutrition.* 2017;11:131-140.

10. Institute of Medicine (US) Committee to Review Dietary Reference Intakes for Vitamin D and Calcium; Ross AC, Taylor CL, Yaktine AL, et al, eds. *Dietary Reference Intakes for Calcium and Vitamin D.* National Academies Press; 2011.

11. National Institutes of Health, Office of Dietary Supplements. *Calcium: dietary supplement fact sheet for health professionals.* Published March 26, 2020. https://ods.od.nih.gov/factsheets/Calcium-HealthProfessional/

12. Andersson K. *Dietary Intake Estimations of Phosphorus: Based on Swedish Market Basket Data 1999-2015. Second Cycle, A2E.* SLU, Department of Molecular Sciences; 2018.

13. Jeong J, Kim JH, Shim JH, Hwang NS, Heo CY. Bioactive calcium phosphate materials and applications in bone regeneration. *Biomater Res.* 2019;23(1):1-11. doi:10.1186/s40824-018-0149-3

14. Takeda E, et al. The regulation and function of phosphate in the human body. *Biofactors.* 2004;21(1-4):345-355. doi:10.1002/biof.552210167

15. Institute of Medicine (US) Standing Committee on the Scientific Evaluation of Dietary Reference Intakes. *Dietary Reference Intakes for Calcium, Phosphorus, Magnesium, Vitamin D, and Fluoride.* National Academies Press (US); 1997. doi:10.17226/5776

16. Paleologos M, Stone E, Braude S. Persistent, progressive hypophosphataemia after voluntary hyperventilation. *Clin Sci (Lond).* 2000;98(5):619-625.

17. Lewis JF, Hodsman AB, Driedger AA, Thompson RT, McFadden RG. Hypophosphatemia and respiratory failure: prolonged abnormal energy metabolism demonstrated by nuclear magnetic resonance spectroscopy. *Am J Med.* 1987;83(6):1139-1143. doi:10.1016/0002-9343(87)90956-9

18. Håglin L, Burman LA, Nilsson M. High prevalence of hypophosphataemia amongst patients with infectious diseases. A retrospective study. *J Intern Med.* 1999;246(1):45-52. doi:10.1046/j.1365-2796.1999.00540.x

19. Tucker KL, Morita K, Qiao N, Hanna MT, Cupples LA, Kiel DP. Colas, but not other carbonated beverages, are associated with low bone mineral density in older women: the Framingham Osteoporosis Study. *Am J Clin Nutr.* 2006;84(4):936-942.

20. Bankir L, Bichet D, Morgenthaler NG. Vasopressin: physiology, assessment and osmosensation. *J Intern Med.* 2017;282(4):284-297. doi:10.1111/joim.12645

21. Murray D, Miller KC, Edwards JE. Does a reduction in serum sodium concentration or serum potassium concentration increase the prevalence of exercise-associated muscle cramps? *J Sport Rehabil.* 2016;25(3):301-304. doi:10.1123/jsr.2014-0293

22. Migdal KU, Bwabcock MC, Robinson AT, et al. The impact of high dietary sodium consumption on blood pressure variability in healthy, young adults. *Am J Hypertens.* 2020;33(5):422-429. doi:10.1093/ajh/hpaa014

23. Oria M, Harrison M, Stallings VA. *Sodium: Dietary Reference Intakes Based on Chronic Disease. Dietary Reference Intakes for Sodium and Potassium.* National Academies Press (US); 2019. Available from: https://www.ncbi.nlm.nih.gov/books/NBK538102/. doi:10.17226/25353

24. Leahy M. The sodium conundrum: evolving recommendations and implications. *Nutrition Today.* 2019;54(1):31-41.

25. Griep LMO, Elliott P. Cardiovascular diseases: sodium and blood pressure. *Public Health Nutrition.* 2017;214.

26. Glasdam S-M, Glasdam S, Peters GH. The importance of magnesium in the human body: a systematic literature review. In: Makowski GS, ed. *Advances in Clinical Chemistry.* Elsevier; 2016:169-193.

27. Zamboni CB, Oliveira LC, Kovacs L, Metairon S. Ca and Mg determination from inhabitants of Brazil using neutron activation analysis. *J Radioanal Nucl Chem.* 2012;291(2):389-393.

28. Yang SJ, Hwang SY, Baik SH, et al. Serum magnesium level is associated with type 2 diabetes in women with a history of gestational diabetes mellitus: the Korea National Diabetes Program study. *J Korean Med Sci.* 2014;29(1):84-89. doi:10.3346/jkms.2014.29.1.84

29. Abdulsahib HT. Determination of magnesium in whole blood and serum of ischemic heart disease (IHD) patients by flame atomic absorption spectrometry. *Am J Analytic Chem.* 2011;2(08):996. doi:10.4236/ajac.2011.28117

30. Insel P. *Nutrition.* 4th ed. Jones & Bartlett Learning; 2010.

31. Zafar MSH, Wani JI, Karim R, Mir MM, Koul PA. Significance of serum magnesium levels in critically ill-patients. *Int J Appl Basic Med Res.* 2014;4(1):34.

32. Rude R, Singer FR. Magnesium deficiency and excess. *Annu Rev Med.* 1981;32:245-259. doi:10.1146/annurev.me.32.020181.001333

33. Rude RK. Magnesium deficiency: a cause of heterogenous disease in humans. *JBMR.* 1998;13(4):749-758. doi:10.1359/jbmr.1998.13.4.749

34. Rayana MCB, et al. Guidelines for sampling, measuring and reporting ionized magnesium in undiluted serum, plasma or blood: International Federation of Clinical Chemistry and Laboratory Medicine (IFCC): IFCC Scientific Division, Committee on Point of Care Testing. *Clin Chem Lab Med.* 2005;43(5):564-569. doi:10.1515/CCLM.2005.098

35. Barbagallo M, Di Bella G, Brucato V, et al. Serum ionized magnesium in diabetic older persons. *Metabolism.* 2014;63(4):502-509. doi:10.1016/j.metabol.2013.12.003

36. Ringer J., Bartlett Y. The significance of potassium. *Pharmceut J.* 2007;278(7449):497–500.

37. World Health Organization. Diet, nutrition and the prevention of chronic diseases. *World Health Organization;* 2003;916(i-viii).

38. World Health Organization. Guideline: potassium intake for adults and children. *World Health Organization;* 2012:48.

39. Aburto NJ, Hanson S, Gutierrez H, Hooper L, Elliott P, Cappuccio FP. Effect of increased potassium intake on cardiovascular risk factors and disease: systematic review and meta-analyses. *BMJ.* 2013 Apr 3;346:f1378. doi:10.1136/bmj.f1378

40. Berend K, van Hulsteijn LH, Gans RO. Chloride: the queen of electrolytes? *Eur J Intern Med.* 2012;23(3):203-211. doi:10.1016/j.eji

41. Powers F. The role of chloride in acid-base balance. *J Intraven Nurs.* 1999;22(5):286-291.

42. Westen EA, Prange HD. A reexamination of the mechanisms underlying the arteriovenous chloride shift. *Physiol Biochem Zool.* 2003;76(5):603-614. doi:10.1086/380208

43. Insitute of Medicine of the National Academies. *Dietary Reference Intakes for Water, Potassium, Sodium, Chloride, and Sulfate.* The National Academies Press; 2005.

44. Lieu PT, Heiskala M, Peterson PA, Yang Y. The roles of iron in health and disease. *Mol Aspects Med.* 2001;22(1-2):1-87. doi:10.1016/s0098-2997(00)00006-6

45. Ganz T, Nemeth E. Iron homeostasis in host defence and inflammation. *Nat Rev Immunol.* 2015;15(8):500-510. doi:10.1038/nri3863

46. Drakesmith H, Prentice AM. Hepcidin and the iron-infection axis. *Science.* 2012;338(6108):768-772. doi:10.1126/science.1224577

47. Gozzelino R, Arosio P. Iron homeostasis in health and disease. *Int J Mol Sci.* 2016;17(1):130. doi:10.3390/ijms17010130

48. Wright JA, Richards T, Srai SKS. The role of iron in the skin and cutaneous wound healing. *Front Pharmacol.* 2014;5:156. doi:10.3389/fphar.2014.00156

49. Zhang D-L, Ghosh MC, Rouault TA. The physiological functions of iron regulatory proteins in iron homeostasis-an update. *Front Pharmacol.* 2014;5:124. doi:10.3389/fphar.2014.00124

50. Sim M, Garvican-Lewis LA, Cox GR, et al. Iron considerations for the athlete: a narrative review. *Eur J Appl Physiol.* 2019;119(7):1463-1478. doi:10.1007/s00421-019-04157-y

51. Al-Fartusie FS, Mohssan SN. Essential trace elements and their vital roles in human body. *Indian Journal of Advances in Chemical Science.* 2017;5(3):127-136.

52. Parks RB, Hetzel SJ, Brooks MA. Iron deficiency and anemia among collegiate athletes: a retrospective chart review. *Med Sci Sports Exerc.* 2017;49(8):1711-1715. doi:10.1249/MSS.0000000000001259

53. Mertz W. Chromium in human nutrition: a review. *J Nutr.* 1993;123(4):626-33. doi:10.1093/jn/123.4.626

54. Cefalu WT, Hu FB. Role of chromium in human health and in diabetes. *Diabetes Care.* 2004;27(11):2741-2751. doi:10.2337/diacare.27.11.2741

55. Russell R, Beard JL, Cousins RJ, et al. Dietary reference intakes for vitamin A, vitamin K, arsenic, boron, chromium, copper, iodine, iron, manganese, molybdenum, nickel, silicon, vanadium, and zinc. A report of the panel on micronutrients, subcommittees on upper reference levels of nutrients and of interpretation and uses of dietary reference intakes, and the standing committee on the scientific evaluation of dietary reference intakes food and nutrition board. *Institute of Medicine.* 2001;797.

56. Anderson RA, Bryden NA, Polansky MM. Dietary chromium intake. *Biol Trace Elem Res.* 1992;32:117-121. doi:10.1007/BF02784595

57. Mann J, Truswell AS. *Essentials of Human Nutrition.* Oxford University Press; 2017.

58. Baj T, Sieniawska E. Vitamins. In: *Pharmacognosy.* Academic Press; 2017:281-292.

59. Linster CL, Van Schaftingen E. Vitamin C. *The FEBS Journal.* 2007;274(1):1-22. doi:10.1111/j.1742-4658.2006.05607.x

60. Lukaski HC. Vitamin and mineral status: effects on physical performance. *Nutrition.* 2004;20(7-8):632-644. doi:10.1016/j.nut.2004.04.001

61. Lee JH, O'Keefe JH, Bell D, Hensrud DD, Holick MF. Vitamin D deficiency: an important, common, and easily treatable cardiovascular risk factor? *J Am Coll Cardiol.* 2008;52(24):1949-1956. doi:10.1016/j.jacc.2008.08.050

62. Looker AC, Pfeiffer CM, Lacher DA, Schleicher RL, Picciano MF, Yetley EA. Serum 25-hydroxyvitamin D status of the US population: 1988–1994 compared with 2000–2004. *Am J Clin Nutr.* 2008;88(6):1519-1527. doi:10.3945/ajcn.2008.2618263

63. Holick MF, Chen TC. Vitamin D deficiency: a worldwide problem with health consequences. *Am J Clin Nutr.* 2008;87(4):1080S-1086S. doi:10.1093/ajcn/87.4.1080S64

64. Powers SK, Jackson MJ. Exercise-induced oxidative stress: cellular mechanisms and impact on muscle force production. *Physiol Rev.* 2008;88(4):1243-1276.

65. Food and Agriculture Organization of the United Nations, World Health Organization. Human vitamin and mineral requirements. Report of a joint FAO/WHO expert consultation, Bangkok, Thailand. *FAO Rome.* 2001:235-247.

66. Wu S, Chen X, Jin D-Y, Stafford DW, Pedersen LG, Tie J-K. Warfarin and vitamin K epoxide reductase: a molecular accounting for observed inhibition. *Blood.* 2018;132(6):647-657. doi:10.1182/blood-2018-01-830901

67. Miller KC. Exercise-associated muscle cramps. In: Adams W, Jardine J, eds. *Exertional Heat Illness.* Springer; 2020.

Chapter 4

Energy Systems

Sarah Snyder, MS, RD, CSSD, LD, CSCS

Commission on Accreditation of Athletic Training Education *2020 Standards*

This chapter addresses the following *2020 Standards for Accreditation of Professional Athletic Training Programs*:

- Standard 54: The professional program requires prerequisite classes in biology, chemistry, physics, psychology, anatomy, and physiology at the postsecondary level.
- Standard 55: Students must gain foundational knowledge in statistics, research design, epidemiology, pathophysiology, biomechanics and pathomechanics, exercise physiology, nutrition, human anatomy, pharmacology, public health, and health care delivery and payor systems.

Learning Objectives

After reviewing this chapter, readers will be able to:

- Identify the aerobic and anaerobic energy systems and the distinctions between them.
- Describe the role of the mitochondria during energy production.
- Understand the role of lactic acid formed during anaerobic energy systems.
- Explain various energy systems used in sport.

Knoblauch M, ed. *Clinical Nutrition in Athletic Training* (pp 41-48).
© 2023 Taylor & Francis Group.

Introduction

Energy in humans comes from food, or more specifically macronutrients, which are used to fuel movement as well as to provide for the body's various functions (eg, metabolism). Macronutrients are absorbed within the intestine into the blood for transport to the cell, where there are 3 existing energy systems. These 3 energy systems ultimately provide the body's principal fuel source for movement, adenosine triphosphate, or ATP. ATP is also necessary to fuel tissue growth and vital bodily functions. The 3 energy systems that function to replenish ATP in muscle are the creatine phosphagen system or CrP system,[1] anaerobic glycolysis[2] or lactic acid system[3] aerobic glycolysis. The CrP system is used for short bursts of power and speed. The duration lasts between 1 and 10 seconds.[3] ATP is rapidly resynthesized but in limited amounts.[3] The anaerobic glycolysis system or lactic acid system is utilized for increased intensity for longer duration when creatine phosphate is not available. Glycogen is broken down in a series of chemical reactions to produce ATP. The aerobic energy system is used during intensities lasting longer than 1 minute that are lower in intensity.[3] Each energy system can operate at any time depending on oxygen availability, but a particular energy system may be activated to a higher degree at any time based on the exercise type, intensity, or duration. Despite their varying levels of activation, the overall purpose of the 3 energy systems during exercise is to increase the production of ATP, as ATP directly fuels muscle contractions.

Adenosine Triphosphate

Energy comes in forms of chemical, mechanical, and heat and can be transferred between the different forms known as the law of thermodynamics. Mechanical energy is characterized by motion or position of an object, while heat energy is the result of movement. Chemical energy is stored in bonds also known as "chemical bond energy." Chemical bond energy is stored in macronutrients (eg, carbohydrate, protein, fats). The movement of the muscle transfers chemical energy into mechanical energy. Heat energy dissipates as a result of the movement of muscle. The chemical energy is stored in different forms such as carbohydrate, protein, and fat. Broken down further into fatty acids, glucose, or muscle glycogen, these substrates (along with creatine phosphate) produce ATP.

Creatine phosphate is a phosphorylated creatine molecule containing high energy that is released once broken down into a creatine and a phosphate group to produce ATP (see Figure 4-6). Creatine phosphate aids in the resynthesis of ATP by contributing an inorganic phosphate group to ADP.[3]

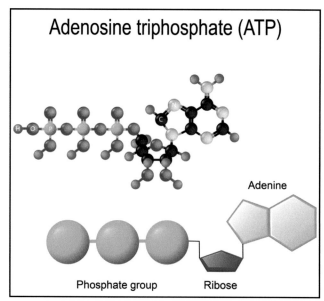

Figure 4-1. Structure of ATP. (Designua/Shutterstock.com.)

In activities where the intensity exceeds the amount of oxygen necessary to meet energy demands in which breathing is taxed, anaerobic glycolysis becomes the major pathway for glycogen to break down into glucose to produce ATP. Glycogen will break down to glucose during lower intensity where oxygen is available to produce ATP but is able to produce more ATP.

Triglycerides are stored in adipose cells or fat cells. They can also be found in muscle cells. Both are available as an energy source for the body. When fat is burned as a source of energy, the stored triglycerides are broken down to fatty acids and glycerol molecule.[4] Each fatty acid is broken down further and goes through cellular processes to generate ATP. The process is known as "oxidation," which requires the cells to have ample oxygen and breathing is not taxed during exercise.[4]

Protein is not a preferred source of energy, but can go through a process called gluconeogenesis to form glucose from protein. Once in the form of glucose, glycolysis can occur to produce energy.

ATP is made of adenine and ribose linked to 3 phosphates (Figure 4-1). The bonds that link the 2 phosphates are high-energy bonds and they release a large amount of energy during hydrolysis, a process in which these high-energy bonds break apart. During hydrolysis, the phosphagen bond of ATP is broken. ATP is broken down to adenosine diphosphate (ADP), a nucleotide, and an inorganic phosphate group (Figure 4-2).

Energy Storage in the Body

The body stores a small amount of ATP—enough to sustain activity for a few seconds (Table 4-1). However, ATP is continuously generated and reformed. When metabolic

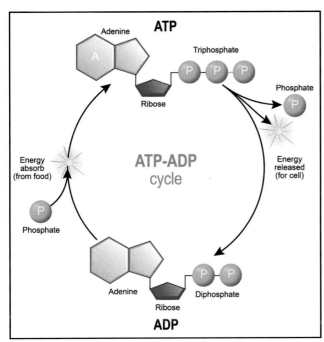

Figure 4-2. ATP-ADP cycle. (Designua/Shutterstock.com.)

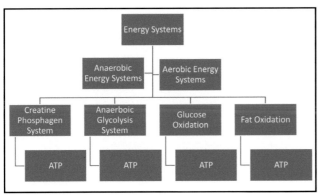

Figure 4-3. Overview of energy systems.[3]

demands increase, the demand for ATP increases. ATP is produced from the 3 energy systems to fuel cells, which involves the storage of energy in large molecules such as glycogen, fatty acids, and (rarely) amino acids (broken down from protein).

Sensitive control systems are in place to signal the cell's energy needs, including current energy demands, the initiation of exercise, depleted sources and substrates (like creatine and ATP), and/or the accumulation of byproducts. In order to sustain continual muscle contraction, ATP needs to be regenerated at a rate that meets the muscle's demand for energy.

The Three Energy Systems

The 3 energy systems used to produce ATP are activated in response to the degree of exercise intensity (Figure 4-3). A cell shifts from one energy system to another based on the

Table 4-1

Energy Source and Storage

ENERGY SOURCE	ENERGY STORAGE
ATP/creatine phosphate	Various tissues
Carbohydrate	Blood glucose, glycogen (in the liver and muscle)
Fat	Serum-free fatty acids, serum triglycerides, muscle triglycerides, adipose tissue
Protein	Muscle

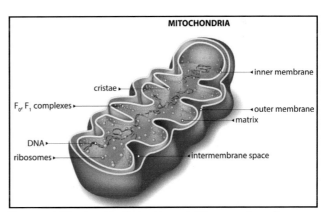

Figure 4-4. Mitochondria. (EreborMountain/Shutterstock.com.)

demands and substrate availability. When creatine phosphagen becomes depleted, anaerobic glycolysis or the lactic acid system will be the driver to produce ATP. If the accumulation of byproduct reaches high levels, the shift in energy systems moves to aerobic systems.[1]

Mitochondria are essential in energy production and play a central role to where reactions take place (Figure 4-4). Mitochondria are double-membrane-bound organelles found in most eukaryotic cells. The outer membrane of the mitochondria encloses another membrane, the inner mitochondrial membrane, creating a space in between referred to as the "inner mitochondrial space." The cristae space and the matrix space are contained inside the 2 membranes. The 3 energy systems take place in various parts of the mitochondria. Mitochondria are equipped with chemicals that break down waste products and recycle others to save energy.[1]

A training adaption that takes place at the cellular level includes a higher number of mitochondria with increased exercise, improving overall production of energy.[1]

The 3 systems differ by the following:
- Ability to function with or without oxygen
- Capacity of total energy

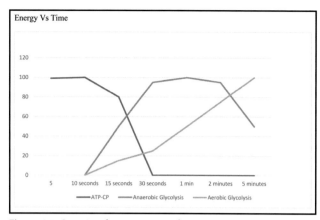

Figure 4-5. Capacity of energy systems.[3]

- Duration of energy system (Figure 4-5)
- Substrates utilized
- Byproducts produced
- Speed of ATP regeneration

Creatine Phosphagen System or Phosphagen System

The CrP system is utilized during explosive movement (Figure 4-6). When the body's supply of ATP is exhausted, which occurs within a few seconds, additional ATP needed to sustain muscle contraction is created from the breakdown of a high-energy compound called phosphocreatine (Sidebar 4-1).

The CrP system functions when the intensity of exercise or activity exceeds the capacity to bring enough oxygen into the system to meet energy demands and breathing is labored during the exercise. Phosphocreatine splits to lend a phosphate group and releases energy in the process. ATP also splits to lend a phosphate group and releases energy. The reactions are reversible in that the phosphate group and creatine form PCr.[3] ATP is reformed from ADP joining with a phosphate group. PCr breakdown is catalyzed buy the enzyme creatine kinase.[3] The energy from PCr breakdown drives ADP to be phosphorylated to make ATP.

ATP supplies the muscle with fuel for a short period of time and fuels activities that are 5 to 6 second fast-twitch muscle contractions.[3] Sports that require intense movements rely heavily on the phosphagen system and include football, baseball, softball, weightlifting, track and field, swimming (sprint events), and tennis.[3]

Anaerobic Glycolysis or Lactic Acid System or Lactate System

Anaerobic glycolysis occurs during high-intensity activity in which the intensity exceeds the capacity to bring enough oxygen into the system to meet energy demands. Glycolysis is the breakdown of glucose. After glycogen is broken down

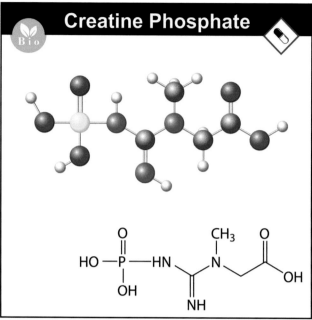

Figure 4-6. Phosphocreatine molecule, creatine phosphate structure. (chromatos/Shutterstock.com.)

Sidebar 4-1

If an athlete supplements with creatine monohydrate, these stores can be increased for more repetitive explosive movements. Creatine monohydrate is available in small quantities in foods like red meat (approximately 1 g per serving of red meat), but can also be taken as a supplement (3 to 5 g a day) to aid the body's phosphocreatine energy systems.

in the muscle, it produces energy through glycolysis. Glucose is converted to pyruvate, and a net gain of 2 ATPs is rapidly produced.[3] Pyruvate is converted into acetyl CoA in what is known as the "citric acid cycle" (or TCA cycle or Krebs cycle) or broken down further to produce lactate. Pyruvate forms lactate or lactic acid as the end-product (Figure 4-7).

Anaerobic glycolysis delivers ATP during intense, 10-second to 2-minute activity bouts.[3] Due to the ongoing demand for energy within the muscles when exercise continues beyond 10 seconds, the anaerobic glycolysis system is initiated to provide energy without lapse by quickly mobilizing glucose.[3]

Lactic Acid

Lactic acid is an organic acid produced in muscle tissues (Figure 4-8). When oxygen level in the body is low, lactic acid is released from the breakdown of glucose during anaerobic glycolysis (Figure 4-9). Strenuous exercise that lasts up to a few minutes may promote blood lactate to accumulate, correlating with the intensity and duration of exercise.

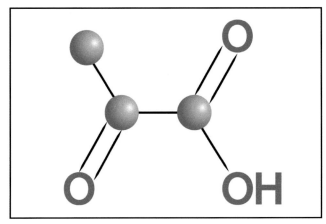

Figure 4-7. Pyruvate. (lyricsai/Shutterstock.com.)

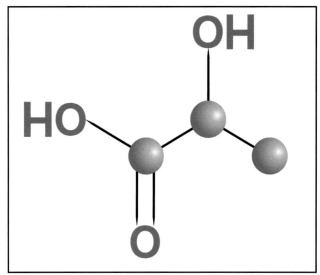

Figure 4-8. Lactic acid. (lyricsai/Shutterstock.com.)

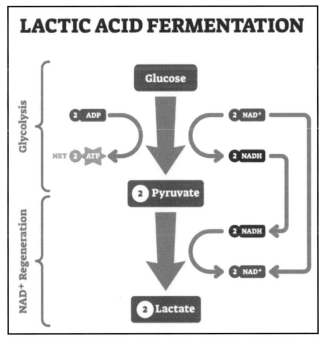

Figure 4-9. Stages with glucose, pyruvate, and lactate regeneration system. (VectorMine/Shutterstock.com.)

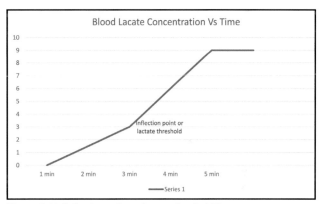

Figure 4-10. Inflection point or lactate threshold.[3]

Lactate is released into the blood stream and metabolized by muscle cells. If lactate is produced at a higher rate than it can be cleared, lactate will accumulate in the blood. Accumulation of lactic acid is associated with increased acidity in the muscles due to hydrogen ion accumulation.[3] Lactate threshold or lactate inflection point is the exercise level at which an imbalance occurs between lactate production and lactate clearance (Figure 4-10).

Tactics have been studied to alleviate the hydrogen ion build-up in the muscle such as the as the ingestion of sodium bicarbonate. Prior to exercise, ingestion of sodium bicarbonate ($NAHCO_3$) can increase the buffering of H^+ and the rate of H^+ coming from the active muscles, meaning lowering the hydration ion concentration and buffering the present concentration of hydration ions can delay the increased acidity

in the muscle.[2] Because sodium bicarbonate can cause adverse reactions such as vomiting and diarrhea once ingested, the side effects often outweigh any performance benefit.[2] Recently, companies have begun exploring topical delivery of sodium bicarbonate in order to help avoid the negative gastrointestinal side effects that can occur.[5]

Niacin containing nicotinamide adenine dinucleotide, or NAD^+, is the coenzyme component of dehydrogenase. NADH forms when NAD^+ gains hydration and 2 electrons and reduces to NADH. NADH carries electrons that can easily transfer. Pyruvate is converted to lactate and the production of lactate allows for the regeneration of NAD^+ from NADH.[3] NAD^+ is a compound that assists the path of glucose through glycolysis. The transfer of electrons between NADH and NAD^+ is known to be part of the electron transport chain, where a series of electrons are transferred to release energy (Figures 4-11 and 4-12).

If an athlete is taxed to breathe during an endurance event or activity, the anaerobic glycolysis provides the means to regenerate ATP for the few minutes it will take to prevent fatigue. When the body shifts from using the anaerobic glycolysis system as the dominant ATP producer back to

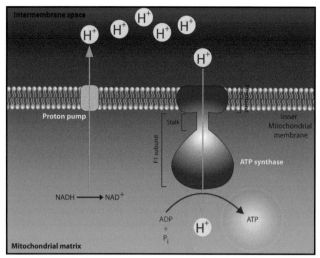

Figure 4-11. NADH lends electron to NAD⁺. (Meletios Verras/Shutterstock.com.)

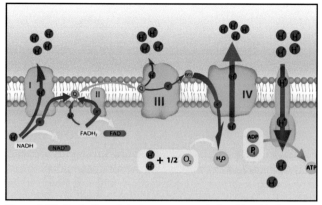

Figure 4-12. Illustration of electron transport chain with oxidative phosphorylation. (extender_01/Shutterstock.com.)

using the aerobic system, there could be overlap of 30 seconds.[3] The anaerobic glycolysis system can make a relatively small amount of ATP compared to aerobic energy systems. Basketball, hockey, lacrosse, soccer, some non-sprint swimming events lasting 2 minutes or under, and some track and field events lasting between 15 to 120 seconds rely on anaerobic glycolysis.[3]

Aerobic Glycolysis or Aerobic System or Oxidative Phosphorylation or Cellular Respiration

The aerobic system includes breakdown of carbohydrates, fatty acids, or (rarely) proteins—all in the presence of oxygen. The aerobic glycolysis system is capable of providing the body with the largest supply of ATP. The series of reactions include the citric acid cycle or TCA cycle, the Krebs cycle, and the electron transport chain (Figure 4-13). Aerobic glycolysis is the process by which glycogen is broken down to pyruvate.[3]

Pyruvate moves into the mitochondria where it enters the citric acid cycle.

Two compounds are produced, NADH and flavin adenine dinucleotide ($FADH_2$).[3] $FADH_2$ is like NADH in its function to transfer electrons easily. These compounds then enter the electron transport chain, a series of oxidation-reduction reactions.

During these reactions, an H^+ gradient is formed, and diffusion of these molecules causes energy to be released and captured in the formation of ATP molecules. Oxygen accepts the electrons and is reduced to form H_2O, water.[3]

Aerobic activity is characterized as low-intensity workload and can be sustained for long periods of time as the athlete breathes easily, supplying oxygen to the cells. Aerobic glycolysis includes more reactions and pathways relative to the other 2 energy systems and relies on the presence of oxygen causing this system to produce ATP at a slower rate relative to ATP-PC or anaerobic glycolysis systems. Athletes who engage in activity that relies on this energy system heavily will have a higher number of mitochondria in type 1 muscles fibers as an adaptation to maximize aerobic capacity.[1] The aerobic system supplies energy for activity or exercise lasting more than 2 minutes. This system is also the pathway that provides ATP to fuel the body's metabolic needs, including building and repairing tissues, digestion, and thermoregulation.

Energy transfer during exercise occurs using the 3 energy systems which use high energy substrates that are broken down to execute movement. The 3 energy systems maintain a continuous energy supply through the production of ATP. Track and field and football will show how the creatine phosphagen is highly utilized. Soccer and basketball show a combination of endurance and stop and go running, and will rely on all 3 systems to produce continual supply of energy.

Track and Field

Repeated sprints in a game or event do not always allow for enough recovery time for the CrP system. During an event like the 400-meter sprint, the production of ATP relies on all 3 energy systems and primarily on anaerobic glycolysis. From the start of the race, the phosphate energy system aids an explosive start off the blocks (Figure 4-14).

After 4 to 10 seconds, the primary system involved in ATP generation shifts to anaerobic glycolysis.[3] Glycogen from the muscle is used to produce ATP, allowing the muscles to continually contract. The working muscles require a quick source of ATP, more than can be produced through anaerobic metabolism. The pyruvic acid left over from anaerobic glycolysis is converted into lactic acid, along with an increase in hydrogen ion concentration.

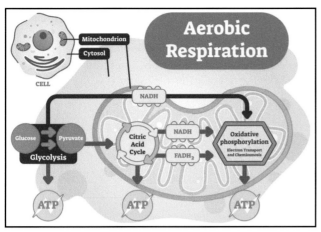

Figure 4-13. Aerobic glycolysis. (VectorMine/Shutterstock.com.)

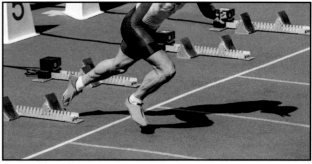

Figure 4-14. Sprinter start running on track race. (sportpoint/Shutterstock.com.)

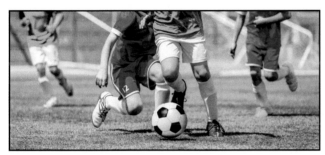

Figure 4-15. Soccer player. (matimix/Shutterstock.com.)

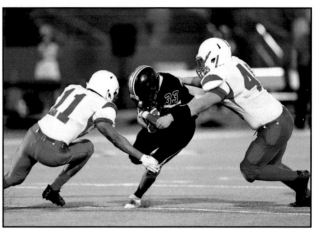

Figure 4-16. Football player making a tackle during a game. (JoeSAPhotos/Shutterstock.com.)

Soccer

An outfield male player can run up to 13 km in a game, including high-speed running, low-intensity running, and walking—showing the need for all 3 energy systems in the game of soccer (Figure 4-15).[6]

Much of soccer relies on the aerobic system with an average heart rate of around 85% of maximal values and peak heart rates approaching 98% of maximal values.[6] The intense intermittent efforts that occur during a game lead to a high rate of CrP breakdown, which resynthesizes during the intermittent low-intensity efforts.[6]

Basketball

Basketball is like soccer in that it also requires the aerobic system. Basketball is a stop-and-go sport where energy demands of the players are constantly changing due to intermittent high-intensity movement including repeated sprints, jumps, and changes in direction.[7] Players may be completely stopped during various times throughout the game, and players spend time walking or jogging on the court. The ability to play at a high level requires aerobic and anaerobic systems at a high capacity. Because of the nature of the sport, CrP can be used up repetitively and regenerated due to periods of lighter activity and rest. Plays lasting 15 to 60 seconds during the games use anaerobic glycolysis to support continual energy supply.[7]

Football

In contrast to basketball and soccer, the game of American football is not continuous, as it consists of a series of plays. The duration of each play can vary from 2 to 13 seconds with an average of 5 seconds.[8] The rest interval between each play varies and maxes out at 25 seconds in duration.[8] Power, strength, speed, endurance, and agility need to be optimal for contacting, tackling, and running downfield (Figure 4-16). Much of the same energy system requirements from CrP system and anaerobic system are seen and the need for sufficient energy stores from carbohydrates is necessary. The anaerobic system may be initiated for a series of plays when there is little rest time between plays.[8] Carbohydrate intake needs to be adequate and therefore available as glycogen. Sufficient carbohydrates are needed to tap into full glycogen stores for each energy system used. Fast-digesting and easily absorbed carbohydrates from sports drinks or chews can deliver carbohydrates to maintain energy levels. Creatine monohydrate may be beneficial for repetitive explosive movement used by these positions for a series of plays.

Endurance

Endurance events or races rely on the aerobic energy system for prolonged energy supply. Due to the longer duration in activity required for endurance events, the production of a steady supply of ATP for the muscles during sustained activities like walking, distance running, distance swimming, or cycling is necessary.

The source of ATP required for endurance-type events is found within the body's carbohydrate and fat stores. In some cases, small amounts of protein may be used as a source of energy during extremely prolonged endurance activities (eg, marathon running), but the amount of energy supplied via protein is not significant. The fuel the body selects and utilizes depends on variables including training status, pre- and post-workout fuel, intensity and duration of the activity, and hormones. For example, muscle glycogen normally provides glucose to be broken down into ATP; however, if glycogen is depleted from a recent bout of long-duration exercise or if the individual is engaged in a low-carbohydrate diet, the availability of glycogen can become limited. In addition to the glycogen found within muscle stores, glycogen can also be found in the liver.

During less intense endurance activities, hormones start to signal fat cells known as "adipocytes" to release fatty acids into the blood. Like glycogen, these free fatty acids can be used by the muscle as energy.[4]

Even though the aerobic system is primarily used during endurance events, the anaerobic energy system can often be used at the start of a race before the aerobic system takes over. The anaerobic energy system also can kick in whenever intensity increases, including running uphill or sprinting to the finish line.

Conclusion

Food that is consumed is broken down to basic macronutrients, carbohydrates, fat, and proteins that provide energy to fuel movement and provide for the body's vital functions.

The complexity of each energy system within the cell and within the mitochondria promotes each energy system to produce and sustain energy. The range of physical activities that humans participate in calls for a mix of energy systems, and the body has the extraordinary ability to effortlessly shift between these systems in response to the type and intensity of physical activity in which it is engaged. The CrP system provides a rapid supply of energy, but is short-term. Some sports like football and track and field rely heavily on CrP to produce quick and intense power outputs. The anaerobic glycolysis system can produce energy for longer periods of time, therefore sustaining high-intensity activity that lasts up to 2 minutes. Aerobic glycolysis functions to provide ATP to sustain endurance activity utilizing the citric acid cycle and electron transport chain. The 3 systems are well coordinated to ensure there is not a shortage of energy.

Discussion Questions

1. What would you expect to see if a deconditioned athlete does not eat breakfast before running a timed conditioning test of a 150-yard shuttle?

2. What ramifications do you see occurring in athletes who follow patterns of a low carbohydrate diet?

References

1. Holloway GP. Nutrition and training influences on the regulation of mitochondrial adenosine diphosphate sensitivity and bioenergetics. *Sports Med.* Published March 22, 2017. Accessed February 20, 2020. https://rd.springer.com/article/10.1007%2Fs40279-017-0693-3

2. Pigozzi F, Giombini A, Fagnani F, Parisi A. The role of diet and nutritional supplements. *Clinical Sports Medicine. Medical Management and Rehabilitation.* Published 2007. Accessed February 20, 2020. https://www.sciencedirect.com/book/9781416024439/clinical-sports-medicine

3. Baker JS, McCormick MC, Robergs RA. Interaction among skeletal muscle metabolic energy systems during intense exercise. *J Nutr Metab.* Published December 6, 2010. Accessed February 20, 2020. doi:10.1155/2010/905612

4. Watt MJ, Heigenhauser GJ, Dyck DJ, Spriet LL. Intramuscular triacylglycerol, glycogen and acetyl group metabolism during 4 h of moderate exercise in man. *J Physiol.* 2002;541:969-978.

5. Misell L, Kern M, Ordille A, Alm M, Salewske B. Double-blind, placebo controlled, randomized crossover pilot study evaluating the impacts of sodium bicarbonate in a transdermal delivery system on delayed muscle onset soreness. *Medicine & Science in Sports & Exercise.* Published May 2018. Accessed April 23, 2020. https://journals.lww.com/acsmmsse/Fulltext/2018/05001/Double_blind,_Placebo_Controlled,_Randomized.1968.aspx

6. Bangsbo J. Physiolgial demands of football. *GSSI SSE 125.* Published June 2014. Accessed February 1, 2020. https://www.gssi-web.org/sports-science-exchange/article/sse-125-physiological-demands-of-football

7. Ransone J. Physiologic profile of basketball athletes. *GSSI SSE 163.* Published February 2017. Accessed February 1, 2020. https://www.gssiweb.org/sports-science-exchange/article/physiologic-profile-of-basketball-athletes

8. Hoffman JR. Physiological demands of American football. *GSSI SSE 143.* Published April 2015. Accessed February 1, 2020. https://www.gssiweb.org/sports-science-exchange/article/sse-143-physiological-demands-of-american-football#articleTopic_9

Chapter 5

Fluid Loss and Hydration

Melanie Clark, MS, RD, CSSD, LD
Kyla Cross, MS, MPH, RD, LD
Brett Singer, MS, RD, CSSD, LD

Commission on Accreditation of Athletic Training Education *2020 Standards*

This chapter addresses the following *2020 Standards for Accreditation of Professional Athletic Training Programs*:

- Standard 72: Perform or obtain the necessary and appropriate diagnostic or laboratory tests—including (but not limited to) imaging, blood work, urinalysis, and electrocardiogram—to facilitate diagnosis, referral, and treatment planning.
- Standard 82: Develop, implement, and supervise comprehensive programs to maximize sport performance that are safe and specific to the client's activity.
- Standard 83: Educate and make recommendations to clients/patients on fluids and nutrients to ingest prior to activity, during activity, and during recovery for a variety of activities and environmental conditions.

Learning Objectives

After reviewing this chapter, readers will be able to:

- Describe the different factors involved in fluid balance.
- Identify signs, symptoms, and opportunities for measuring hypohydration and hypernatremia.
- Describe strategies for improving performance through cooling techniques.
- Calculate fluid needs for more accurate recommendations.

Knoblauch M, ed. *Clinical Nutrition in Athletic Training* (pp 49-59).

Introduction

Water is vital for nearly every function in an individual's daily life. It helps with the production of food and agriculture and serves a vital role in cleaning one's hands, body, and clothes. As scientists search the universe for signs of potential life, a common theme remains the question of whether water exists within any new discovery, recognizing that survival cannot occur without it. Take away water from daily life for just a few hours, and it becomes obvious just how challenging life can be to function without it. When looking at the human body and how it performs in various environments, it is easy to see how imperative water can be for health and human performance.

Water accounts for about 60% of total body mass in the human body, with lean tissue such as muscle made up of about 75% water and adipose tissue being as low as approximately 5% water.[1,2] Body water is distributed into 2 main compartments. Intracellular fluid, which accounts for nearly two-thirds of body water, and extracellular fluid, including both intravascular and interstitial fluid, accounts for the remaining one-third of total body water.[1]

Fluid Balance

As will be noted throughout this chapter, there are numerous factors that will alter fluid needs within a given day of activity or competition. To attempt to paint a broad brush over all populations with an exact fluid recommendation would be nearly impossible. The 2004 Dietary Reference Intake (DRI) has recommended the adequate intake for water at 3.7 L/day in men and 2.7 L/day in women.[3] However, these recommendations account for minimum fluid needs within the general population and do not take other factors into account, such as environment, physical activity, or the size of the individual.

Fluid balance, or euhydration, is achieved when fluid gain is equal to fluid loss. Fluid loss can be the result of several different factors including respiration, skin, feces, and urine. In a temperate environment, a sedentary adult may expect to lose approximately 600 mL/day through the skin, 100 mL/day within feces, and 800 to 1600 mL/day in the form of urine.[2] Factors such as environment and activity level have the ability to alter respiration and skin losses dramatically. Fluid gains can come in the form of fluid intake such as water, tea, or juices, as well as the consumption of high-water-content foods such as fruits and vegetables. In addition to consumption of fluids, water is also produced to a small degree through the oxidation of macronutrients. The oxidation of carbohydrate, for example, produces 15 mL of water per 100 calories (kcal) of metabolized energy, while protein and fat contribute 10.5 mL/100 kcal and 11.1 mL/100 kcal respectively.[3] Specific to fluid balance, if fluid gain exceeds that of which has been lost, a state of hyperhydration occurs. If fluid loss exceeds what has been gained through consumption and metabolic production, a state of hypohydration occurs. Both hypohydration and hyperhydration will be discussed in further detail later in this chapter.

Thermoregulation

When exercising, heat production causes a rise in core temperature and a subsequent effort by the body to remove heat in order to mitigate the rise in core temperature. If core temperature rises too significantly, heat-related injury can occur. During exercise, the body attempts to find a balance between heat produced from exercise and gained from the environment versus heat removed by the body. This regulatory process is known as "thermoregulation." In addition to heat production within the body, heat can also be gained from the environment depending on temperature, humidity, wind, and radiation. Within a hot environment, heat can be gained through convection, conduction, and radiation. Heat can also be removed through evaporative cooling, as well as conduction, convection, and radiation. Convection heat transfer occurs between the body and fluid or air.[4] If, for example, someone with an elevated skin temperature were placed into a cold tub, heat would be transferred to the water, removing heat from the body. Conversely, if an athlete were to sit in an excessively hot tub, heat transfer to the body would occur. Conduction heat transfer occurs between the body and a solid surface. Imagine an athlete coming inside and sprawling out onto their cold tile floor after a long strenuous workout under the hot sun. As their skin rests on the cold tile, heat is given off from the skin to the floor, resulting in conductive heat transfer.[4]

Sweat Loss

While convection and conduction are potential forms of heat transfer, athletes are primarily dependent on evaporative cooling for heat transfer, or removal of heat, during exercise. During exercise, particularly in hot environments, heat is removed through evaporation of sweat from the skin. Several variables can impact sweat rates, including environment, the size of the athlete, clothing, intensity and duration of activity, and numerous other factors. Sweat evaporation can be impaired due to humid environments (Sidebar 5-1) as well as clothing worn by the athlete, resulting in a less efficient evaporation.

With excessive equipment, as may be seen with a football player in helmet and pads, permeability of that equipment may be poor, resulting in an inability for sweat to evaporate. In this scenario, sweat may simply drip off the athlete, failing to evaporate. This prevents heat from being removed from the body. When evaporative cooling is less efficient, such as in the example of a football player in heavy equipment, core temperature continues to rise. The body fights

Sidebar 5-1

You may ask the question, why are fluid needs higher in a humid environment in comparison to a dry environment? Consider the idea of when warm skin touches a cold surface, the warm skin gives off heat to the colder surface. Sweat evaporation is a similar concept. The larger the difference between the water vapor pressure within a given environment, the easier for sweat to evaporate off the skin into the environment. When water vapor pressure is high (eg, in a humid environment), the gradient is minimal and sweat is less able to evaporate off of the skin. If the humidity is 100%, sweat will not evaporate and will merely drip off skin, rendering it ineffective for heat removal.

Sidebar 5-2

What is in your sweat? Similar to sweat rates, electrolyte losses within sweat will vary widely. Sodium and chloride are the 2 electrolytes primarily lost within sweat, thus they are the 2 most common electrolytes you will find in most sports drinks. Potassium, calcium, and magnesium are also lost in sweat, but at much lower levels. These electrolytes may also be included in sports drinks, but are rarely required during activity.

Sidebar 5-3

Acclimatization and acclimation are 2 terms that are often mentioned interchangeably, but they actually have 2 different meanings.

Acclimatization occurs when the body adapts to the actual type of environment the athlete will be competing in, such as an athlete training at altitude or traveling to Hawaii weeks in advance to adapt to the heat and humidity of the environment.

Acclimation is an artificial stimulus to help the body adapt to a given environment. Examples of heat acclimation are an athlete training in an environmental chamber, wearing extra layers of clothing during exercise to increase core temperature, or sitting in a hot bath following exercise. Each of these tactics have the ability to induce heat adaptation, despite the fact that the athlete is not actually training within the specific environment.

In this chapter we will strictly use the phrase *acclimation,* despite it referencing both acclimatization and acclimation.

to overcome the rise in core temperature and poor sweat evaporation by continuing to increase the sweat rate in order to provide a greater opportunity for sweat evaporation and heat removal. This process of high sweat rates (Sidebar 5-2), poor sweat evaporation, and heat removal increases the likelihood of hypohydration due to excessive fluid loss, as well as an elevated core temperature and heat-related illness. In addition to clothing and environment, factors such as acclimatization may also play a role in altered sweat rates and thermoregulation.

Acclimatization

Imagine an athlete from Alaska preparing for an upcoming outdoor summer triathlon in Texas. While training in Alaska would still prepare the athlete to complete the race, most coaches and athletes recognize this race would be a significant challenge due to the drastic difference in climate. The athlete might benefit by spending a few weeks training in Texas shortly before the race.

Acclimatization (Sidebar 5-3) is the process of an athlete training in a unique environment such as a high altitude or in hot and humid weather that will prepare their body to handle that environment in a future competition. Acclimating to a hot environment produces unique physiological adaptations such as a lower resting and active heart rate, an increased sweat rate, and a reduced sweat sodium concentration.[4,5] Once an athlete has acclimatized to hot environments, sweating initiates earlier during activity and is sustained at higher levels, resulting in improved removal of heat from the body. There are several benefits related to acclimatization, including increased blood volume, skin blood flow, and size of sweat glands.[2,5] These factors help acclimatized athletes maintain a lower skin and core temperature, resulting in improved performance. Acclimatization typically requires 10 to 14 days of training at least 60 minutes per session within a similar environment, although benefits can be seen within a few days.

Even with the best intentions, athletes can still run into hydration-related complications. It may not always be possible for athletes to consume enough fluid to match excessive sweat loss seen in extreme environments such as hot and humid climates. When fluid intake cannot match fluid loss during activity, hypohydration (often also referenced as dehydration) may occur.

Dehydration

Hydration status is affected by several factors, including duration, type, and intensity of exercise. These factors can impact the amount of sweat lost during exercise. With higher temperatures, extra gear, or in humid weather, sweat rate is further increased.[6-10] Training status and level of physical fitness also impact sweat rate. If fluid lost through sweat is not replaced, over time dehydration occurs. "Dehydration" refers to the loss of body water, whereas "hypohydration" refers to body water content deficits. The term dehydration will be used throughout this chapter to describe the body water loss.

Sweat-induced dehydration is defined as losing 2% or more of body mass in sweat (Sidebar 5-4). When sweat loss exceeds 2%, a decline in performance may occur. To briefly explain the risk for declined performance, in a dehydrated state the body will have less intracellular and extracellular water available for important bodily functions. Less water within the body can lead to less fluid available for circulation to the brain, cardiovascular system, and to facilitate thermal functions. Sweat-induced dehydration can then lead to reduced cardiovascular function and thermal capacity. These effects can be prevented with adequate fluid intake. This section will describe the signs and symptoms of dehydration, impacts on health and performance, as well as tactics for reducing the risk of dehydration.

Signs and Symptoms

Awareness of the signs and symptoms of dehydration can help prevent decreased performance and more importantly, prevent serious health consequences. Signs of dehydration include dark urine, infrequent urination, unusual rapid heart rate, poor skin turgor, and sunken eyes. Symptoms of dehydration include thirst, unusual fatigue, and dry mucous membranes. Thirst can be a symptom of dehydration, however it is not always the most reliable indicator. For instance, during exercise there are many distractions that make it easy to ignore thirst. Second, athletes may not always have fluid readily available, thus they may have to ignore this cue. Lastly, a significant amount of body water must be lost before thirst is perceived, so sweat-induced dehydration may have already occurred by the time thirst is triggered.

Signs and symptoms of dehydration:
- Dark urine
- Infrequent urination
- Unusual rapid heart rate
- Poor skin turgor
- Sunken eyes
- Thirst
- Unusual fatigue
- Dry mucous membranes

Physiological Implications of Dehydration

Dehydration can result in negative effects on physiological functions (Table 5-1). The degree of physiological strain that is occurring to a body can be measured by factors that include core temperature, heart rate, and perceived exertion. As body water loss increases, physiological strain also increases.[11] Dehydration decreases total blood volume, resulting in cardiovascular strain due to an increased workload.[12] Additionally, reduced blood volume results in reduced blood flow to tissues, such as muscle, throughout the body. When high-intensity exercise is performed, heart rate is increased to circulate blood flow to the muscles, thus providing oxygen and substrates to the working muscles. Blood flow to the skin is also necessary to remove heat.[13] Furthermore, when heart rate is elevated, stroke volume is lessened. Subsequently, less blood is pumped with each beat to the muscle, brain, and skin—if the heart counters the lower stroke volume with faster beats, blood flow remains adequate though the heart works harder. Reduced blood flow during whole-body exercise results in reduced oxygen supply and increased body temperature. Ultimately, reduction in work capacity (VO_2max) and fatigue occurs.[12]

Decreased blood flow to the brain may be partially responsible for cognitive impairments (eg, worsened accuracy, attention, coordination, memory, reaction time).[14,15] Higher-order cognitive functions, such as attention and coordination, appear to be the most susceptible cognitive functions impaired by dehydration.[15]

Performance Effects

Along with potentially diminishing blood flow, dehydration can also cause reduced alertness[16-19] and increased perceived effort.[20-22] Each of the dehydration-related challenges referenced previously can result in a reduction in performance. The extent of decreased performance will depend on the individual factors, such as physical fitness, heat acclimatization, duration, and intensity of performance. Additionally, depending on dehydration severity and length of time left untreated, physical and cognitive performance effects may occur. For example, in a 2017 study from the United Kingdom, the impact of hydration status on endurance cycling performance was assessed in the heat in untrained cyclists.[18] Participants were blinded to their hydration status (hypohydrated or euhydrated) and fluids were delivered through an intragastric tube. Unique to this study, participants could drink fluids orally and perceived thirst was measured. In those participants who started the

Table 5-1

Negative Effects of Dehydration on the Physiological Functions of the Brain, Cardiovascular System, Muscle, and Skin

This table shows how the body's physiologic functions are altered when dehydration occurs. Dehydration negatively impacts the brain, cardiovascular, muscular, and thermal systems in the body. Because different physiologic functions rely on adequate body water, severe dehydration can potentially be life-threatening.

BRAIN	• Increased perceived effort • Increased thirst sensation • Reduced cerebral blood flow
CARDIOVASCULAR SYSTEM	• Reduced blood volume of about 5% and lowered stroke volume[12] • Increased heart rate and blood pressure • Reduced blood flow to limbs[19]
MUSCLE	• Muscle fatigue • Impaired muscle blood flow[19] • Elevated muscle glycogen usage[23]
SKIN	• Reduced skin blood flow • Reduced skin turgor • Increased skin temperature • Increased core temperature

performance test hypohydrated (2.4% body mass), endurance performance was reduced by 8.1%. When hypohydrated, participants had significantly lower plasma volume and thirst was greater ($P<.05$). Therefore, researchers concluded that starting exercise activity in a dehydrated state results in decreased endurance performance.

Monitoring Hydration Status

Hydration needs are individualized based on the athlete's sweat rate and exercise environment and should not be measured during periods of rehydration. Urine specific gravity and urine osmolality are quantifiable measures. Urine specific gravity at or below 1.020 indicates euhydration.[23] Urine osmolality indication of euhydration includes values at or less than 700 mOsmol. Urine color and urine volume are subjective measures that can also be utilized.

Individuals can monitor their own hydration status using body weight and urine color. Measuring body weight after voiding in addition to measuring urine concentration can provide insight into hydration status. When measuring weight first thing in the morning after voiding and with minimal clothing, body weight should be stable with less than 1% fluctuation. Three consecutive measurements should be

logged as a baseline euhydrated status.[23] Urine color is a simple method of measuring hydration status throughout the day. Dark urine color may indicate dehydration (Figure 5-1).

Change in body weight from before to after exercise is a simple and accurate method used to calculate sweat rate. To measure whole-body sweat rate, athletes are weighed before and after exercise after toweling off existing sweat. Weights are collected nude or with minimal clothing to avoid measuring sweat trapped in clothing. Fluid losses and fluid intake during exercise such as urine and stool output, and food or fluid intake should be measured and tracked to avoid overestimation of sweat loss. Sweat rate testing should be conducted in a setting similar to event (eg, race, game) heat conditions.

Sweat Loss Calculation

1. Record weight before and after exercise in minimal clothing and after drying off
2. Record fluid consumed during training
3. Determine change in body mass before and after using the bathroom
4. Sweat loss (mL) = change in body mass (g) + fluid intake (mL) – urine losses (mL)

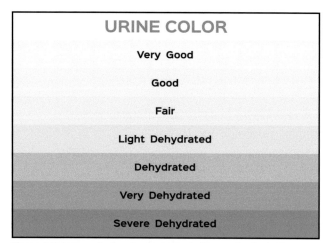

URINE COLOR

Very Good

Good

Fair

Light Dehydrated

Dehydrated

Very Dehydrated

Severe Dehydrated

Figure 5-1. Urine color is a simple method of measuring hydration status. (gritsalak karalak/Shutterstock.com.)

Fluid Recommendations

Recognizing the impact that dehydration can have on health and performance, the importance of meeting fluid demands before, during, and after activity becomes abundantly clear. It is recommended to begin exercise well hydrated by correcting sweat-induced dehydration prior to exercising. Taking in fluids and maintaining euhydration during some sports, such as endurance open water swimming, laser sailing, triathlon, or some team sports, can be extraordinarily difficult due to limited access to fluids. In scenarios where meeting fluid needs during activity is challenging, it can be especially important to work with the athlete and coach on pre-exercise hydration tactics to ensure they begin activity in a euhydrated state. It may also require working with the athlete to identify opportunities to carry and consume fluids during the activity as well.

When providing fluid recommendations, individualization may be necessary, especially when working with endurance-based sports that do not have half-time breaks or time outs. For example, laser sailing is a unique sport in which the athlete is on a very small sailboat alone and the athlete's hands are being used throughout the entire race to control the boat. Boats are not designed with hydration needs in mind! Instead, sailors must rely on grabbing fluids from their coach's boat as opportunities permit. Due to the nature of the sport, dehydration is likely to occur during competition, magnifying the importance of starting competition hydrated.

In the hours leading up to exercise, consuming fluids as well as foods containing water—such as fruits and vegetables—can help achieve hydration goals. In preparation for competition, athletes should practice their pre-event hydration strategy during training to learn how to prevent over- or underhydrating. Overconsuming fluids may result in frequent urination and interrupt exercise or competition. Additionally, excess fluid can result in an acute increase in body mass and hyponatremia. There are several simple pre-exercise fluid recommendations athletes can follow, which include:

- It is recommended to consume 5 to 7 mL of fluid per kg of body mass about 4 hours before exercise starts. Carry a water bottle throughout the day of competition to encourage frequent sipping.
- If no urine is produced or urine color is dark, consume an additional 3 to 5 mL of fluid per kg of body mass in the final 2 hours before exercise.
- During prolonged exercise when thirst is suppressed, include sodium-containing foods and beverages to promote thirst and retain fluids.[24-26]

During exercise, the goal is to prevent a loss of greater than 2% body mass from sweat. In endurance exercise that lasts longer than 3 hours, the fluid replacement plan should be established prior to starting exercise.[27] In order to develop a hydration strategy, knowledge of individual sweat rates is necessary. Think back to the previous hydration calculation described earlier in this chapter. If an athlete lost 1 kg of body weight during 2 hours of exercise, this would be equal to the loss of 1 L of sweat. This indicates that the athlete would need to consume 500 mL of fluid each hour during a 2-hour training session to maintain euhydration. Monitoring sweat and body weight losses periodically throughout a training cycle can assist the practitioner and providing a more concrete recommendation on how much fluid an athlete should consume.

During endurance events, fluids should be consumed regularly throughout the duration of the event. However, taking into account the ambient temperature as well as the intensity of the activity can help determine the amount of fluids needed. In cold weather or when intensity is low, frequent drinking could result in overhydration and hyponatremia, whereas high-intensity exercise in the heat may require additional fluids.[28]

During exercise, some sports face challenges with maintaining hydration. For instance, during ultra-endurance open water swimming, spotters have been utilized to ride in a boat alongside the swimmer to provide fluids. For example, Sarah Thomas is a marathon swimmer who swam across the English Channel 4 times nonstop and had a unique hydration plan. She stayed hydrated with the support of her team and family. They would pass her a water bottle that was tied to a rope while she stayed in the water and when she was finished rehydrating they would pull in the water bottle and place it back inside the support boat. Whereas in laser sailing competitions, athletes do not take any water bottles with them due to a lack of space as well as wanting to avoid carrying extra weight, therefore putting themselves at risk of dehydration. In Ironman races, athletes often elect to carry 6 to 8 hours' worth of hydration with them on their bike. In unique sport scenarios, it is helpful for a sports dietitian to work with the athlete to help them find ways to ensure they have a method to hydrate during exercise and competition.

Athletes can utilize sports beverages to replace electrolytes lost in sweat. A sports beverage includes: 20 to 30 mEq/L sodium, 2 to 5 mEq/L potassium, and 5% to 10% carbohydrates.[29] A sports dietitian will recommend a sports beverage for prolonged exercise in hot weather. The sodium within a sports drink stimulates thirst, improves the retention of fluid, and adds to the palatability of the beverage. Many sports drinks will also contain carbohydrates to help delay the onset of fatigue and improve performance. While it is not a strict guideline, a simple method to help athletes remember when they should utilize a sports beverage is with the 3 "Hs" of hydration: when exercise takes place in a hot environment, at a high intensity, and for longer than an hour—then a sports beverage may be beneficial.

After exercise, athletes should focus on rehydrating, especially if significant fluid losses have occurred or if they are competing in other events within the same day, such as when in a tournament. The current guidelines for fluid replacement recommend replacing 150% of body mass losses postexercise.[23] This is the equivalent of consuming approximately 1.5 L of fluids to replace 1 kg of body weight lost during physical activity. Consuming fluids in small doses periodically over time is a more effective strategy for rehydration in comparison to one large dose of fluid, which often leads to greater urine production and delayed rehydration. Additionally, including sodium either within the beverage or in the form of food can also help with retention of fluid and improved hydration status. A proper recovery meal with fluids, as discussed in Chapter 10, can help not only with recovery but also with rehydration.

While avoiding the potential risks of dehydration is a common focal point for many practitioners and athletes, there is also the potential for athletes to go too far on the other end of the extremes. As discussed next, consuming excessive amounts of fluid can present its own performance detriments and health complications.

Hyponatremia

Hyponatremia was first described in the early 1980s as a result of low sodium blood levels in marathon, ultramarathon, and triathlon competitions. Hyponatremia is a rare condition that occurs when the level of sodium in the blood is too low (<135 mmol/L; normal = 135 to 145 mmol/L). A sustained decrease in plasma sodium concentration can, in severe cases, disrupt the osmotic balance across the blood-brain barrier, resulting in a rapid influx of water into the brain.[30] This can cause brain swelling and a cascade of increasingly severe neurological responses that can eventually lead to death.[30] More specifically, exercise-associated hyponatremia (EAH) describes hyponatremia after sustained physical exertion and can occur in 10% to 20% of athletes.[31] It is important to note that while athletes may present with symptoms in conjunction with low serum sodium levels, it is possible they may also appear to be asymptomatic. Even though hyponatremia is rare, data continue to accumulate showing that it can be a greater risk for athletes than dehydration, due to the severe clinical implications.[31] Understanding the pathophysiology, who is at risk, signs and symptoms, and the treatment of hyponatremia is essential in working with athletes.

Pathophysiology

In a normal euvolemic, euhydrated state, the renal and hormonal systems maintain plasma osmolality (with 1% to 2% variation) through a variety of mechanisms and pathways.[32] The development of hyponatremia (usually in the setting of hypo-osmolality) reflects either defects in these hormonal and renal control mechanisms or water ingestion that overwhelms them. In the specific instance of EAH, defects in renal diluting mechanisms, hormonal control of water excretion, excessive sodium losses, and excessive water intake all contribute to the development of hypo-osmolality.[32]

Overdrinking is clearly the most important causative factor in the development of EAH.[33] Thirst or conditioned behaviors are the main drivers for this excessive oral intake of hypotonic fluids. However, due to the maximal water excretory capacity of the kidneys (between 750 and 1500 mL/hour), it is evident there may be other causative factors driving hyponatremia. Another potential factor is excessive sodium loss within sweat, which is worsened when replacing lost water with hypotonic fluids.[34] With sweat generating a variable amount of sodium loss (usually between 15 and 60 mEq/L, with highly fit sport athletes at a concentration around 30 to 40 mEq/L),[35] the consumption of electrolytes with water, and most importantly the avoidance of excessive fluid intake, should be prioritized to prevent EAH.

In addition to altered metabolic water production, an inability to mobilize sodium stores and/or impaired renal water excretion are physiological factors that can contribute to hyponatremia.[36] Impaired renal water excretion can be due to increased arginine vasopressin levels, impaired diluting capacity via decreased glomerular filtration rate, decreased renal blood flow, or decreased distal filtrate delivery.[37] During exercise, especially in the heat, urine production declines 20% to 60% due to a decrease in kidney blood flow that results in a decreased rate of urine production.[36] Meanwhile, the kidneys reabsorb water and electrolytes due to an exercise-induced increase in aldosterone. As a result of this increase, there is a reduced capacity to excrete water from the kidneys. In addition, exercising in a hot environment can lead to the secretion of antidiuretic hormone, which tells the kidneys how much water to conserve and further compounds the effects of exercising in the heat. The secretion of antidiuretic hormone may lead to excess sweat loss, increased heart rate, as well as increased blood pressure. Lastly, the abuse of nonsteroidal anti-inflammatory drugs (NSAIDs), which may alter kidney function and decrease urine production, can also cause hyponatremia. Hyponatremia involves multiple pathways that include both environmental and physiologic systems, and recognizing the risk factors, signs, and symptoms is crucial to prevent morbidity and mortality in athletes.

Risk Factors

Hyponatremia no longer only affects ultra-runners[31] and Ironman triathletes.[35] In general, athletes who drink too much before and during prolonged exercise in warm, humid climates and those who lose an abnormally high amount of sodium through sweat are at risk for developing hyponatremia. In addition, athletes participating in prolonged exercise events can develop hyponatremia if they lose a significant amount of sodium in their sweat and also drink excessive quantities of hypotonic solutions to replace what they lost in sweat.[31] For example, 9 cases of hyponatremia among US Marine recruits occurred on a single day in the summer of 1995 as a result of each soldier drinking 10 to 22 quarts of water over a few hours, with no electrolytes.[38] Their plasma sodium concentrations ranged from 114 to 133 mmol/L.[38] Fortunately, medical treatment was available, but this example demonstrates the importance of hydrating with more than just hypotonic solutions.

Gender has been thought to be a predictor of hyponatremia. However, many arguments surround hormones and the control of vasopressin and the amount of fluid consumed related to the size of women compared to men. More research is needed to determine if gender does play a role in hyponatremia.

Other risk factors for hyponatremia include drinking >1.5 L/hour, starting an athletic event overhydrated, having an extremely low or high BMI, and participating in an event where the athlete is inexperienced.[33] Some event-related (high fluid availability, >4 hours activity duration, extreme hot or cold temperatures, change in normal/expected weather pattern) factors can also play a role in hyponatremia.

Signs and Symptoms

Clinical symptoms are often neurological (eg, EAH-encephalopathy, confusion, seizures, coma) but can include a variety of other symptoms. Generally, athletes are expected to lose weight during exercise through sweat loss. However, when weight gain occurs during activity, this may be an indication of hyperhydration and the potential for hyponatremia. With small decreases in plasma sodium concentration of 125 to 135 mmol/L, athletes can present with modest symptoms such as bloating and mild nausea, or with no symptoms at all. When levels drop <125 mmol/L, the symptoms will be more severe and include headaches, vomiting, difficulty breathing, swollen hands and feet, restlessness, fatigue confusion, and disorientation.[39] Plasma sodium levels below 120 mmol/L present with the most severe symptoms: seizures,

respiratory arrest, coma, permanent brain damage, and death become more likely. However, blood levels are not always indicative of symptoms, as some athletes have died exhibiting a plasma sodium level of around 125 mmol/L and others have survived when dropping below 118 mmol/L.[39] Early recognition of hyponatremia is essential and can help prevent severe and permanent neurological damage to the athlete.

Treatment and Supplementation

As noted previously within this chapter, athletes are expected to lose weight during activity through the loss of sweat. Gaining weight as a result of fluid intake exceeding fluid lost through sweat increases the risk of hyponatremia. The risk of hyponatremia can be reduced by making certain that fluid intake does not exceed sweat loss, and by ingesting sodium-containing beverages or foods to help replace sodium lost in sweat. Due to the deadly nature of hyponatremia, it is of utmost importance to determine the extent of symptoms in order to lower the risk of severe neurological damage. In the case of mild EAH, fluid restriction (no electrolyte-free fluids during recovery) and observation until diuresis will be the first line of treatment. In severe EAH, when plasma sodium is <125 to 120 or they are symptomatic (encephalopathy or pulmonary edema), the athlete will need to be hospitalized. A hypertonic saline IV will allow for rapid correction and blood levels should be monitored in order to restore serum sodium.

Summary

Proper hydration is a major benefit for health, performance, and the body's physiological functions. Excessive fluid and low sodium can potentially create a life-threatening situation. Because overdrinking is the primary cause of hyponatremia, it is imperative that practitioners continue to educate our athletes about proper hydration guidelines and the potential warning signs of hyponatremia.

Cooling Tactics— A Performance Strategy Beyond Proper Hydration

In addition to maintenance of fluid balance to reduce the risk of performance complications from dehydration or hyponatremia, there are other fluid-related tactics that can be utilized by athletes to get the most out of their performance in the heat. Whether psychological or physiological, athletes can struggle with the demands of competition in warm environments. Providing tools, such as appropriate fluid recommendations as well as techniques for staying cool, may help the athlete excel. Cold baths for conduction heat transfer, ice cold fluids for internal cooling, or simply exercising in the shade rather than direct sunlight all offer a potential opportunity to minimize the effects of heat. The incorporation of cooling tactics into team hydration protocols may offer another opportunity for athletic trainers, exercise physiologists, and sports dietitians to improve athletic performance in the heat.

Cooling Defined

Athletes compete in high temperature and humid environments, which are known to impact performance. Exercise-induced increases in core body temperature can lead to heat-related illness, thus preventing the athlete from competing at the highest level. Some 70% to 80% of energy during exercise is released as heat. When this heat production exceeds the capacity to lose and dissipate heat, core temperature rises.[40] Cooling interventions have the potential to impact performance by increasing heat storage capacity, attenuating the exercise induced increase in core temperature, and accelerating recovery following intense exercise.[41]

Methods of Cooling

There are several cooling techniques used throughout the literature. Surface area, the effect of cooling on core body temperature, and applicability in the field are the main indicators to determine which technique is most successful in cooling the athlete.[42]

Cooling vests and ice vests can be used as "pre-" (before exercise) and "per-" (during exercise) cooling techniques. They cover a large part of the body, but are often heavy and difficult to transport to the field. Cold water ingestion and ice slurry ingestion can be used for pre- and per-cooling, and have a direct effect on core body temperature. Both cover a small part of the body (digested internally) and are easily applicable in field-based settings. Menthol cooling can also be used for pre- and per-cooling and can be easily used in the field, but the best application of menthol is still unknown. Facial wind and/or water spray is a common pre- and per-cooling technique—it can often be seen on TV in professional football with players sitting in front of large fans that mist water. This technique covers a large part of the body and can aid with evaporative cooling, but can be difficult in the majority of field-based settings. Cooling packs or ice towels are also used for pre- and per-cooling and can be easily used. This covers a small part of the body, and is not logical to use while playing as it could be restrictive or interfere with the activity. Cold water immersion and cryotherapy are most often used in pre- and per-cooling as they cover the largest body surface. However, cryotherapy can be expensive and have some limitations as far as exposure.

It is important to note that utilizing a combination of cooling methods has been found to be the most effective to enhance exercise performance, as it can target a larger surface area of the body. Techniques that are more feasible, easier to implement in field-based settings, and cover a larger part of the body can be utilized by athletic trainers to cool athletes more effectively.

Components of Cooling

Pre-Cooling

Pre-cooling is the rapid removal of heat from the body before exercise to create a larger heat storage capacity.[43] Cold water immersion, cold water/ice slurry ingestion, cooling packs, and cooling vests have been the most effective pre-cooling strategies used to enhance performance. The effectiveness of pre-cooling is dependent on the ambient temperature; during mild and cold temperatures techniques are not as effective as compared to hot temperatures (>80 °F).[44] Pre-cooling is also shown to have a greater benefit in endurance athletes than for intermittent sprint athletes. This increased benefit can potentially be explained by various thermoregulatory factors, muscle temperature, and anaerobic metabolism demands of sprint versus endurance exercise. Pre-cooling will largely depend on the strategy, exercise setting, and ambient conditions, but overall the most optimal cooling strategy is one that covers a major part of the body and is used during endurance exercise in hot and humid conditions.[41]

Per-Cooling

The effects of pre-cooling normally diminish after 20 to 25 minutes of exercise, so per-cooling has been found to extend the duration of the performance benefits of a cooling intervention. Per-cooling can be defined as any opportunity to reduce thermal stress during an exercise performance trial.[41] Per-cooling can be challenging due to the nature of the athletic event, but many methods have been shown to be effective such as an ice vest, cold water/ice slurry ingestion, and cooling packs. As in pre-cooling, ambient temperature also affects per-cooling, as greater performance benefits have been seen in moderate conditions compared to hot or cold. In addition, a combination of pre- and per-cooling has been mentioned in the literature to improve exercise performance and time to exhaustion. However, many studies have been inconsistent related to cooling effects on performance. Cuttell et al found a 16.7% improvement in time to exhaustion by utilizing an ice vest during cycling[45]; Luomala et al also found a 21.5% improvement in time to exhaustion during a 70-minute cycling trial while using an ice vest.[46] However, many studies found no difference in time to exhaustion or no time trial difference utilizing similar methods.[47-49] In addition, one study found that hand cooling had an 11.6% impairment of exercise time to exhaustion while running.[50]

Overall, endurance-based activities (eg, cycling, running, team sports) have had the most positive performance benefits from utilizing per-cooling strategies. However, the discrepancy among many studies indicates that more per-cooling studies are needed to confirm the most effective strategy.

Post-Cooling

Post-cooling can be defined as any opportunity to reduce the core, skin, and/or muscle temperature directly after exercise to enhance recovery and to reduce exercise-induced muscle soreness. Cold water immersion is the most frequently used post-cooling technique, along with cryotherapy. Cold water immersion entails the athlete sitting in a cold tub (5 to 15 °C) for 10 to 12 minutes, with most of the body submerged. In post-cooling, total body cryotherapy involves exposure to extremely cold dry air (-100 °C) for short periods of time (2 to 4 minutes).[51] During exposure, athletes wear minimal clothing (eg, gloves; a headband covering the ears, nose, and mouth; dry shoes and socks) to reduce the risk of cold injury.

Outcomes of cold water immersion and cryotherapy have been classified as both subjective and objective in terms of recovery. Post-cooling directly after exercise improves subjective recovery due to the decrease in soreness and reduced rate of perceived exertion 24 hours after exercise. Cryotherapy has been shown to reduce the degree of delayed onset muscle soreness in athletes, but unlike cold water immersion, it was objectively found to reduce the inflammatory response after exercise and increase maximal muscle strength.[52] No differences in biomarkers of muscle damage and inflammation were found after cold water immersion.

In summary of post-cooling techniques, cold water immersion has been found as the most effective in reducing delayed onset muscle soreness and is a feasible method that can be used in field-based settings, as compared to total body cryotherapy, which can be expensive and inapplicable to most athletic settings.

Conclusion

Hydration is a fascinating and complex topic. As soon as a practitioner feels they have grasped the latest concepts, another variable most certainly will come into play and change the entire dynamic. It is incredible to think that despite decades of research, there are still frequent cases of hydration complications at even the highest of levels of athletics. Educating the athlete on the importance of hydration, as well as some of the clear signs and symptoms of dehydration and hyponatremia, is a great starting point. This sets the foundation for the athlete's and practitioner's ability to adjust strategies on the fly based on their interpretation of these warning signs. It also hopefully places the athlete as the primary stakeholder regarding their hydration status, rather than placing that responsibility on the health care practitioner. While broad pre, per, and post activity hydration recommendations are not perfect, they can offer an excellent framework in determining best recommendations. Certainly as long as environment, sport, and the human body changes, so too will hydration tactics. That's part of what makes the role of the sports medicine and performance staff so unique and interesting, isn't it?

Discussion Questions

1. Can you think of other potential examples of conduction and convection heat transfer?

2. For a high school football player in Texas preparing to begin fall camp in August, how could you strategically help build a training schedule in July to help the athlete acclimatize and prepare him for the upcoming training camp, while also avoiding entering camp fatigued from excessive training?

3. An athlete starts their soccer practice at 75 kg and ends the 3-hour practice at 73 kg. They brought their own personal water bottle that contained 500 mL of fluid and consumed all of it. How much fluid would they need to consume in future training sessions to maintain euhydration?

References

1. Baker LB, Jeukendrup AE. Optimal composition of fluid-replacement beverages. *Comprehensive Physiology*. 2014;575-620. doi:10.1002/cphy.c130014

2. Jeukendrup AE, Gleeson M. *Sport Nutrition*. Human Kinetics; 2019.

3. Institute of Medicine. *Dietary Reference Intakes for Water, Potassium, Sodium, Chloride, and Sulfate*. The National Academies Press; 2005. doi:10.17226/10925

4. Tyler CJ. *Maximising Performance in Hot Environments: A Problem-Based Learning Approach*. Routledge; 2019.

5. Périard JD, Travers GJ, Racinais S, Sawka MN. Cardiovascular adaptations supporting human exercise-heat acclimation. *Autonomic Neuroscience*. 2016;196:52-62. doi:10.1016/j.autneu.2016.02.002

6. Gonzalez-Alonso J, Mora-Rodriguez R, Below PR, Coyle EF. Dehydration reduces cardiac output and increases systemic and cutaneous vascular resistance during exercise. *J Appl Physiol (1985)*. 1995;79(5):1487-1496.

7. Cheung SS, McLellan TM. Heat acclimation, aerobic fitness, and hydration effects on tolerance during uncompensable heat stress. *J Appl Physiol (1985)*. 1998;84(5):1731-1739.

8. Ebert TR, Martin DT, Bullock N, et al. Influence of hydration status on thermoregulation and cycling hill climbing. *Med Sci Sports Exerc*. 2007;39(2):323-329.

9. Kenefick RW, Cheuvront SN, Palombo LJ, Ely BR, Sawka MN. Skin temperature modifies the impact of hypohydration on aerobic performance. *J Appl Physiol (1985)*. 2010;109(1):79-86.

10. Sawka MN. Physiological consequences of hypohydration: exercise performance and thermoregulation. *Med Sci Sports Exerc*. 1992;24(6):657-670.

11. American College of Sports Medicine, Sawka MN, Burke LM, et al. American college of sports medicine position stand. Exercise and fluid replacement. *Med Sci Sports Exerc.* 2007;39(2):377-390.

12. Trangmar SJ, Gonzalez-Alonso J. Heat, hydration and the human brain, heart and skeletal muscles. *Sports Med.* 2019;49(Suppl 1):69-85.

13. McCubbin AJ, Allanson BA, Caldwell Odgers JN, et al. Sports dietitians Australia position statement: nutrition for exercise in hot environments. *Int J Sport Nutr Exerc Metab.* 2020:1-16.

14. Ganio MS, Wingo JE, Carrolll CE, Thomas MK, Cureton KJ. Fluid ingestion attenuates the decline in VO2 peak associated with cardiovascular drift. *Med Sci Sports Exerc.* 2006;38(5):901-909.

15. Wittbrodt MT, Millard-Stafford M. Dehydration impairs cognitive performance: a meta-analysis. *Med Sci Sports Exerc.* 2018;50(11):2360-2368.

16. Ganio MS, Armstrong LE, Casa DJ, et al. Mild dehydration impairs cognitive performance and mood of men. *Br J Nutr.* 2011;106(10):1535-1543.

17. Adan A. Cognitive performance and dehydration. *J Am Coll Nutr.* 2012;31(2):71-78.

18. James LJ, Moss J, Henry J, Papadopoulou C, Mears SA. Hypohydration impairs endurance performance: a blinded study. *Physiol Rep.* 2017;5(12). doi:10.14814/phy2.13315

19. Gonzalez-Alonso J, Teller C, Andersen SL, Jensen FB, Hyldig T, Nielsen B. Influence of body temperature on the development of fatigue during prolonged exercise in the heat. *J Appl Physiol (1985).* 1999;86(3):1032-1039.

20. Nybo L, Nielsen B. Hyperthermia and central fatigue during prolonged exercise in humans. *J Appl Physiol (1985).* 2001;91(3):1055-1060.

21. Saltin B. Circulatory response to submaximal and maximal exercise after thermal dehydration. *J Appl Physiol.* 1964;19:1125-1132.

22. Beetham WP, Jr, Buskirk ER. Effects of dehydration, physical conditioning and heat acclimatization on the response to passive tilting. *J Appl Physiol.* 1958;13(3):465-468.

23. American College of Sports Medicine, Sawka MN, Burke LM, et al. American College of Sports Medicine position stand. Exercise and fluid replacement. *Med Sci Sports Exerc.* 2007;39(2):377-390.

24. Sawka MN, Coyle EF. Influence of body water and blood volume on thermoregulation and exercise performance in the heat. *Exerc Sport Sci Rev.* 1999;27:167-218.

25. Ray ML, Bryan MW, Ruden TM, Baier SM, Sharp RL, King DS. Effect of sodium in a rehydration beverage when consumed as a fluid or meal. *J Appl Physiol.* 1998;85:1329-1336.

26. Maughan RJ, Leiper JB, Shirreffs SM. Restoration of fluid balance after exercise-induced dehydration: effects of food and fluid intake. *Eur J Appl Physiol.* 1996;73:317-325.

27. Montain SJ, Cheuvront SN, Sawka MN. Exercise associated hyponatraemia: quantitative analysis to understand the aetiology. *Br J Sports Med.* 2006;40(2):98-105; discussion 98-105.

28. Coyle EF. Fluid and fuel intake during exercise. *J Sports Sci.* 2004;22(1):39-55.

29. Institute of Medicine (US) Committee on Military Nutrition Research, Marriott BM, eds. *Fluid Replacement and Heat Stress.* National Academies Press (US);1994.

30. Backer HD, Shopes E, Collins SL. Hyponatremia in recreational hikers in Grand Canyon National Park. *J Wilderness Med.* 1993;4:391-406.

31. Frizzell RT, Lang GH, Lowance DC, Lathan SR. Hyponatremia and ultramarathon running. *JAMA.* 1986;255(6):772-774. doi:10.1001/jama.1986.03370060086025

32. Rosner MH, Kirven J. Exercise-associated hyponatremia. *Clinical Journal of the American Society of Nephrology.* 2007;2(1):151-161.

33. Hew-Butler T, Loi V, Pani A, Rosner MH. Exercise-associated hyponatremia: 2017 update. *Front Med.* 2017;4:21.

34. Rose BD, Post TW. *Clinical Physiology of Acid-Base and Electrolyte Disorders.* McGraw Hill; 2001:285-296.

35. Speedy DB, Noakes TD, Rogers IR, et al. Hyponatremia in ultra-distance triathletes. *Med Sci Sports Exerc.* 1999;31(6):809-815. doi:10.1097/00005768-199906000-00008

36. Zambraski EJ. Renal regulation of fluid homeostasis during exercise. In: Gisolfi CV and Lamb DR, eds. *Perspectives in Exercise Science and Sports Medicine. Vol. 3, Fluid Homeostasis During Exercise.* Benchmark Press; 1990:247-280.

37. Pham PCT, Pham PMT, Pham PTT. Vasopressin excess and hyponatremia. *Am J Kidney Dis.* 2006;47(5):727-737.

38. Gardner JW. Death by water intoxication. *Military Med.* 2002;5:432-434.

39. Adrogué HJ, Madias NE. Hyponatremia. *N Engl J Med.* 2000;342:1581-1589.

40. Ament W, Verkerke GJ. Exercise and fatigue. *Sports Med.* 2009;39(5):389-422.

41. Bongers CC, Hopman MT, Eijsvogels TM. Cooling interventions for athletes: an overview of effectiveness, physiological mechanisms and practical considerations. *Temperature.* 2017;4(1):60-78.

42. Quod MJ, Martin DT, Laursen PB. Cooling athletes before competition in the heat. *Sports Med.* 2006;36(8):671-682.

43. Ross M, Abbiss C, Laursen P, Martin D, Burke L. Precooling methods and their effects on athletic performance a systematic review and practical applications. *Sports Med.* 2013;43:207-225. doi:10.1007/s40279-012-0014-9

44. Wegmann M, Faude O, Poppendieck W, Hecksteden A, Frohlich M, Meyer T. Pre-cooling and sports performance: a meta-analytical review. *Sports Med.* 2012;42:545-564. doi:10.2165/11630550-000000000-00000

45. Cuttell SA, Kiri V, Tyler C. A comparison of 2 practical cooling methods on cycling capacity in the heat. *J Athl Train.* 2016;51:525-32. doi:10.4085/1062-6050-51.8.07

46. Luomala MJ, Oksa J, Salmi JA, et al. Adding a cooling vest during cycling improves performance in warm and humid conditions. *J Therm Biol.* 2012;37:47-55.

47. Barwood MJ, Corbett J, Thomas K, Twentyman P. Relieving thermal discomfort: effects of sprayed L-menthol on perception, performance, and time trial cycling in the heat. *Scand J Med Sci Sports.* 2015;25:211-218.

48. Eijsvogels TM, Bongers CC, Veltmeijer MT, Moen MH, Hopman M. Cooling during exercise in temperate conditions: impact on performance and thermoregulation. *Int J Sports Med.* 2014;35:840-846. PMID:24771132

49. De Carvalho MV, De Andrade MT, Ramos GP, et al. The temperature of water ingested ad libitum does not influence performance during a 40-km self-paced cycling trial in the heat. *J Sports Med Phys Fitness.* 2015;55:1473-1479.

50. Scheadler CM, Saunders NW, Hanson NJ, Devor ST. Palm cooling does not improve running performance. *Int J Sports Med.* 2013;34:732-735.

51. Costello JT, Baker PR, Minett GM, et al. Whole-body cryotherapy (extreme cold air exposure) for preventing and treating muscle soreness after exercise in adults. *Cochrane Database Syst Rev.* 2015:CD010789. doi:10.1002/14651858.CD010789

52. Banfi G, Melegati G, Barassi A, et al. Effects of whole-body cryotherapy on serum mediators of inflammation and serum muscle enzymes in athletes. *J Therm Biol.* 2009;34:55-59. doi:10.1016/j.jtherbio.2008.10.00

Chapter 6

Dietary Supplements

Christina Curry King, MS, RD, CSSD, LD

Commission on Accreditation of Athletic Training Education *2020 Standards*

This chapter addresses the following *2020 Standards for Accreditation of Professional Athletic Training Programs*:

- Standard 55: Students must gain foundational knowledge in statistics, research design, epidemiology, pathophysiology, biomechanics and pathomechanics, exercise physiology, nutrition, human anatomy, pharmacology, public health, and health care delivery and payor systems.
- Standard 62: Provide athletic training services in a manner that uses evidence to inform practice.
- Standard 83: Educate and make recommendations to clients/patients on fluids and nutrients to ingest prior to activity, during activity, and during recovery for a variety of activities and environmental conditions.

Learning Objectives

After reviewing this chapter, readers will be able to:

- Discuss the composition and role of sports foods and sports drinks in training and competition.
- Explain the efficacy and uses of various common performance supplements.
- Describe the role of third-party testing for supplement safety.

Knoblauch M, ed. *Clinical Nutrition in Athletic Training* (pp 61-72).
© 2023 Taylor & Francis Group.

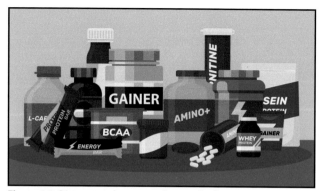

Figure 6-1. Dietary supplements and sports foods come in all shapes and sizes. (KittyVector/Shutterstock.com.)

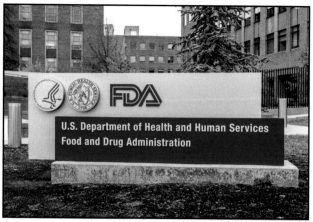

Figure 6-2. The FDA provides guidelines for regulation of supplements on the market. (JHVEPhoto/Shutterstock.com.)

Introduction

The dietary supplement industry is a billion-dollar industry, with new products and new manufacturers entering the market every year. Dietary supplements can serve many different purposes for the athlete. For instance, supplementation with a vitamin or mineral may be indicated to treat a deficiency. Female athletes may regularly supplement with iron, while a vegetarian or vegan athlete would likely require B_{12} and calcium supplements. Dietary supplements may also be used by athletes to improve performance or enhance athlete recovery from training or competition. There is no shortage of supplements claiming to have benefits for athletes; however, only a handful are actually effective. These ergogenic aids will be discussed in detail during this chapter.

Due to high usage rates among athletes and low regulatory standards, it is important that the athletic trainer have a working knowledge of common sports supplements, their efficacy, and safe usage. In-depth coverage of *all* available supplements is beyond the scope of this text. Instead, the purpose of this chapter is to familiarize the athletic trainer with the supplements and sports foods available on the market that have sufficient research supporting their use and efficacy. Additionally, this chapter will also discuss the steps needed to ensure the athlete remains protected from harmful and banned substances while using supplements (Figure 6-1).

What Is a Supplement and Who Uses Them?

In the United States, dietary supplements and dietary ingredients fall under the jurisdiction of the US Food and Drug Administration (FDA), and safety regulations are outlined in the Dietary Supplement Health and Education Act (DSHEA) of 1994. According to DSHEA, a dietary supplement

> is a product intended to supplement the diet that bears or contains one or more of the following dietary ingredients: a vitamin; mineral; herb or

Sidebar 6-1

FDA labeling. You may have noticed disclaimers on your supplement's labels. Supplement manufacturers are limited on what can be printed on product labels. They cannot legally claim a supplement can diagnose, treat, or cure a disease. If a supplement label contains a Structure/Function or Health claim (eg, "supports healthy joints," "may reduce the risk of osteoporosis") they are required by law to include a disclaimer on the label that states "These statements have not been evaluated by the FDA. This product is not intended to diagnose, treat, cure, or prevent any disease." This text is required to be in boldface type on a box that is linked to the claim, usually by an asterisk. Essentially, this disclaimer only demonstrates that the supplement manufacturers have followed the law, not that their product is truly effective and backed by science.

other botanical; amino acid; dietary substance for use by humans to supplement the diet by increasing the total dietary intake; or a concentrate, metabolite, constituent, extract, or combination of the preceding substances.[1]

Conversely, according to the FDA a drug is defined as a substance intended to diagnose, treat, or prevent disease. Practitioners should note that, unlike drugs, supplements do not undergo extended clinical testing for efficacy and do not require FDA approval before being placed on the market. The DSHEA outlines that supplement manufacturers cannot make claims to "treat, diagnose, prevent, or cure diseases" (Figure 6-2, Sidebar 6-1).

According to the 2018 CRN Consumer Survey on Dietary Supplements, 69% of adults aged 18 to 34 years use dietary supplements, with the top reasons for supplement use being overall wellness and filling nutrient gaps.[1] A review conducted by Garthe and Maughan found high supplement use among athletes as well, as up to 46% of collegiate athletes and 59% of elite athletes reported using dietary supplements. Elite athletes were found to have higher supplement usage than nonelite athletes, and those who competed in endurance-based sports had the highest usage rates.[2] Most of the supplements used by athletes in this study were sport supplements. For the purposes of this chapter, supplements will be categorized as either sports foods and sports drinks (eg, sports gels and confectionaries, electrolyte replacement and protein supplements) or performance supplements (eg, caffeine, nitrates, sodium bicarbonate, beta-alanine, creatine). For further information on supplements for deficiency, please see Chapter 3 on micronutrients.

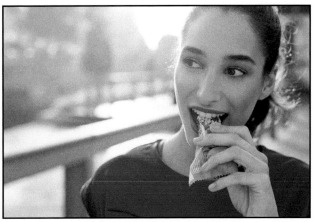

Figure 6-3. Sports foods provide athletes with essential nutrients like protein and carbohydrates in easy-to-consume and convenient packages. (Rido/Shutterstock.com.)

Sports Foods

Sports foods are products that are specifically designed to provide needed nutrients when it may be unrealistic to consume whole foods. Sports foods can be found in powder, liquid, or gel form, or even made into confectionaries like bars and waffles. There are many different combinations and varieties of sports foods in the market, but this chapter will focus on the composition, efficacy, and uses of the more commonly used sports drinks and electrolyte replacements, sports gels and confectionaries, and protein supplements (Figure 6-3).

Sports Drinks and Electrolyte Replacements

Sports drinks and electrolyte replacements options have evolved a long way from early formulations of Gatorade (PepsiCo). Sports drinks are often found in liquid or powdered form, contain electrolytes like sodium and potassium, and may or may not contain carbohydrates. Many athletes turn to sports drinks before, during, or after training and competition to improve hydration status, and often to provide a quick energy source via easily digestible carbohydrates like glucose, dextrose, and maltodextrin. For drinks that do contain carbohydrates, it is important that the formulation remain hypotonic (ie, lower concentration of carbs and electrolytes than the blood) to avoid gastrointestinal distress while exercising. If the sports drink is hypertonic, water will be pulled from the body into the gut to dilute the solution, which may lead to nausea, cramping, and potentially diarrhea. Most sports drinks on the market typically range from 4% to 8% carbohydrate, falling into this hypotonic range and allowing for an appropriate rate of gastric emptying.[3]

For athletes training or competing at a high intensity and/or in warm climates for at least 90 minutes, it is recommended that they consume some form of carbohydrate. Due to the higher calorie and high sugar content, sports drinks that contain carbohydrates are appropriate for these athletes as a way of meeting their needs when whole foods may not be accessible or appropriate. For those athletes or exercisers that are looking to improve hydration without the added sugar, most sports drink companies have increased their product lines beyond the traditional high carbohydrate formulas and now offer lower calorie formulations that contain less carbohydrates or no carbohydrates at all. For example, Gatorade's line includes not only their traditional formula but a 50% reduced carbohydrate formula, zero calorie formula, and electrolyte-infused water.

In addition to sports drinks, athletes and exercisers now have more options to replace electrolytes lost through sweat. Common forms of electrolyte supplementation include powders to be mixed into water, pills, and chewable tablets. The primary electrolyte lost in sweat is sodium, with small amounts of potassium and chloride lost as well. When exercising for prolonged periods of time, it is important to replace sodium and avoid an overconsumption of water, both of which can help prevent hyponatremia. The amount of sodium lost during exercise varies widely from athlete to athlete and depends greatly on the environment. Due to this wide range, uniform recommendations for sodium supplementation do not exist. If an athlete is exercising for 2 or more hours, sodium should be consumed in the form of a food, supplement, or sports drink. On average, sports drinks will contain approximately 400 to 500 mg of sodium per liter, and other electrolyte replacement supplements range from 300 to 700 mg per serving.

It is not uncommon to see an extremely high intake of sodium and electrolytes by endurance and ultra-endurance athletes during training and in competition. While it is not necessarily harmful to consume large amounts of electrolytes while exercising, there is doubt in whether or not it actually enhances performance. In a study of athletes competing in the ultra-endurance Ironman race in Cape Town, South Africa, the authors found that additional supplemental

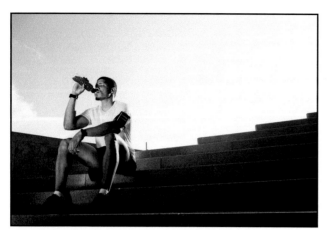

Figure 6-4. Sports drinks can provide athletes with easy to digest carbohydrates, electrolytes, and fluid to enhance their performance. (GaudiLab/Shutterstock.com.)

sodium intake via tablets was not necessary to maintain plasma sodium concentration throughout the 12-hour competition.[4] Despite consuming an extra 3600 mg of sodium, there was no difference in serum sodium levels, weight, and performance outcomes when compared to those consuming a placebo. The authors concluded that the sodium intake from sports drinks, gels, and food was sufficient for safe and effective performance in an ultra-endurance event.

Another common misconception surrounding electrolyte supplementation is its relationship to exercise-associated muscle cramps (EAMC). Initially it was thought that electrolyte imbalances were a primary contributor to EAMC, however this relationship has not been consistently shown in the literature. Rather, scientists have begun to lean more toward the belief that the primary cause of EAMC may be more related to muscle fatigue and overload, which in turn causes localized muscle cramping.[5] While hypohydration can still negatively impact muscle performance, acute treatment with electrolyte replacement supplements have not been shown to be effective.

Gatorade is no longer the only choice when it comes to picking a sports drink or electrolyte replacement. There are countless formulations and flavors available on the market. When recommending a sports drink or electrolyte replacement, the athletic trainer should take into consideration the types of electrolytes provided, sodium being most important, and match the carbohydrate content to the environment, intensity, and goals of the individual athlete (Figure 6-4).

Sports Gels and Confectionaries

It is recommended that athletes take in carbohydrates during training if exercising for longer than 90 minutes. Sports drinks are often used as carbohydrate vehicles in these circumstances; however, sports gels and other confectionaries like chews or bars may be utilized when the athlete does not wish to consume the amount of fluid from a sports drink necessary to ingest appropriate amounts of carbohydrate. For example, it is generally recommended to take in 30 to 60 g of carbohydrate per hour when exercising continuously for more than 2 hours, equating to approximately 16 to 30 ounces of sports drink over that same time in order to ingest the appropriate amount of carbohydrate. Similarly, a sports gel generally contains 20 to 25 g of carbohydrate in a 1- to 1.2-ounce formulation (along with several electrolytes), making sports gels an attractive option for those situations when ingesting higher volumes of fluid may be unappealing or impractical (ie, during an endurance race). Like sports drinks, these gels and confectionaries often contain easy-to-digest carbohydrates like the monosaccharides glucose and fructose and polysaccharides like maltose and dextrose (chain of glucose molecules).

When athletes engage in training or competition that lasts more than 3 hours, it is recommended to consume up to 90 g of carbohydrate per hour to meet energy demands. The maximal rate of the monosaccharide glucose's uptake into the cells is 60 g/hour; therefore, in order to meet the 90 g/hour recommendation, athletes must consume additional monosaccharides like fructose that utilize different cell transporters.[6] Fructose is often found in sports gels in combination with glucose or with maltodextrin. In addition to the use during continuous exercise, sports drinks and gels may also be effective performance enhancers when consumed during intermission or half-times of competitions. Athletes who consumed carbohydrates at these times saw improvements in blood glucose levels, sprint performance, and sport-related skills.[7,8]

Sports gels and confectionaries provide needed carbohydrates in convenient formulations for athletes training and competing for extended periods of time. The athletic trainer should consider the total time of training and available formulations when choosing the appropriate product.

Protein Supplements

While carbohydrates are the primary energy source for exercising muscle, proteins are the building blocks of muscle. Protein supplements may be appropriate for athletes or exercisers who are trying to build or maintain lean mass and have short time frames between training sessions or other responsibilities like work or a busy class schedule. Common forms of protein supplements include powders and liquids and are the primary ingredient in protein bars. When choosing a protein supplement, it is important to consider the source. The most common source of protein within supplements is whey protein. Whey is derived from milk, and has been shown to be effective for increasing muscle hypertrophy as well as strength. The benefit of whey protein is thought to be due in part to its high content of essential amino acids, specifically the branched-chain amino acid leucine.[9] Leucine is an important modulator of muscle protein synthesis. When the leucine threshold is met, approximately 2.5 to 3 g in a meal, muscle protein synthesis is activated within the myofiber, thereby allowing for muscle fiber growth and repair.[10] This leucine threshold is easily met in a 20 to 25 g whey protein supplement, making it an excellent option for those looking to build muscle.

For athletes who are dairy intolerant or prefer non-animal-based protein, a plant-based protein supplement may be a more favorable option. When choosing plant-based protein options, it is important to consider leucine content. Pea protein has been shown comparable to whey for stimulating similar rates of muscle protein synthesis.[11]

Protein supplements can provide a concentrated source of nutrition to support muscle growth and repair, and are ideal for athletes who must transition quickly from training to class, work, or their next activity without time to consume a full meal (Figure 6-5).

When added to a well-balanced diet, sports foods and drinks can provide necessary nutrients for athletes that are packaged in convenient forms. Nutrients like carbohydrates, proteins, fluids, and electrolytes are often required in specific doses at specific times for the enhancement of performance and recovery. Protein supplements can be favorable options to support overall protein intake and muscle protein synthesis. Sports foods like gels and confectionaries or sports drinks can help the athlete support the energy requirements of their exercise with ease and convenience. An important role of the athletic trainer is to help guide the athlete to appropriate usage of sports foods and drinks for optimum performance and recovery.

Performance Supplements

Caffeine

Caffeine has been widely studied as an ergogenic aid. In a recent meta-analysis, caffeine was found to be effective in enhancing performance across a variety of athletic endeavors.[12] Caffeine is readily available in common beverages like coffee and tea, and can also be found in specially formulated sports or energy drinks. The ubiquity of caffeine in food and drink products makes it an accessible ergogenic aid for most athletes; however, dosage and timing of caffeine ingestion is important for actual improvement in performance.

Mechanism of Action

Caffeine's mechanism of action exists within the central nervous system as well as peripherally in the muscle. It is absorbed relatively quickly, with peak plasma levels occurring approximately 1 hour after consumption, and it can cross the blood-brain barrier.[13] Caffeine's primary action is as an adenosine antagonist leading to decreased levels of perceived exertion and pain, as well as increased alertness.[9,14] In the muscle, caffeine has been shown to modulate substrate utilization, by increasing free fatty acid mobilization and

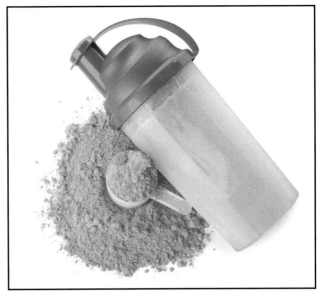

Figure 6-5. Protein powders can be an easy addition to an athlete's diet to ensure they are meeting their protein intake and timing goals. (Africa Studio/Shutterstock.com.)

oxidation and decreasing glycogen use.[14] This glycogen sparing early on in a race or competition can delay muscle fatigue and lead to performance improvements. The effective dose of caffeine ranges from 3 to 6 mg/kg, with higher doses generally not being more effective than 6 mg/kg and potentially producing negative side effects such as dizziness, insomnia, or gastrointestinal distress.[15] In most studies this dosage has been provided as caffeine anhydrous in a powdered form, and less is known about caffeine from food-based sources like coffee and sports gels or gums.[16] More research is needed to better understand the effectiveness of caffeine in the different sports food products (Sidebar 6-2). Caffeine contents in coffee vary widely depending on the type of bean, the roast, and how it is brewed as coffee, with medium roast cold brew coffee typically yielding the highest amounts of caffeine.[17]

Initially, it was thought that athletes should avoid caffeine due to the potential diuretic effects and subsequent risk for dehydration. Recent research, however, has concluded that this dehydration concern is unwarranted when caffeine is consumed at recommended intakes. Furthermore, beverages containing caffeine up to 6 mg/kg are not believed to contribute negatively to hydration status overall.[13] A recommendation of 2 cups of coffee (~200 mg of caffeine) about an hour before activity for the average-sized athlete weighing ~70 kg would be close to the described ergogenic range of 3 mg/kg.

Efficacy

Caffeine is one of the most studied ergogenic aids, and most athletes can benefit from caffeine supplementation in some form. The majority of the research has found caffeine to be beneficial in endurance sports when taken in moderate doses of 2 to 3 mg/kg before and during the event.[15] Recently, more research has come out to support the use of caffeine for increased muscular strength and power, and caffeine use (4 to 6 mg/kg) in team sports has been found to improve performance, especially in elite athletes.[12,13] When counseling an athlete on caffeine use and performance, it is important to consider dose and frequency, as well as potential negative impacts. When working with endurance athletes, it may be beneficial to dose several times throughout the race, with emphasis on the end of the race to potentially reduce rates of perceived exertion. In a team sport athlete, a moderate dose of caffeine approximately 60 minutes before game start would be appropriate. In a tournament setting it is also important to consider potential negative impacts on sleep with caffeine usage, as it may prolong alertness and wakefulness during sleeping hours that are crucial for recovery between games or matches. It may be advisable to allow for additional time to rest the following day.

More recently there has been investigation into genetic variability in an athlete's response to caffeine. The genotype of an athlete's CYP1A2 gene, which encodes the enzyme responsible for around 95% of caffeine metabolism, will determine whether they are a "fast" or slow metabolizer of caffeine.[19] Athletes who are fast metabolizers tend to see performance benefits with lower doses of caffeine, while athletes who are slow metabolizers have longer caffeine clearance times. These long clearing times lead to higher instances of negative side effects and may actually cause decreases in performance.[20] It has been suggested that slower metabolizers may require more time between caffeine ingestion and exercise to see performance benefit.[21] Due to the high cost and limited availability outside of research purposes, genetic testing for caffeine response may only be available to the most elite athletes.

Caffeine can be a cheap and effective source of performance enhancement in a variety of sporting events. When counseling athletes on caffeine usage, it is important to emphasize the correct dosage and timing to prevent negative effects like jitteriness and poor sleep post competition. It may also be advisable to choose caffeine sources that have measured amounts of caffeine as opposed to the variability found in beverages like coffee and tea.

Buffers

Like caffeine, supplements that help to manage acid base balance in the muscle can help delay fatigue for athletes participating in intense exercise. During high-intensity exercise the primary energy pathway utilized by muscle is anaerobic glycolysis. As the use of this energy system is prolonged, the byproduct of lactic acid dissociates into lactate and hydrogen ions (H^+), eventually overcoming the muscle's inherent buffering capacity and lowering the pH of the muscle. This increase in acidity (ie, lowered pH) is thought to be the main driver of muscle fatigue. The increase in acidity in the muscle may also lead to disruption of the muscle's energy systems (ie, creatine phosphate re-phosphorylation, glycolysis energy pathway) and muscle contraction mechanisms, leading to an increase in perception of effort during exercise.[22] Supplementation with buffers is typically recommended for athletes competing in events that require high-intensity bouts of exercise lasting from 1 to 8 minutes. Such athletes include track and field sprinters and middle-distance runners, as well as swimmers and cyclists. There may also be an indication for buffer supplementation in competition that requires repeated bouts of sprinting, such as in team sports like basketball or soccer. Sodium bicarbonate and beta-alanine are 2 dietary supplements that can enhance the muscle's buffering capacity and potentially improve high-intensity exercise improvement.

Sodium Bicarbonate

Sodium bicarbonate ($NaHCO_3$) is commonly found in one's pantry as baking soda. Baking soda was identified for its potential buffering capacity as early as the 1930s, but studies to determine the ergogenic capacity of sodium bicarbonate did not begin until the 1970s[23] (Figure 6-6).

Mechanism of Action

When supplemented orally, sodium bicarbonate acts as an extracellular buffer. Upon reaching the intestines, sodium bicarbonate absorbs into the blood and increases bicarbonate concentration from 25 mmol at rest to 30 mmol in the extracellular matrix surrounding the muscle. This increase in the pH surrounding the muscle draws the hydrogen ions out of the muscle cell and into the extracellular matrix, where they bind to bicarbonate to form carbonic acid and are eventually neutralized to carbon dioxide (CO_2) and water (H_2O).

Initially the acute dosage to optimize buffering capacity was identified as 0.3 g/kg 60 to 120 minutes before competition; however, this large dose may cause increased CO_2 production in the stomach leading to gastrointestinal distress like nausea, vomiting, and diarrhea that outweighs any ergogenic benefit.[24] For an athlete that weighs 150 pounds, 0.3 g/kg of sodium bicarbonate would be approximately 1 tablespoon, although the most common form of supplementation is as a capsule. Sodium bicarbonate is also effective when taken in consecutive days, making it an appropriate recommendation for athletes competing over multiple days.[25] In

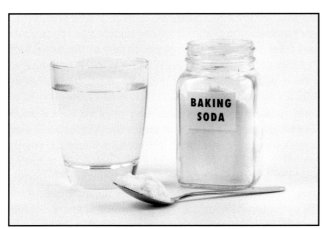

Figure 6-6. Baking soda, a common baking ingredient, can be used as an effective buffer for athletes. (TY Lim/Shutterstock.com.)

order to reduce the potential for gastrointestinal symptoms, it has been recommended to consume the appropriate dose earlier—about 2 to 2.5 hours before competition with a small meal.[26] Even with adjustments to the dosage schedule, some athletes may still experience negative symptoms of sodium bicarbonate supplementation; therefore, it is always recommended to trial supplementation before competition.[27]

Efficacy

According to a meta-analysis by Carr et al,[26] under laboratory conditions, 0.3 g/kg improved performance of a 60-second sprint by almost 2%. However, the authors also found that the sprint performance benefits were lost after 10 minutes of continuous exercise.[26] There are several studies that suggest a greater magnitude of improvement from supplementation in repeated bouts of sprinting-type activity as well as a potential benefit in sports like judo, boxing, or water polo.[24,28] One study compared results from judo testing and an upper-body Wingate protocol after supplementing with 0.3 g/kg sodium bicarbonate and placebo. The athletes who were given sodium bicarbonate saw improved performance in later bouts of the judo protocol as well as increased mean and peak power in the Wingate testing.[29]

While there have been some studies that have shown promising results and significant improvement in sport or exercise performance after acute and chronic supplementation, the research protocols and dosages have been inconsistent in the literature—making a scientific consensus difficult to achieve. A recent meta-analysis by Hadzic et al found the duration of exercise to be essential in determining dosage and timing; however, there is currently too much heterogenicity in the current literature to state a consensus. The authors call for further research into potential benefits for truly elite athletes, as well as determining acute versus chronic supplementation effects.[30] When it comes to the efficacy of sodium bicarbonate supplementation, the bottom line is that acute supplementation of 0.3 g/kg of sodium bicarbonate can be effective in sprint performance ranging from 1 to 8 minutes; however, due to inconsistencies in the research, less

is known about longer events and chronic supplementation. Sodium bicarbonate supplementation should always be trialed before competition due to the potential risk of adverse gastrointestinal side effects.

Beta-Alanine

Beta-alanine is an amino acid that can be synthesized in the liver or taken in exogenously via foods like meat and poultry. Beta-alanine supplements are often found in tablets or powder form. On its own, beta-alanine provides little performance-enhancing benefit; however, when it combines with L-histidine it becomes the intracellular buffer carnosine.

Mechanism of Action

Beta-alanine, when combined with the amino acid L-histidine, forms the molecule carnosine that acts as an intracellular buffer in muscle. Beta-alanine is the rate-limiting step in this reaction, meaning without appropriate amounts of beta-alanine present carnosine cannot be synthesized. Like sodium bicarbonate, carnosine acts as a buffer by sequestering hydrogen ions to delay acidosis in muscle. This action takes place within the muscle cell, preceding the effects of sodium bicarbonate's buffering in the extracellular matrix (Sidebar 6-3). When supplementing, the recommended dosage of beta-alanine is 4 to 6 g/day, which can lead to a 64% increase in muscle carnosine content after 4 weeks and as much as 80% after 10 weeks.[31]

It is recommended that individuals interested in supplementing with beta-alanine undergo a loading phase for at least 4 weeks in order to increase muscle carnosine levels. During this loading phase, the athlete should consume 4 to 6 g total of beta-alanine per day, dividing this amount into separate doses of 2 g or less. Consuming the beta-alanine with a meal may optimize muscle carnosine storage.[31] It is hypothesized that the release of insulin after a meal improves the uptake of beta-alanine and storage of carnosine in the muscle.[33] The most common side effect to beta-alanine supplementation is paresthesia or tingling in the face, neck, and back of hands. This sensation is nonharmful and normally subsides after 60 to 90 minutes. Furthermore, this side effect has been reduced as a result of a sustained-release beta-alanine formulation.

Efficacy

A recent meta-analysis published in 2017 concluded that the most important factor influencing efficacy of beta-alanine supplementation was exercise duration. The authors found that supplementation with beta-alanine was most effective in exercises lasting 0.5 to 10 minutes, and there was no effect found for exercise activity lasting less than 0.5 minutes.[34] The researchers also suggested that more benefit was found in untrained or nonelite athletes who supplement with beta-alanine. Examples of activity that can be improved by beta-alanine include the 800 m sprint, 1000 to 2000 m running, rowing, or combat sports where rounds last between 1 to 10 minutes.[35]

Interestingly, there are a few studies that show an increased benefit from combining beta-alanine and sodium bicarbonate supplementation for both intracellular and extracellular buffering. These results show a potential to increase cycling capacity and rowing performance with dual supplementation of beta-alanine and sodium bicarbonate over beta-alanine supplementation alone.[36,37]

Buffers like beta-alanine and sodium bicarbonate can be effective for athletes competing in events lasting 10 minutes or less. Testing these buffers before competition will be important, as both have potential side effects that could negatively impact performance. It will also be pertinent for the athletic trainer to guide athletes in proper timing and dosage of these supplements to see benefits.

Creatine

Creatine is one of the most popular supplements used by athletes and exercisers today, with more than $400 million in sales annually.[38] While found in supplements, it is also present in food sources like fish and meat and is synthesized by the body in the liver and kidneys. Creatine has also been declared to be the most effective ergogenic aid for athletes by several organizations, including the International Society of Sports Nutrition, American College of Sports Medicine, Academy of Nutrition and Dietetics, and the Dietitians of Canada.

Approximately 95% of creatine is stored in the muscle, while the other 5% can be found in the brain. The upper limit of creatine storage in the muscle is around 160 mmol/kg of muscle, while the average found in most humans is around 120 mmol/kg—and even lower levels of 110 mmol/kg are found in vegetarians.[39] These existing suboptimal levels of creatine allow for the high rates of efficacy found in supplementation with creatine.

Mechanism of Action

The main role of creatine during exercise is to aid in the rapid resynthesis of adenosine triphosphate (ATP), the energy molecule needed for muscle contraction, via the creatine-phosphate energy pathway. The mechanism of action is as follows: The third phosphate group in ATP is cleaved, which releases energy and allows for the muscle fiber to contract and leave adenosine diphosphate (ADP) as the byproduct. In order to be an effective energy source, ADP must bind to a third phosphate group. A molecule of creatine combines with a phosphoryl group via the creatine kinase enzyme to form creatine phosphate. Creatine phosphate then donates its phosphate group to ADP to synthesize ATP, and it is used again for muscle contraction. The creatine phosphate energy system is utilized during maximal exercise efforts lasting only 1 to 10 seconds. Additionally, creatine supplementation may improve the shuttling of ATP from the mitochondria to the cytosol, enhancing not only the anaerobic energy system but also the efficiency of the energy system.[40]

Efficacy

The supplemental form of creatine is available in different formulations including creatine monohydrate, creatine citrate, creatine ethyl ester, and creatine nitrate; however, none of these products have been found to be as effective in the uptake and storage of creatine as creatine monohydrate.[41] For the fastest increase in muscle creatine levels, it is suggested to "load" with 0.3 g/kg body weight (approximately 5 g) 4 times daily for the first 5 to 7 days followed by a maintenance dose of 3 to 5 g per day. The timing of the maintenance dose is less important than in the loading protocol; however, it is often recommended to take post-training alongside a recovery meal. Like with beta-alanine, creatine uptake is improved when consumed alongside carbohydrates and protein, as the release of insulin improves creatine uptake in muscle.[42]

Creatine supplementation has been proven to be effective in increasing muscle levels of creatine, which in turn provides an added energy source for acute and repeated maximal effort strength training or sprinting activity. Several studies have shown that creatine is effective in increasing muscle mass when combined with strength training.[43] This gain in muscle mass is a result of the increase in the muscle's capacity for exercise due to the elevated levels of phosphocreatine, which in turn leads to faster ATP resynthesis. In addition to increases in muscle mass, creatine supplementation may be effective in improving sport performance, particularly in sprinting and intermittent team sport activities.

More recently, studies have uncovered additional uses for creatine beyond performance alone. For example, there may be a potential for enhanced muscle recovery with creatine supplementation. In one study, creatine supplementation decreased markers of muscle damage and allowed for faster muscle strength recovery after intense exercise.[44] In endurance racers, creatine loading decreased markers of inflammation and muscle soreness as compared to controls.[45]

Due to the osmotic properties of creatine, it is effective in improving body water retention and inducing a state of hyperhydration. A study by Kilduff et al found that intracellular water levels were elevated following supplementation, and heart rate and rectal temperatures we lower during prolonged exercise in the heat in the creatine supplementation group.[46] For athletes that suffer injuries that require immobilization, creatine supplementation may help decrease the rate of atrophy and improve muscle growth during rehabilitation.[47] Perhaps the most promising potential use for creatine is for improving brain health after a head injury. For obvious ethical reasons, most of the studies of creatine's effect on traumatic brain injury (TBI) has been done in rodents. It has been found that TBI may result in mitochondrial dysfunction and a subsequent reduction in supply of ATP.[48] When supplemented with creatine prior to injury, rodents displayed increased ATP levels alongside smaller brain lesions and reduced reactive oxygen species.[49] In the very limited human TBI studies that have been conducted, there seems to be improvement in cognition, dizziness, and headaches in the 6 months after TBI when the patients were supplemented with 0.4 g/kg creatine daily.[48] While more studies are needed, especially in the instances of concussion, the relative safety and low cost of creatine makes it an attractive option for those seeking relief from symptoms of brain injury. And contrary to popular belief, there is no evidence that creatine usage, even when consumed over long periods of time, increases incidences of dehydration, muscle cramping or injuries, or renal disfunction.[39]

Creatine has been consistently proven to be effective for improving sprint and intermittent high-intensity exercise performance as well as muscle growth and retention. It also has potential capabilities for improved hydration status and recovery from musculoskeletal and brain injury. Fortunately, it is relatively inexpensive and extremely safe when used in appropriate doses, making it a viable supplement option for almost every athlete.

Nitrates

Dietary nitrates can be found in high amounts in green leafy vegetables like spinach, celery, arugula, and lettuce, as well as in beetroot. Still, the amount of nitrates present in food is extremely variable; therefore, consuming the necessary amount of food in order to attain nitrate levels at a high enough level to impact performance may require an unrealistic volume of whole foods. Beetroot extract is the most common source for nitrate supplementation in sports. It may be found as a juice, concentrate, or powder mixture. A recent study by Gallardo and Coggan examined the nitrate content of several sports supplements and juices on the market and found several to have suboptimal levels of nitrate[50] (Figure 6-7).

Mechanism of Action

Dietary nitrates (NO_3) are consumed via foods or supplementation, and then anaerobic bacteria residing on the tongue reduces the inorganic nitrate to nitrite (NO_2). After this conversion, some of the nitrite is further reduced to nitric oxide (NO) in the stomach; however, some NO_2 will

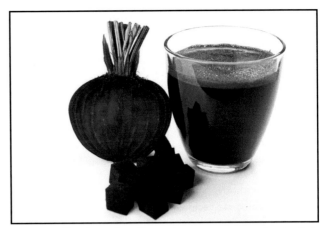

Figure 6-7. The nitrates found in supplements are commonly extracted from beetroot. (Africa Studio/Shutterstock.com.)

enter the blood stream before being reduced. Once in the blood stream, the nitrite is delivered to tissues that possess reducing capability. In normal environments, muscle is able to generate NO via reduction of L-arginine; however, without the presence of oxygen, this production of NO is greatly diminished. For example, hypoxia is induced in exercising muscle, and the endogenous production of NO is limited. In such cases, the increase in NO availability from the ingestion of dietary nitrates may serve as another source of NO production when the normal pathways are disabled. This "back-up" source of dietary nitrate may improve exercise capacity due to increased blood flow to the exercising muscle, increased mitochondrial ATP production, or a reduced cost of ATP (measured by less oxygen consumed per ATP molecule generated) for muscle contraction.[51]

Efficacy

Nitrate supplementation has been shown to be most effective in prolonged submaximal exercise, as well as high-intensity, intermittent, short-duration exercise.[52] It is recommended that 300 to 500 mg or 5 to 9 mmol of nitrate in about 500 mL of juice be ingested approximately 2 to 3 hours before training or competition.[53] There does not seem to be any benefit in supplementing beyond ~500 mg. Effects may be seen with acute supplementation; however, intake for 3 days or more seems to be beneficial as well.[54] Supplementation in endurance events may extend time to exhaustion by 4% to 25%, while use in high-intensity, intermittent, and team sport settings garners the biggest benefit in events that last 12 to 40 minutes.[55,56] In one study by Thompson and colleagues, male team sport athletes were given 6.4 mmol nitrate or a non-nitrate-containing beverage for 5 days before completing a series of sprint testing and cognitive tasks. The authors found that the group supplementing with nitrate-containing beetroot juice saw improved sprint times as well as improvement in total distance covered in a set time, along with improvements in cognitive tasks at rest when compared to placebo.[54]

For athletic trainers planning to employ nitrate supplementation with their athletes, it is important to consider other habits that may impact the sensitive microbiome of the mouth that is necessary for the reduction of nitrates to nitrites. For example, gum chewing, use of alcohol-containing mouthwash, or use of tobacco products may disrupt the presence of the bacteria needed for nitrate-to-nitrate conversion and render the supplementation ineffective. Due to the potential high cost of prolonged nitrate supplementation, it will be important to address oral hygiene habits and compliance beforehand.

Nitrates have become a popular supplement among endurance and team sport athletes. Nitrates can be found in food sources, though it can be hard to determine the correct dosage supplied via various foods. Using beetroot juice supplements can be an effective way to take in the necessary 300 to 500 mg of nitrates, but the brand of the supplement and the oral hygiene practices of the athlete must be considered before implementation.

Supplement Safety

As mentioned previously in this chapter, there is very little testing required before a supplement goes to market. In addition, there is limited oversight of supplement companies and formulations allowed on the market. According to DSHEA, it is the responsibility of the supplement company to ensure the safety and quality of the product. Many athletes may be subject to drug testing and tainted supplements may lead to an anti-doping violation or a loss of eligibility, championships, or suspension from competition. A list of banned substances can be found on the World Anti-Doping Agency's website, or if the athlete is competing in the National Collegiate Athletic Association the banned list can be found on their website and is updated yearly.[57,58]

Unfortunately, the presence of banned substances, as specified by the World Anti-Doping Agency, in supplements used in sport may be as high as 12% to 58%.[59] In order to prevent a potential violation due to contamination, several companies offer "third-party" testing for banned substances in sports supplements. A consensus statement released by representatives from the US Anti-Doping Agency, Major League Baseball, Ultimate Fighting Championship, and the Consortium for Health and Military Performance in 2019 details the best practices for third-party testing programs.[60] The authors' complete recommendations are beyond the scope of this chapter, but it is essential that the third-party testing companies operate independently from both supplement companies and drug testing agencies.

NSF Certified for Sport

One third-party testing agency that meets the recommended criteria is NSF International Certified for Sport. A supplement bearing this label is certified to not contain any banned substances, ensures that the contents of the

supplement match what is printed on the label, ensures that there are not unsafe levels of contaminants in the product, and outlines that the product is manufactured in a facility that is both Good Manufacturing Practice (GMP) certified and is audited twice annually for quality and safety by NSF International.[61]

Informed Sport

Informed Sport testing is another third-party agency that tests supplements for banned substances. According to the Informed Sport website, any supplement bearing the Informed Sport label undergoes product evaluation including formulation, label claims, nutritional labeling, contaminant test, and raw material evaluation at each production site. The certification also includes a review of accreditations held by the manufacturing and packing facility, quality system and standard operating procedure review for raw material storage, handling, production, and packaging, as well as raw material supplier assessment and evaluation of finished goods storage and distribution.[62]

NSF Certified for Sport and Informed Sport labeling are trusted by collegiate and professional sports organizations and athletes worldwide to aid in the safe and legal intake of supplements and ergogenic aids. Unfortunately no label can completely guarantee safety and efficacy of a supplement, but these third-party companies can offer a needed level of protection for athletes looking to utilize supplements. It is important that the athletic trainer be able to identify these third-party testing labels and help athletes choose the supplement brand that is least likely to lead to a doping infraction.

Conclusion

The supplements covered in this chapter are considered effective according to scientific consensus, but are only a fraction of the ones found in the market. Athletic trainers should have a working knowledge of the effective compounds, the mechanisms, and dosing recommendations of the more widely used and researched supplements that can positively affect performance. Athletic trainers should also be able to recommend the appropriate sports foods and drinks to complement the athlete's training and diet. An athlete's future, reputation, and livelihood can depend on their athletic performance. As such, it is highly important that an athlete or individual not acquire an anti-doping violation as a result of using supplements. Perhaps the most important factor in choosing the correct supplement is whether or not it has undergone third-party testing for harmful or banned substances. The athletic trainer, in conjunction with the multidisciplinary athlete care team, should work to provide recommendations for the most effective and highest quality supplements to ensure the safety and performance of the athlete.

Discussion Questions

1. Out of the supplements covered, which supplement(s) will benefit athletes of all types, ages, and abilities?
2. When guiding an athlete on the use of sports foods or supplements, what factors should the athletic trainer take into consideration?

References

1. Council for Responsible Nutrition. Dietary supplement use reaches all time high—Available-for-purchase consumer survey reaffirms the vital role supplementation plays in the lives of most Americans. https://www.crnusa.org/newsroom/dietary-supplement-use-reaches-all-time-high-available-purchase-consumer-survey-reaffirms

2. Garthe I, Maughan RJ. Athletes and supplements: prevalence and perspectives. *Int J Sport Nutr Exerc Metab.* 2018;28(2):126-138. doi:10.1123/ijsnem.2017-0429

3. American Dietetic Association, Dietitians of Canada, American College of Sports Medicine, Rodriguez NR, Di Marco NM, Langley S. American College of Sports Medicine position stand. Nutrition and athletic performance. *Med Sci Sports Exerc.* 2009;41(3):709-731. doi:10.1249/MSS.0b013e31890eb86

4. Hew-Butler TD, Sharwood K, Collins M, Speedy D, Noakes T. Sodium supplementation is not required to maintain serum sodium concentrations during an Ironman triathlon. *Br J Sports Med.* 2006;40(3):255-259. doi:10.1136/bjsm.2005.022418

5. Jahic D, Begic E. Exercise-associated muscle cramp: doubts about the cause. *Mater Socio-Medica.* 2018;30(1):67-69. doi:10.5455/msm.2018.30.67-69

6. Triplett D, Doyle JA, Rupp JC, Benardot D. An isocaloric glucose-fructose beverage's effect on simulated 100-km cycling performance compared with a glucose-only beverage. *Int J Sport Nutr Exerc Metab.* 2010;20(2):122-131. doi:10.1123/ijsnem.20.2.122

7. Kingsley M, Penas-Ruiz C, Terry C, Russell M. Effects of carbohydrate-hydration strategies on glucose metabolism, sprint performance and hydration during a soccer match simulation in recreational players. *J Sci Med Sport.* 2014;17(2):239-243. doi:10.1016/j.jsams.2013.04.010

8. Russell M, Benton D, Kingsley M. Influence of carbohydrate supplementation on skill performance during a soccer match simulation. *J Sci Med Sport.* 2012;15(4):348-354. doi:10.1016/j.jsams.2011.12.006

9. Devries MC, Phillips SM. Supplemental protein in support of muscle mass and health: advantage whey: whey, body composition, and muscle mass. *J Food Sci.* 2015;80(S1):A8-A15. doi:10.1111/1750-3841.12802

10. Duan Y, Li F, Li Y, et al. The role of leucine and its metabolites in protein and energy metabolism. *Amino Acids.* 2016;48(1):41-51. doi:10.1007/s00726-015-2067-1

11. Babault N, Païzis C, Deley G, et al. Pea proteins oral supplementation promotes muscle thickness gains during resistance training: a double-blind, randomized, placebo-controlled clinical trial vs. Whey protein. *J Int Soc Sports Nutr.* 2015;12(1):3. doi:10.1186/s12970-014-0064-5

12. Grgic J, Trexler ET, Lazinica B, Pedisic Z. Effects of caffeine intake on muscle strength and power: a systematic review and meta-analysis. *J Int Soc Sports Nutr.* 2018;15(1):11. doi:10.1186/s12970-018-0216-0

13. Goldstein ER, Ziegenfuss T, Kalman D, et al. International society of sports nutrition position stand: caffeine and performance. *J Int Soc Sports Nutr.* 2010;7(1):5. doi:10.1186/1550-2783-7-5

14. Ganio MS, Klau JF, Casa DJ, Armstrong LE, Maresh CM. Effect of caffeine on sport-specific endurance performance: a systematic review. *J Strength Cond Res.* 2009;23(1):315-324. doi:10.1519/JSC.0b013e31818b979a

15. Burke LM. Caffeine and sports performance. *Appl Physiol Nutr Metab.* 2008;33(6):1319-1334. doi:10.1139/H08-130

16. Wickham KA, Spriet LL. Administration of caffeine in alternate forms. *Sports Med.* 2018;48(S1):79-91. doi:10.1007/s40279-017-0848-2

17. Fuller M, Rao NZ. The effect of time, roasting temperature, and grind size on caffeine and chlorogenic acid concentrations in cold brew coffee. *Sci Rep.* 2017;7(1):17979. doi:10.1038/s41598-017-18247-4

18. McCusker RR, Goldberger BA, Cone EJ. Caffeine content of specialty coffees. *J Anal Toxicol.* 2003;27(7):520-522. doi:10.1093/jat/27.7.520

19. Womack CJ, Saunders MJ, Bechtel MK, et al. The influence of a CYP1A2 polymorphism on the ergogenic effects of caffeine. *J Int Soc Sports Nutr.* 2012;9(1):7. doi:10.1186/1550-2783-9-7

20. Guest N, Corey P, Vescovi J, El-Sohemy A. Caffeine, CYP1A2 genotype, and endurance performance in athletes. *Med Sci Sports Exerc.* 2018;50(8):1570-1578. doi:10.1249/MSS.0000000000001596

21. Pickering C, Kiely J. Are the current guidelines on caffeine use in sport optimal for everyone? Inter-individual variation in caffeine ergogenicity, and a move towards personalised sports nutrition. *Sports Med Auckl Nz.* 2018;48(1):7-16. doi:10.1007/s40279-017-0776-1

22. Hobson RM, Saunders B, Ball G, Harris RC, Sale C. Effects of β-alanine supplementation on exercise performance: a meta-analysis. *Amino Acids.* 2012;43(1):25-37. doi:10.1007/s00726-011-1200-z

23. Siegler JC, Marshall PWM, Bishop D, Shaw G, Green S. Mechanistic insights into the efficacy of sodium bicarbonate supplementation to improve athletic performance. *Sports Med - Open.* 2016;2(1):41. doi:10.1186/s40798-016-0065-9

24. Lancha Junior AH, de Salles Painelli V, Saunders B, Artioli GG. Nutritional strategies to modulate intracellular and extracellular buffering capacity during high-intensity exercise. *Sports Med.* 2015;45(S1):71-81. doi:10.1007/s40279-015-0397-5

25. Mueller SM, Gehrig SM, Frese S, Wagner CA, Boutellier U, Toigo M. Multiday acute sodium bicarbonate intake improves endurance capacity and reduces acidosis in men. *J Int Soc Sports Nutr.* 2013;10(1):16. doi:10.1186/1550-2783-10-16

26. Carr AJ, Slater GJ, Gore CJ, Dawson B, Burke LM. Effect of sodium bicarbonate on [HCO3−], pH, and gastrointestinal symptoms. *Int J Sport Nutr Exerc Metab.* 2011;21(3):189-194. doi:10.1123/ijsnem.21.3.189

27. Saunders B, Sale C, Harris RC, Sunderland C. Sodium bicarbonate and high-intensity-cycling capacity: variability in responses. *Int J Sports Physiol Perform.* 2014;9(4):627-632. doi:10.1123/ijspp.2013-0295

28. Price M, Moss P, Rance S. Effects of sodium bicarbonate ingestion on prolonged intermittent exercise. *Med Sci Sports Exerc.* 2003;35(8):1303-1308. doi:10.1249/01.MSS.0000079067.46555.3C

29. Artioli GG, Gualano B, Coelho DF, Benatti FB, Gailey AW, Lancha AH. Does sodium-bicarbonate ingestion improve simulated judo performance? *Int J Sport Nutr Exerc Metab.* 2007;17(2):206-217. doi:10.1123/ijsnem.17.2.206

30. Hadzic M, Eckstein ML, Schugardt M. The impact of sodium bicarbonate on performance in response to exercise duration in athletes: a systematic review. *J Sports Sci Med.* 2019;18(2):271-281.

31. Trexler ET, Smith-Ryan AE, Stout JR, et al. International society of sports nutrition position stand: beta-alanine. *J Int Soc Sports Nutr.* 2015;12(1):30. doi:10.1186/s12970-015-0090-y

32. Klebanov GI, Teselkin YuO, Babenkova IV, et al. Effect of carnosine and its components on free-radical reactions. *Membr Cell Biol.* 1998;12(1):89-99.

33. Stegen S, Blancquaert L, Everaert I, et al. Meal and beta-alanine co-ingestion enhances muscle carnosine loading. *Med Sci Sports Exerc.* 2013;45(8):1478-1485. doi:10.1249/MSS.0b013e31828ab073

34. Saunders B, Elliott-Sale K, Artioli GG, et al. β-alanine supplementation to improve exercise capacity and performance: a systematic review and meta-analysis. *Br J Sports Med.* 2017;51(8):658-669. doi:10.1136/bjsports-2016-096396

35. Bagchi D, Nair S, Sen CK. *Nutrition and Enhanced Sports Performance: Muscle Building, Endurance, and Strength.* Academic Press; 2018.

36. Sale C, Saunders B, Hudson S, Wise JA, Harris RC, Sunderland CD. Effect of β-alanine plus sodium bicarbonate on high-intensity cycling capacity. *Med Sci Sports Exerc.* 2011;43(10):1972-1978. doi:10.1249/MSS.0b013e3182188501

37. Hobson RM, Harris RC, Martin D, et al. Effect of beta-alanine, with and without sodium bicarbonate, on 2000-m rowing performance. *Int J Sport Nutr Exerc Metab.* 2013;23(5):480-487. doi:10.1123/ijsnem.23.5.480

38. Butts J, Jacobs B, Silvis M. Creatine use in sports. *Sports Health Multidiscip Approach.* 2018;10(1):31-34. doi:10.1177/1941738117737248

39. Kreider RB, Kalman DS, Antonio J, et al. International Society of Sports Nutrition position stand: safety and efficacy of creatine supplementation in exercise, sport, and medicine. *J Int Soc Sports Nutr.* 2017;14(1):18. doi:10.1186/s12970-017-0173-z

40. Wallimann T, Tokarska-Schlattner M, Schlattner U. The creatine kinase system and pleiotropic effects of creatine. *Amino Acids.* 2011;40(5):1271-1296. doi:10.1007/s00726-011-0877-3

41. Jäger R, Purpura M, Shao A, Inoue T, Kreider RB. Analysis of the efficacy, safety, and regulatory status of novel forms of creatine. *Amino Acids.* 2011;40(5):1369-1383. doi:10.1007/s00726-011-0874-6

42. Steenge GR, Simpson EJ, Greenhaff PL. Protein- and carbohydrate-induced augmentation of whole body creatine retention in humans. *J Appl Physiol Bethesda Md 1985.* 2000;89(3):1165-1171. doi:10.1152/jappl.2000.89.3.1165

43. Buford TW, Kreider RB, Stout JR, et al. International Society of Sports Nutrition position stand: creatine supplementation and exercise. *J Int Soc Sports Nutr.* 2007;4(1):6. doi:10.1186/1550-2783-4-6

44. Cooke MB, Rybalka E, Williams AD, Cribb PJ, Hayes A. Creatine supplementation enhances muscle force recovery after eccentrically-induced muscle damage in healthy individuals. *J Int Soc Sports Nutr.* 2009;6:13. doi:10.1186/1550-2783-6-13

45. Santos RVT, Bassit RA, Caperuto EC, Costa Rosa LFBP. The effect of creatine supplementation upon inflammatory and muscle soreness markers after a 30km race. *Life Sci.* 2004;75(16):1917-1924. doi:10.1016/j.lfs.2003.11.036

46. Kilduff LP, Georgiades E, James N, et al. The effects of creatine supplementation on cardiovascular, metabolic, and thermoregulatory responses during exercise in the heat in endurance-trained humans. *Int J Sport Nutr Exerc Metab.* 2004;14(4):443-460. doi:10.1123/ijsnem.14.4.443

47. Hespel P, Op't Eijnde B, Van Leemputte M, et al. Oral creatine supplementation facilitates the rehabilitation of disuse atrophy and alters the expression of muscle myogenic factors in humans. *J Physiol.* 2001;536(Pt 2):625-633. doi:10.1111/j.1469-7793.2001.0625c.xd

48. Riesberg LA, Weed SA, McDonald TL, Eckerson JM, Drescher KM. Beyond muscles: the untapped potential of creatine. *Int Immunopharmacol.* 2016;37:31-42. doi:10.1016/j.intimp.2015.12.034

49. Sullivan PG, Geiger JD, Mattson MP, Scheff SW. Dietary supplement creatine protects against traumatic brain injury. *Ann Neurol.* 2000;48(5):723-729.

50. Gallardo EJ, Coggan AR. What is in your beet juice? Nitrate and nitrite content of beet juice products marketed to athletes. *Int J Sport Nutr Exerc Metab.* 2019;29(4):345-349. doi:10.1123/ijsnem.2018-0223

51. Williams M. Nitrate supplementation and endurance performance. *Marathon & Beyond.* 2012;16(5):16.

52. Maughan RJ, Burke LM, Dvorak J, et al. IOC consensus statement: dietary supplements and the high-performance athlete. *Int J Sport Nutr Exerc Metab.* 2018;28(2):104-105.

53. Lundberg JO, Larsen FJ, Weitzberg E. Supplementation with nitrate and nitrite salts in exercise: a word of caution. *J Appl Physiol.* 2011;111(2):616-617. doi:10.1152/japplphysiol.00521.2011

54. Thompson C, Vanhatalo A, Jell H, et al. Dietary nitrate supplementation improves sprint and high-intensity intermittent running performance. *Nitric Oxide.* 2016;61:55-61. doi:10.1016/j.niox.2016.10.006

55. Bailey SJ, Varnham RL, DiMenna FJ, Breese BC, Wylie LJ, Jones AM. Inorganic nitrate supplementation improves muscle oxygenation, O2 uptake kinetics, and exercise tolerance at high but not low pedal rates. *J Appl Physiol.* 2015;118(11):1396-1405. doi:10.1152/japplphysiol.01141.2014

56. Wylie LJ, Bailey SJ, Kelly J, Blackwell JR, Vanhatalo A, Jones AM. Influence of beetroot juice supplementation on intermittent exercise performance. *Eur J Appl Physiol.* 2016;116(2):415-425. doi:10.1007/s00421-015-3296-4

57. wada_2020_english_prohibited_list_0.pdf. Accessed March 8, 2020. https://www.wada-ama.org/sites/default/files/wada_2020_english_prohibited_list_0.pdf.

58. 2019-20NCAA_BannedSubstances.pdf. Accessed March 8, 2020. https://ncaaorg.s3.amazonaws.com/ssi/substance/2019-20NCAA_BannedSubstances.pdf

59. Martínez-Sanz JM, Sospedra I, Mañas Ortiz C, Baladía E, Gil-Izquierdo A, Ortiz-Moncada R. Intended or unintended doping? A review of the presence of doping substances in dietary supplements used in sports. *Nutrients.* 2017;9(10). doi:10.3390/nu9101093

60. Eichner AK, Coyles J, Fedoruk M, et al. Essential features of third-party certification programs for dietary supplements: a consensus statement. *Curr Sports Med Rep.* 2019;18(5):5.

61. Certified for Sport. *What our mark means.* Accessed March 9, 2020. https://www.nsfsport.com/our-mark.php

62. Informed Sport. *About Informed Sport.* Accessed March 9, 2020. https://www.informed-sport.com/about

Chapter 7

Nutrition and Weight Management

Layci Harrison, PhD, LAT, ATC

Commission on Accreditation of Athletic Training Education *2020 Standards*

This chapter addresses the following *2020 Standards for Accreditation of Professional Athletic Training Programs*:

- Standard 59: Communicate effectively and appropriately with clients/patients, family members, coaches, administrators, other health care professionals, consumers, payors, policy makers, and others.
- Standard 61: Practice in collaboration with other health care and wellness professionals.
- Standard 83: Educate and make recommendations to clients/patients on fluids and nutrients to ingest prior to activity, during activity, and during recovery for a variety of activities and environmental conditions.
- Standard 84: Educate clients/patients about the effects, participation consequences, and risks of misuse and abuse of alcohol, tobacco, performance-enhancing drugs/substances, and over-the-counter, prescription, and recreational drugs.

Learning Objectives

After reviewing this chapter, readers will be able to:

- Identify the differences in physiology of weight loss between general and active populations.
- Understand how weight restriction and dieting affect sport performance.
- Recognize different cultures of weight-restricted and weight-sensitive sports.

Knoblauch M, ed. *Clinical Nutrition in Athletic Training* (pp 73-87). © 2023 Taylor & Francis Group.

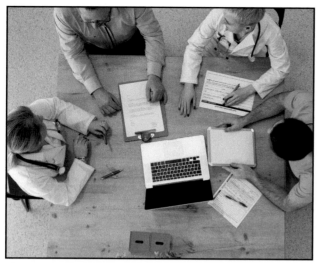

Figure 7-1. Health care team. (Micolas/Shutterstock.com.)

Introduction

Many sports have created a culture in which weight loss is viewed as a requirement for success or enhanced performance. Reasons include mechanical advantages (eg, skiing), placement in certain weight classes (eg, wrestling), or achieving a specific body type (eg, cheerleading). Such weight loss is often rapid because athletes are trying to follow competition schedules and they typically regain weight between competitions without being aware of the associated risk. Furthermore, athletes and coaches may rely on incorrect or outdated information such as online blogs, websites, and social media that put the client at risk of developing unhealthy behaviors. Such rapid weight loss can lead to changes in physiological responses to exercise resulting in increased resting and exercise heart rate and, in turn, decreased performance.

To guide the client safely through a healthy weight loss protocol, the athletic trainer should assemble a multidisciplinary team including coaches, administrators, and other health care providers such as registered dietitians. This team should advocate for the best interest of the client by providing resources for weight loss accompanied by strategies for health and success in sport. The health care team should be well versed on the culture of the sport as it is helpful in building relationships with all team stakeholders. Learning about the sport and the goals of the athlete will allow for open communication, education, and training (Figure 7-1, Sidebar 7-1).

The Process of Weight Loss

Weight loss is a complex process influenced by a wealth of variables. Although equating energy intake to energy expenditure, known as the "energy balance equation," can provide some insight to determining caloric needs for weight

Sidebar 7-1

Although I grew up in a town where wrestling was emphasized more than other sports, as an athletic trainer I was unfamiliar with wrestling weight loss strategies—most of which are very unhealthy. By talking to coaches, athletes, and parents I quickly became aware of the vast weight loss techniques used by wrestlers. Although understanding the common methods of weight loss did not mean I accepted or supported every strategy, it did make me more understanding of why athletes employ these methods. Learning about the culture allowed me to build relationships and have valuable conversations about health, performance, and injury prevention with the team.

While working with wrestling I also provided health care for cross country and cheer and dance athletes. While I thought I knew everything I needed to know about weight loss, I quickly realized weight loss for aesthetics or performance, as is associated with these sports in particular, differed greatly from wrestling. These sports do not have the weight-loss safety restrictions that are utilized in wrestling. I again spent time learning about each sport from the athletes, coaches, and families. This gave me a better understanding of the reasoning inherent to these sports, specific to weight loss, which then helped me safely guide the athletes through the process of weight loss when applicable.

Through these experiences, I learned about weight loss for both weight-restricted and aesthetic sports through on-the-job experience and published research. Although you may not be working with weight-restricted or weight sensitive individuals, you will certainly work with some type of active individual at some point who will want to lose weight for various reasons. Education is the best tool to keep your athletes, patients, and clients safe. Understanding the culture of the sport or activity and building a rapport with coaches and clients will help you promote safe weight loss.

loss, manipulation of the equation does not account for all factors associated with the process. In a very basic explanation, weight gain is caused by energy intake (ie, caloric intake) being higher than energy expenditure, while weight loss results from energy intake being less than energy expenditure. Therefore, with the energy balance equation in mind, weight loss can be achieved in 3 ways: reduction of caloric intake below daily energy expenditure, maintaining normal caloric intake and increasing energy expenditure, or combining both methods,[1] but not everyone responds the same to caloric restriction and increased physical activity due to a variety of variables.[2] These variables include things such as appetite, physical activity level, body composition, and sleep, all of which can skew the equation (caloric intake versus caloric expenditure), making caloric calculations complicated.[3,4] These factors can vary significantly between individuals, thereby making generic weight loss plans ineffective. For example, in weight-bearing exercise there is a relationship between the weight of the person and caloric expenditure during exercise. A heavier person will burn more calories walking than a lighter person,[1] making it difficult to generalize weight loss. Considering the energy balance equation along with potential confounding variables is a great starting point to assist an individual in reaching weight loss goals (Figure 7-2).

It has been pointed out that it is not a change in caloric intake but a decrease in physical activity that is causing weight gain in Americans[1]; therefore, recognizing fluctuations in total daily energy expenditure (TDEE) will provide a better understanding of weight loss for an active population such as athletes. The energy needed for all chemical reactions in the body can be quantified by calculating TDEE. Three factors influence TDEE: the metabolic needs required to maintain life, which includes both resting metabolic rate (RMR) and basal metabolic rate (BMR), thermogenic effect of food, and energy expended during physical activity and recovery. The body requires energy to maintain basic functionals (BMR)[4] and requires slightly more during rest (termed RMR) to maintain normal body functions. This RMR energy requirement (which encompasses BMR), can account for up to 75% of TDEE.[1] The body uses energy to digest and absorb food, as well as to stimulate metabolism using the sympathetic nervous system. These factors together are the thermogenic effect of food. Lastly, physical activity and recovery can account for 15% to 30% of TDEE.[1] Each of these factors vary considerably by individual and with participation in sport. For example, the energy needs for sedentary adults may only be 1.5 times the minimal energy needed for basic functions, known as BMR, while the energy needs of an active adult can be more than twice the individual's BMR.[5]

Caloric intake is determined by the drive to eat, and the drive to eat is influenced by hunger and appetite. Appetite is influenced by internal or nonenvironmental cues, such as body composition.[6] The role of body composition on appetite makes the energy balance equation even more complicated for the active population, as these individuals may be manipulating body composition for performance reasons. It was previously understood that caloric intake is affected by fat mass, but new information shows it may actually be controlled by fat-free, or lean, mass.[6] As lean mass increases so does total daily energy intake,[6] but it appears that individuals with high levels of lean mass (fat-free mass) are able to balance intake with differences in satiety after meals as compared to those with higher percentages of fat mass. Individuals with a higher lean mass experience increased appetite leading up to a meal due to the additional needs of the

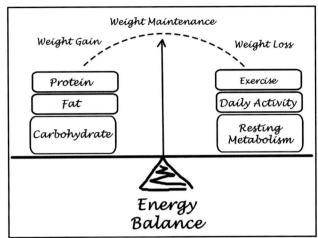

Figure 7-2. Energy balance. (arka36/Shutterstock.com.)

lean mass,[6] but interestingly those individuals feel satisfied after the meal as compared to those with a higher percentage fat mass who may still feel hungry after a meal.[6] The initial increase in appetite in those with large amounts of lean mass may be explained by the energy needed to maintain fat-free mass and further explain why those with decreased fat-free mass, or muscle mass, such as older adults, have decreased appetite.[6]

Due to the excessive energy output of athletes as compared to the general population, the balance between caloric intake and caloric expenditure (the energy equation) is constantly shifting throughout training. For example, increased activity can increase appetite[7] due to carbohydrate utilization, causing a decrease in leptin. Leptin, a hormone that inhibits the need to eat, will decrease with carbohydrate utilization causing an increase in appetite. As the athlete increases caloric output with physical activity, the body is receiving signals from decreased leptin levels to increase caloric intake and as a result can equalize energy intake and energy expenditure in the energy balance equation. Conversely, an effect of long-term exercise training is reduction in reliance upon carbohydrates. Physical activity with reduced utilization of carbohydrates then reduces the effect of leptin fluctuations that generally accompany increased energy expenditure.[3]

The appetite variations between the general population and highly active individuals continues beyond basic caloric intake. Highly active individuals can balance their energy intake throughout multiple meals. For example, if an active individual consumes a high-calorie meal for breakfast, it is likely that they will experience satiety after a low-calorie lunch or dinner. On the other hand, individuals who participate in lower levels of activity do not experience this same moderation. For example, if an individual who records low levels of physical activity consumes a high-calorie breakfast, they may not experience satiety after a low-calorie lunch and may continue to increase caloric intake over caloric expenditure throughout the day.[8] This suggests highly active individuals can adapt and balance the energy equation by not craving or eating additional food later in the day, while individuals who participate in lower levels of activity will push the equation toward a positive energy balance[8] that can result in weight gain.

Although physical activity is usually thought of as a typical method of caloric expenditure, calories expended without activity should also be considered. Due to energy needs during rest, sleep can affect TDEE. Individuals who are not getting an adequate amount of sleep may consume more calories during the day to account for the additional energy needed to maintain wakefulness, but more calories are consumed than needed—leading to weight gain. Those who only get 5 hours of sleep per night over a 5-day span tend to increase their caloric intake with after dinner snacks. Interestingly, returning from a poor sleep schedule to an adequate schedule, approximately 9 hours of sleep per night, can result in weight loss due to a decrease in caloric intake.[9]

Although things such as diet, physical activity, and sleep can be manipulated, the body will try to maintain weight at the body's set point. During caloric restriction, there is frequently a decrease in RMR and nonresting energy expenditure, leading to a decrease in TDEE and a plateau in weight loss as compared to those who are not restricting calories for weight loss.[10,11] These adaptations occur by changes in metabolic, neuroendocrine, and autonomic systems.[12] For example, hormonal changes associated with weight loss attempt to defend the body from losing too much weight. Activity of the parasympathetic nervous system may increase as a result of hormonal changes, which in turn reduces RMR.[12] Changes to neuroendocrine and energy systems result in decreases in TDEE,[12] leading to a decrease in caloric expenditure and an unbalancing of the energy equation (caloric intake versus caloric expenditure). Discrepancies in weight loss can be amplified when there are additional fluctuations in energy expenditure, as is often experienced by athletes transitioning to the end of their playing season or sport retirement.

Weight Loss and the Active Population

Clinicians working with an active or athletic population should consider the differences in energy balance compared to those who are overweight or obese when proving guidance for weight loss. Weight loss as low as 3% has been associated with positive changes in chronic disease risk factors.[13] In the general population, this amount can be accomplished by 200 to 300 minutes per week of moderate intensity physical activity.[14] Although the benefits of decreasing risk factors should not be ignored, reducing disease risk is not usually the goal of the athlete. Weight loss in athletics should be managed differently due to possible negative consequences of weight loss on performance. According to the American College of Sports Medicine, there are specific considerations for weight loss in the athletic population, including specialized members of the health care team, macronutrient manipulations, and social influences. First, a qualified sports dietitian should be part of the health care team to assist the client in proper diet manipulation. A sports dietitian will provide expertise to ensure that carbohydrate and protein needs are met throughout the weight loss plan to a degree that still allows for adequate fueling required for the high demands of sport-related physical activity.

Any diet manipulation should be planned with a dietitian, but the athletic trainer, who usually sees patients and clients daily, can assist in daily monitoring of weight loss. For example, the athlete may experience slight decreases in body weight post-training that occurs as a result of dehydration. Dehydration can negatively affect performance when occurring at a higher level; therefore the client should work closely with the athletic trainer to remain hydrated before, during, and after activity,[15] and avoid using dehydration as a mechanism for weight loss. Proper guidance and education in weight loss from the athletic trainer will assist the client in meeting their specific weight loss goals.

While increasing one's physical activity can contribute to weight loss, combining physical activity with caloric restriction can accelerate the process of weight loss.[13] In an athletic population, specifically aesthetic activities or those with speed as a performance goal, the client (although already recording high levels of physical activity) may try to further increase physical activity in combination with decreased caloric intake. Consequently, weight loss is different for highly active individuals because the caloric intake of the client must be high enough to fuel high levels of activity as compared to the nonathlete.[16] The higher caloric intake common to athletes also assists in additional growth and repair of muscle tissue that is associated with athletic activity.[16,17] While trying to reach this delicate balance of weight loss and proper fueling, fat mass should be the target of weight loss while lean mass is preserved, as the preservation of lean mass is important to achieving performance goals. To preserve lean mass, the athlete should not exceed a loss of 1.5% of total body weight or 1 to 2 pounds each week.[18] Although many may want to jump into weight loss by using caloric restriction, a caloric reduction of 1000 kcals is poorly tolerated and decreases energy expenditure,[1] resulting in a leveling of the energy balance equation and limiting weight loss (especially in those with above average caloric expenditure).

Differences in physical activity levels should be considered when manipulating macronutrient intake. While increasing protein intake to 0.8 g protein/kg per day for the general population may assist with weight loss due to increased satiety and thermogenic effect,[19] a highly active individual may benefit from 1 to 3 g protein/kg per day to assist with maintaining performance levels by sparing the loss of lean mass.[20,21] This should include high-quality proteins spread out in 4 meals throughout the day.[22] While limiting carbohydrates should be avoided because carbohydrates are essential to performance,[20] an increase in protein should be coupled with a decrease in lipids to maintain an energy balance directed at weight loss.[20] Furthermore, although frequently debated, there is no evidence to suggest an increase in protein will negatively affect kidney function in those with normal renal function.[20] Coupled with the increase in protein, resistance training has been shown to increase muscle mass and RMR, which will decrease body fat. While the combination of resistance training and increased protein intake can assist with weight loss in the general population, it is an especially beneficial strategy for the active individual who has concurrent goals of weight loss and increased strength.

The clinician should keep in mind that weight loss may not be the client's only goal. Many individuals will want to lose weight while simultaneously achieving performance goals. For example, it is common to have the client or athlete working to decrease body weight, while also trying to increase strength, speed, or power. Unfortunately, training goals can be negatively affected if the client is improperly losing weight while working toward increased strength leading up to competition. This happens in weight-restricted sports such as wrestling or in sports in which body mass restricts performance due to mechanical reasons (eg, wind resistance, gravity) such as running, skiing, cycling, or jumping—leading to decreases in strength and performance. Strength deficits can stem from caloric restriction leading to decreases in insulin like growth factor, insulin, and testosterone—which can lead to decreases in lean body mass[23] and decreased strength and performance. To avoid these negative effects, both the clinician and the client need to ensure proper fueling for performance goals.

Environmental influences of weight loss cannot go unmentioned. In athletics, participants report things such as sport uniforms, time of day, and influences from coaches and teammates can affect caloric intake of the athlete.[24,25] While competition uniforms and times of competitions may not be changed, educating teams about their influence on others' caloric choices may reduce the risk of unhealthy behaviors. Teammates and coaches can have a large effect on an athlete's diet and exercise. For example, an athlete may perceive pressure from a teammate to lose weight, or suspect a teammate is displaying disordered eating patterns—in turn leading to their own body dissatisfaction. The use of unsafe weight loss techniques can spread through a team if the team members believe this behavior is expected or normal.[26] This is especially true if the pressure to lose weight is coming from the coaching staff in the form of playing time restrictions. Weight loss requests from a coach can lead to depression, fatigue, nervousness, and appetite changes.[26] In the case that weight loss requests are coming from within the team, teammates or coaches may be monitoring body weight, when in fact these changes should be assessed by a health care provider. Interestingly, supportive teammate relationships have been shown to contribute significantly to satisfaction of body image and safe exercise and diet behavior.[27]

Assessing Body Composition

Although it is common for individuals to monitor weight loss progress based on a number on the scale, body weight does not account for body composition. Body composition refers to the percentages of fat-free mass (ie, lean body mass) and fat mass. All weight loss goals should consider body composition to avoid unsafe weight loss and preserve lean body mass. During the weight loss process, the athletic trainer, with proper training, should conduct weight and body composition assessments to monitor progress and, when necessary, reevaluate goals and modify the weight loss plan.

The National Athletic Trainers' Association (NATA) provides multiple recommendations for guiding and monitoring athlete weight loss in both weight-restricted and weight-sensitive sports. During weight loss for weight-restricted sports, weight and body composition should be monitored to avoid large weight fluctuations. In sports that require equipment, or those sports requiring training in hot and humid environments, pre- and postpractice weigh-ins are advised. However, for those individual participating in weight-restricted sports or losing weight for aesthetics, weigh-ins should not take place more than once per week.[19] Ideally these weight assessments should only happen every 2 to 3 months, but that is not practical for weight-restricted sports that constantly monitor weight for roster placement. Those participating in weight-restricted sports may have individual weight loss plans outlined by the particular sport's governing body. Although body weight is the deciding factor for competition and will be recorded at weigh-ins prior to events when applicable, sport-specific weight loss guidelines for assigning weight classes were designed to consider body composition and body weight.

When conducting any body mass or body composition assessments, the assessor should be well educated and properly trained on the method of choice. Regardless of the chosen assessment, the athlete should be hydrated. In some cases, such as weight class certifications for wrestling, hydration must be evaluated and confirmed with a refractometer. These assessments are sensitive. Privacy and discretion during the assessments should be considered. As with all medical information, this client information is confidential and should be properly stored. Furthermore, be aware that some weight-restricted sports, such as wrestling, have guidelines for the method of assessing body composition. In the case of National Collegiate Athletic Association (NCAA) wrestling, all coaches and body weight assessors must watch the Wrestling Weight Management presentation from Trackwrestling. Information on competition weight certification is then entered and calculated through an account with the National Wrestling Coaches Association and the Trackwrestling Optimal Performance Calculator.

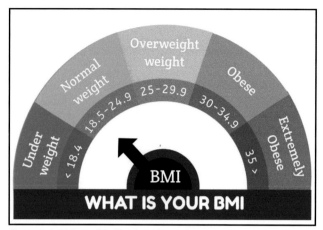

Figure 7-3. BMI graphic. (Pradip Valavai/Shutterstock.com.)

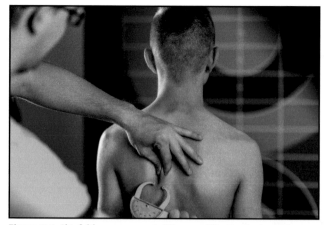

Figure 7-4. Skinfold measurement. (Microgen/Shutterstock.com.)

Sidebar 7-2

Skinfold Equations. Seven-Site Skinfold Formula[19,28]

Men: Body density = 1.112 − 0.00043499 (sum of 7 skinfolds) + 0.00000055 (sum of 7 skinfolds)^2 − 0.00028826 (age)

Women: Body density = 1.097 − 0.00046971 (sum of 7 skinfolds) + 0.00000056 (sum of 7 skinfolds)^2 − 0.00012828 (age)

There are multiple techniques to assess body composition. Although validity should always be considered, the clinician's assessment choice may be based on access to equipment, cost, and time required of the clinician and athlete. When assessing large numbers of people, many clinicians rely on BMI, due to ease of use and low time commitment. This calculation is easily done by dividing an individual's body weight (in kilograms) by height (in meters^2). The athlete can then be categorized based on that number[28] such that a score <18.5 m/kg^2 lists them as underweight, 18.5 to 24.9 m/kg^2 is within normal body weight, 25 to 29.9 kg/m^2 representing overweight. These are followed by 30 to 34.9 kg/m^2, 35 to 39.9 kg/m^2, and ≥40 kg/m^2 representing class 1, 2, and 3 obesity, respectively. BMI, however, does not take into account an individual's body composition (ie, fat-free mass) and has a large standard error when used to estimate percent body fat[28] (Figure 7-3).

When considering low cost, validity, and a small-time commitment, then skinfold measurements are frequently the assessment of choice among athletic trainers. The use of skinfold measurements has been established valid when compared to the reference standard, hydrodensitometry, is cost effective and fairly quick compared to other methods. However, accuracy of the assessment is dependent upon the training of the clinician on skinfold measurement techniques.[28] This training includes an understanding of basic anatomical landmarks and methodology specific to skinfold measurement. A typical skinfold assessment includes the measurement of 7 skinfold locations. These locations include chest, midaxillary, triceps, subscapular, abdomen, suprailiac, and thigh. Skinfold measurements provide a valid assessment of body composition through the assumption that subcutaneous body fat is proportional to total body fat (Figure 7-4).[28] Refer to Sidebar 7-2 for body density calculations using the 7-site skinfold method.

Ideally all athletes will request weight loss guidance from someone on the health care team or refer to their sport's governing body. Unfortunately, many athletes may rely on coaches or teammates. Some athletes and coaches may be getting guidance on weight loss from social media or other unreliable sources. Because some athletes and coaches may not have a background in weight loss and nutritional guidelines, they may believe the number on the scale equates to weight loss success. Therefore, coaches and athletes may benefit from informal educational sessions with the athletic trainer and other members of the health care team.

Educational sessions on weight loss and guidance of weight loss should promote the idea that regardless of weight loss reasons, goals should be built based on body composition and not body weight.[19] Coaches and athletes should also be directed toward the sport's governing body and the NCAA, both of which provide educational resources. For example, the NCAA Sport Science Institute website is a free resource that provides education on weight loss health and safety as it relates to sport.

Weight Loss Guidelines

Multiple organizations have set guidelines for safe weight loss specific to weight-restricted sports, but there is a lack of guidelines for clients attempting to lose weight for performance or for meeting competition expectations such as runners, cyclists, gymnasts, or dancers (Sidebar 7-3). In general, the nutritional needs of the athlete should always be a priority over athletic performance.[18] This is especially important with adolescent athletes and differs between men and women. Male clients should never drop below 7% body fat, and female clients should stay at a body fat percentage that maintains energy requirements for normal menstruation, which may differ by individual.[18] To assist clinicians in guiding safe weight loss practices, many organizations have set guidelines or regulations for weight loss.

Unfortunately, organizations usually set guidelines and rules for weight loss as the result of catastrophic incidents. Due to deaths that occurred in the sport of wrestling in the 1990s, the NCAA established the Wrestling Weight Certification Program (WWCP). Prior to implementation, many wrestlers were starting the season 10 to 20 pounds over their desired weight class and then would purposely lose a substantial amount of weight during the first week of practice to prepare for weight certifications. The implementation of the WWCP required wrestlers to be hydrated, as measured by a refractometer, during the body composition assessment. The WWCP also set regulations for body composition assessments, citing skinfold measurements, underwater weighing, or a BOD POC analysis as the only accepted methods. Following a hydrated assessment, the optimal performance calculator is used to calculate percentage of body fat, fat weight, fat-free weight, and lowest allowable weight. From there, weight class is determined by allowing 1.5% of body weight loss per week from initial assessment to weight certification date. After a full year of the WWCP regulations, weight loss during the first week of the season was decreased, with many wrestlers losing most of their weight during the second half of the season.[29] This was the first successful attempt to break the cycle of historically unhealthy weight culture in wrestling.

To complement these wrestling specific guidelines, multiple organizations have published recommendations outside of sport-specific rules that encourage safe weight loss in all sports.[30] In terms of safety, the American College of Sports Medicine suggests restrictions on the use of sauna suits, laxatives, and diuretics for weight loss in wrestling.[31] The organization also suggests performing daily weigh-ins to monitor and avoid rapid weight loss and replenishing excessive weight loss that occurs during wrestling practice with both food and fluid.[31]

In addition to weight loss guidelines provided by the American College of Sports Medicine, the NATA has guidelines for nutrition during weight loss. Clients should follow guidelines such as those set forth by the NATA suggesting 5 to 7 g/kg/day of carbohydrates and 0.8 to 1 g/kg/day of

Sidebar 7-3

Weight-restricted sports have not always had weight loss guidelines. In the 1990s, 3 wrestlers died within 33 days due to excessive "weight cutting." Their techniques included laxatives, sauna suits, vomiting, and fasting. Reactively, the NCAA wrestling committee modified rules to encourage safe and healthy weight loss. Within a few years the rules extended to the high school level. New regulations included a ban of sauna suits, laxatives, and diuretics. The NCAA also initiated a rule to eliminate exercising in rooms above 75 °F and the use of illegal substances, such as laxatives, that accelerate weight loss. This led to additional preventive measures, including requiring wrestlers having a body fat and hydration assessment to determine their weight class at the beginning of the season. In addition, there are restrictions on the amount and pace at which wrestlers can reduce their weight. Pace of weight loss is monitored by athletic trainers and coaches and regulated by the NWCA throughout the season and at competition weigh-ins. A few athletes have passed away since the release of these rules that were believed to be due to dehydration while trying to lose excessive amounts of weight. As a health care provider, you are obligated to report any illegal or unsafe weight loss practices. More information can be found at Trackwrestling (www.trackwrestling.com), NWCA (http://www.nwcaonline.com/), and NCAA Sport Science Institute (http://www.ncaa.org/sport-science-institute).

protein.[19] This is important as many athletes believe they should limit carbohydrates, which will in fact will negatively affect performance.[32] Furthermore, athletes should be discouraged from deciding on weight loss methods influenced by teammates and seek advice from the health care team on building an individualized weight loss plan (Sidebar 7-4).[33]

Weight Maintenance

To avoid unhealthy weight cycling (ie, weight fluctuations including repeated weight gain and weight loss) often experienced in athletics or seasonal activities, proper nutrition and physical activity should continue to be maintained during the off-season. Since physical activity levels typically decrease during the off-season, and as a result access to the health care team may also be limited, clients should be educated and responsible for their nutrition and weight management. To provide guidance and autonomy in times with limited access to the health care team, the athletic trainer in

Sidebar 7-4

Education is the most important factor for safe weight loss. As mentioned, many athletes rely on coaches for information and many coaches have incorrect or outdated information that has been passed through the culture of the sport. It is not your job as the athletic trainer to set "rules" for athlete weight loss with no explanation. Weight loss, especially in weight-restricted sports, is part of the coach's responsibility. In wrestling, body weight (as far as weight class assignment) is a coaching decision based on regulations from WWCP. Therefore, you should share your knowledge and the knowledge of the health care team with the coach. The athletic trainer is not a registered dietitian and should never try to take the place of other health care professionals. Build a qualified team including the team physician, dietitians, sports psychologists, and strength and conditioning coaches, but remember the client is part of that team. It is impossible for you or the coaching staff to constantly monitor the client. We are constantly flooded with information from social media and other sources. Teach the client what to look for among the flood of information. Teach them how nutrition and weight loss affect performance. Show the clients that they are in control of their health and performance. In my experience, the team approach is the best approach.

collaboration with a dietitian can calculate proper caloric intake by using formulas that include BMR, body composition, age, sex, and energy expenditure. These calculations provide clients with information to monitor their own caloric intake. Unfortunately, these equations are not always accurate and patient adherence may be an issue if the calculation is complicated. There are more direct and accurate methods such as measuring metabolic function and oxygen utilization that would also provide the client with some guiding data, but these methods are time consuming and require equipment that is not always available to the athletic trainer.[19] Therefore, when there is limited access to measures of metabolic function and the health care team would like to provide the client with a plan for times of limited athletic trainer-client interaction, a viable option is the use of the US Department of Agriculture ChooseMyPlate website (www.choosemyplate. gov). Although Board-certified sports dietitians (CSSD) are the best professionals to guide the athlete through a nutritional plan,[19] ChooseMyPlate is a great starting point. This resource allows some autonomy for the individual to build a nutritional plan guided by validated information. Specific to the athlete, ChooseMyPlate can be a helpful tool in times of limited athletic trainer–client interaction, such as the off-season or after sport retirement.

Physical activity is a component of weight maintenance that seems easy to accomplish for the active individual, but activity may need to be prescribed for nonathletes. During the off-season or time of decreased physical activity, the client may experience unwanted weight gain if there is not a coinciding decrease in caloric intake. A supplemental exercise program is a way to mediate unwanted weight gain during times of decreased activity or sport-specific training. This program should be based on the client's weight loss goals. The prescribed activity should include aerobic training, as aerobic activity is suggested to facilitate weight loss,[19] totaling at least 150 minutes per week.[28] The program should be specific to the individual and separate from sport training, ideally in the off-season so as to not interfere with performance goals.

Weight Loss and Performance

Depending on the physiological demands of each sport, weight loss creates different performance challenges. Not all weight loss has negative effects, but any time weight loss exceeds 1% to 2% body weight per week, there is an increased chance for health and performance deficits.[34] Rapid weight loss tends to happen when there are deadlines for weight loss. Weight loss deadlines can include achieving a particular weight class for activities, such as wrestling or obtaining a desired appearance by the competition date, for activities such as cheerleading where participants may feel pressured to have a particular body type. Athletes choose to reduce body weight for multiple reasons. Understanding the nutritional needs of athletes who manipulate body weight for sport performance or aesthetics can assist in building strength and conditioning programs, as well as contribute to injury prevention by creating a wholistic plan that includes both diet and exercise to reach performance goals.[35]

Endurance and Aesthetic Activities

The effects of weight loss for endurance sports and activities are different than the effects of weight loss for power activities, as physiological responses that may not affect the anaerobic system can compromise the aerobic system. Weight loss of 5% body weight achieved by dehydration can hinder aerobic performance to a greater extent than anaerobic activities.[36] Performance deficits are commonly the result of dehydration, which results in a decrease in oxygen transport and muscle glycogen utilization.[36] The changes in oxygen and muscle glycogen lead to challenges in thermoregulation, making it difficult to regulate body temperature and therefore decreasing performance as the body is working hard to lower its temperature.[36]

Power Sports and Activities

Power athletes, those who compete in a mostly anaerobic metabolic state, such as jumpers, sprinters, and power lifters, have different considerations for weight loss than those who perform in a mostly aerobic state. Weight reductions, although believed to be for performance benefits, can negatively affect strength and power. For example, those who practice a slow reduction in body weight, under 0.75% of body weight per week, can concurrently decrease body weight and gain lean body mass and strength.[37] Conversely, those who engage in rapid weight loss while training, such as combative athletes, may limit increases of lean body mass and therefore not achieve strength training goals.[37] To assist with training goals, the addition of high-intensity resistance training 1 hour a day 4 days a week has been shown to preserve lean body mass and RMR during caloric restriction.[38]

Effects of Rapid Weight Loss on Performance

It is not uncommon for clients in sports with weight classes to lose up to 5% body weight within a few days to reach a competition goal. This amount of weight loss, frequently referred to as "rapid weight loss,"[39-41] is part of the culture for many sports. It is achieved with increased exercise and caloric restriction—including the elimination of one or more meals per day[39,40]—dehydration through fluid restriction and sweating,[42,43] and sometimes more dangerous methods such as laxatives and diuretics.[44] Mostly commonly, athletes in weight-restricted sports use a combination of increased exercise and decreased caloric and fluid intake to lose weight rapidly. In weight-restricted sports, weight loss methods typically do not differ by weight class[39] meaning the entire team could be practicing unsafe weight loss practices. The risks and negative effects of unsafe, rapid weight loss usually outweigh any positive performance benefits.

Rapid weight loss, including caloric restriction and dehydration, provides a complex challenge for the body's energy systems. Aerobic performance is affected by as little as 2% body weight loss due to dehydration[34] and decreased glycogen storage, both of which are typically experienced during rapid weight loss. The most common method of rapid weight loss, dehydration,[45] may not affect anaerobic activities (quick powerful movements). For example, peak power may not be affected by rapid weight loss, allowing the athlete the ability to successfully complete powerful and explosive movements.[40] But, as the duration of the competition increases, so does the reliance on the aerobic energy system. For example, average lower body power and fatigue index of both the lower and upper body are affected by rapid weight loss,[40] leading to premature competition fatigue due to dehydration.

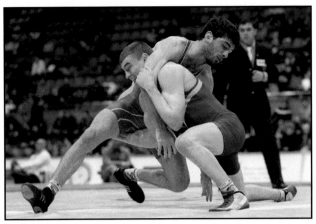

Figure 7-5. Single-leg take down. (StockphotoVideo/Shutterstock.com.)

Due to increased muscle marker damage and decreased glucose availability as a result of rapid weight loss and excessive exercise, decreases in sport-specific strength has been reported.[46] For example, the single-leg take down, a common offensive scoring move for wrestling and other combative sports, is negatively affected by rapid weight loss due to changing the linear maximum velocity, position, and angular maximum velocity of the shoulders, pelvis, and knee.[47] Although the single-leg take down is considered an anaerobic movement, biomechanical changes due to rapid weight loss can lead to performance deficits (Figure 7-5).

Other body systems may be affected by rapid weight loss accompanied by dehydration. Although reaction time is not reduced, which is good for the safety of the athlete,[42] muscle cramping, dizziness, irritability, motor skill performance such as balance, and increased heart rate have been reported by athletes participating in rapid weight loss.[39,48] These physiological changes include increases in both resting and recovery heart rate,[40,43] which can lead to decreased training and competition intensity resulting in long-term performance deficits.

While the long-term relationship between rapid weight loss and anaerobic performance is not clear, some evidence suggests muscular endurance and strength will decrease throughout the season as a result of continued rapid weight loss and weight cycling.[36] For example, force exerted from small muscles, such as those that assist with hand grip, may not be affected by rapid weight loss initially, but a pattern of rapid weight loss throughout a season can result in a regression of strength throughout a competitive season.[36] Similar progressive strength deficits in response to repetitive rapid weight loss have been recorded in elbow flexors and extensors and quadriceps throughout the course of a season.[49,50] This information is important for combative athletes due to the need to reduce weight for competition, as they may not notice a slow decrease in small muscle group strength as it happens not immediately following rapid weight loss but throughout the season. This becomes increasingly important during post-season championships following a season of rapid weight loss and weight cycling, as the longer the season continues the further the strength deficit.

Consequences of Weight Cycling

Frequent rapid weight loss followed by regaining of the lost weight is termed "weight cycling." Weight cycling is common in athletes who participate in weight-restricted sports. Constant fluctuations in weight usually occur when rapid weight loss is used as the primary method to meet competition guidelines. For example, an athlete may rapidly reduce weight to meet weight class requirements or appearance expectations; then, following weigh-in or competition, rapidly increase or regain lost weight, leading to the need for rapid weight loss prior to the next competition. This is especially common in combative sports such as mixed martial arts or wrestling, which have official weigh-ins an hour or more prior to competition. This extended time frame between weigh-ins and competition allows the athlete to regain much of the weight lost during the "weight cutting" phase of competition preparation. The extended time frame between the weigh-ins and competition has implications on health and future weight loss.

Weight cycling that includes rapid weight loss, or losing 4% of body weight in 48 hours, results in many negative consequences to the body. The athlete may experience hormonal changes, such as decreases in testosterone, electrolyte loss, diminished immune system response,[51] or, in the youth athlete, stunting of growth.[36] A long-term effect of weight cycling is a decrease in BMR,[36] which results in a decreased caloric expenditure and requires an increase in caloric restriction to maintain future weight loss. In addition, rapid weight gain after an extreme weight loss will cause the body to store more energy as it is expecting to be in a caloric deficit soon.[36] A decrease in BMR, coupled with an increased tendency for energy storage, will increase the difficulty of future weight loss. Those individuals that participate in weight-restricted sports should consider the long-term effect of weight cycling on health, but sometimes these unhealthy practices are the result of factors outside weight class regulations—such as sport culture and coach and teammate influences.

Steps to Avoid Performance Deficits

There are a few steps the client can take leading up competition to mitigate the negative effects of weight loss on performance. One of the first steps involves training load. In the days leading up to competition, the training volume should decrease as training intensity increases.[52] In addition,

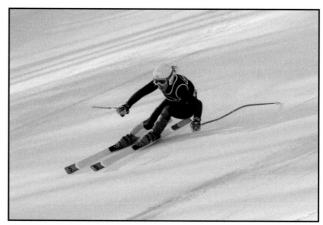

Figure 7-6. Downhill skiing. (PHOTOMDP/Shutterstock.com.)

after weight loss and prior to competition, the client should hydrate and replenish carbohydrates,[52] although this may be difficult for aesthetic activities. This is because unlike combative sports, these individuals may not have time to replenish between weight loss and competition. Although not typically the case for aesthetic activities, recovery time between weight loss and competition could limit performance deficits.[52] Unfortunately, even when allowing recovery time and when weight gain is recorded, the client may still be dehydrated prior to competition.[53] Lastly, clinicians should be aware that while some clients may wish to reduce body weight for performance reasons, such as speed when racing, and others, such as dancers and gymnasts, choose to reduce weight for aesthetic reasons, both reasons create dieting behaviors that frequently lead to disordered eating (Figure 7-6).[54]

Understanding Weight-Restricted Sports

Weight-restricted sport athletes participate in weight cutting (decreasing body weight for competition requirements) to reach their assigned competition weight. Unfortunately, weight-restricted athletes tend to gravitate toward unsafe weight loss practices such as dehydration, dietary restrictions, and disordered eating patterns. Understanding the culture of weight-restricted sports, including sport-specific weight loss practices, will help the athletic trainer identify and educate the athlete on how to avoid unsafe practices.

Combative athletes strive to be at the lowest weight class possible in an attempt to overpower a hopefully smaller competitor. Some combative sports such as boxing and taekwondo require competitors to control their own body as a defensive technique, and in turn use their own body mass to be successful—in which case weight loss may benefit performance. Other combative sports, such as wrestling, rely on the athlete's ability to manipulate and control the opponent's body mass[55]—in which case the competitor will want to gain weight quickly after weigh-ins to overpower the opponent. For example, the wrestler will want to be at the lowest possible weight class at weigh-in, but gain weight back prior to competition in order to compete against a smaller and hopefully weaker opponent. This leads to weight cycling. The different rationales for weight loss result in variations in weight loss goals by sport. Weight cutting can easily have a negative affect if physiological function is impaired due to poor nutrition or dehydration.[1] Sports with weight loss guidelines are attempting to safeguard the athlete, but complications still exist.

Although sports that require participants to compete within a weight class have guidelines for minimal body weight and weight loss, most combative athletes report that their main source of nutritional guidance is their coach.[39] Some athletes even report getting much of their weight loss and nutritional information from social media.[56] Furthermore, competitive athletes often make weight loss decisions without the guidance of a registered dietitian.[56] The abundance of invalid information is why unsafe weight loss behaviors continue to be a part of sport. Not only should the athletic trainer understand the effects of rapid weight loss and weight cycling on athletic performance but with the assistance of a dietitian, athletic trainers should educate coaches and athletes on safe strategies for weight loss. More importantly, they should make it clear where to find valid information to avoid unsafe behaviors.

Choosing a Weight Loss Strategy for Weight-Restricted Sports

The possible effects on performance should be considered when selecting a weight loss method for weight-restricted sport clients. Common weight loss methods for weight-restricted sports include gut content manipulation (manipulation of nutrient intake), dehydration, or a combination of these tactics accompanied by increased physical activity. Gut content manipulation can be done with food restriction, decreased dietary fiber, or laxatives.[55] This type of weight loss can result in a 1% to 2% decrease in body weight within 1 day, but does decrease satiety and cardiovascular exercise intensity,[55] meaning the individual will feel hungry and have a decreased training capacity. Although gut content manipulation is a common weight loss method, it may not be the best option for those competing or trying to reach performance goals as it makes it difficult for the client to continue training intensity and may decrease competition performance.

The client may choose passive or active dehydration to see quick decreases in weight. The use of activity to increase body temperature and induce sweating is considered active dehydration. For example, exercise can increase sweat rate, resulting in active dehydration. Alternately, sauna suits and sauna-like environments may be used to induce passive dehydration, by inducing sweating caused by increased body temperature that is not a result of exercise or activity.

Active sweating from high-intensity exercise may cause delayed muscle soreness and gastrointestinal distress but maintains plasma volume better than passive sweating. In contrast some athletes prefer passive sweating, such as occurs through the use of saunas, due to the possibility of inducing a state of relaxation before competition while being less taxing on the muscles as compared to active sweating, such as occurs through exercise.[55] Although dehydration is a common method for weight loss, restoring fluid balance after an active or passive sweating session can be difficult if a particular weight class must be achieved on the same day as competition. Furthermore, dehydration increases thirst and decreases tolerance to heat and aerobic exercise, thereby making dehydration a questionable method for effective weight loss.

Some consider glycogen depletion a more tolerable method. Glycogen depletion is accomplished by increasing exercise and decreasing carbohydrate intake to manipulate body water. If this is the selected method for weight loss, it is important to note that prior to competition a carbohydrate recovery plan should be created.[55] Glycogen depletion can decrease aerobic performance, but having a carbohydrate recovery plan allows the client to maintain strength for short bouts, making glycogen depletion a preferred method for rapid weight loss. A similar method, utilizing a low-fiber diet with a mild fluid deficit, is an effective acute weight loss strategy to maintain performance because it decreases fluids usually attached to fiber.[57] Both glycogen depletion and decreased fiber consumption assist in decreasing body weight by decreasing water content.[58]

The client, with the assistance of the health care team, should create a refueling plan. The refueling plan should be practiced during mock weigh-ins. A client can conduct a mock weigh-in by going through the weight loss process and diet plan as they would prior to competition. The mock weigh-in can provide valuable information about gastric emptying (how long it takes food to pass through the body) and how refueling will affect the body (eg, gastrointestinal distress). For example, think of a precompetition meal as something the client would eat before a hard practice or training session. The client should then note how this meal affected training and if it caused gastrointestinal distress. If applicable, the client should try to consume a meal 3 hours prior to competition consisting of 1 g/kg carbohydrate. After the competition, the health care team should continue to communicate with the client about what worked and make a plan for the next competition.[55]

Recovery for Weight-Restricted Sports

The negative effects on performance experienced during weight loss, such as cardiovascular strain, gastrointestinal discomfort, and fatigue, may be avoided given an adequate recovery period prior to competition. Although peak power is negatively affected during rapid weight loss, it typically returns to normal after a 12-hour recovery.[40] In the instance of a weight-restricted sports, relative peak power has reportedly increased after 12 hours of recovery, strengthening the theory that competing at a lower weight class is an advantage if the tournament or competition allows proper recovery time, such as in the case of a multiday tournament.[40] The need for recovery is increased after rapid weight loss. For example, following rapid weight loss, the individual may experience symptoms similar to a hypoglycemic state, including decreased short-term memory and mood changes as well as confusion and tension.[41,58,59] Symptoms are usually resolved after 72 hours when food and fluid intake, body weight, plasma volume, and blood glucose return to normal.[58] Unfortunately, many weight-restricted sports do not allow for this amount of recovery time after weigh-ins.

Although according to the literature there is not an exact amount of time needed for recovery, it is imperative to consider the need for some recovery time and monitor changes in performance and symptoms. Some literature shows no difference in anaerobic activities, such as vertical jump or short sprints, when comparing rapid weight loss to gradual weight loss following a 5-hour reloading period.[60] This leads to uncertainty on recovery time due to varying methodology in the research.[36] Furthermore, many studies report no change in lactate, power, or total work after rapid weight loss.[61] Although most of the literature supports no change in anaerobic outcome, such as strength and power with rapid weight loss, rapid weight loss can result in nutrient values being below the recommended values—putting those practicing a hypocaloric diet at risk.[62] The clinician should carefully review research that is applicable to the athlete's specific weight-restricted sport and recovery time.

Why Do Sports Have Weight Restrictions?

Some sports have weight restrictions for biomechanical advantages, safety, or aesthetics. Athletes in combative sports (eg, wrestling, judo, taekwondo, boxing) compete within weight classes and must manipulate body weight without compromising performance. Although some athletes will decrease food and fluid intake during the 2 or 3 weeks leading up to a competition to gradually reach the desired weight class, many weight-restricted sport athletes use more rapid and dangerous weight loss methods, such as intense exercise in sweat suits and saunas.[63,64] In fact, many athletes will engage in their most prominent weight loss 1 to 2 days prior to competition.[63] Reports of these dangerous weight loss techniques, such as rapid weight loss and the use of diuretics and sauna suits, leave many unfamiliar with the sports asking a common question: Why not complete at a higher weight class? To safely guide athletes through sport-related weight loss the clinicians must understand the sport from the athlete's perspective.

For many combative sports, athletes believe rapid weight loss to meet a weight class requirement, followed by rapid regain of weight after the weigh-in prior to competition, leads

to competitive advantages. For example, having a body mass larger than one's opponent can result in increased leverage, reach, and strength.[63] Therefore, some competitors will rapidly decrease their weight in order to qualify for a lower weight class to face smaller or weaker competitors, then regain that lost weight in an attempt to overpower that competitor. Interestingly, according to competitors, those are not the most important justifications for extreme weight loss in combative sports. Rather, 3 attributes have been linked to the theory that weight regulation has a mental benefit to combative athletes. These attributes include (1) a sense of belonging to the team, (2) self-discipline, and (3) self-confidence.[63] Understanding the reasons that weight-restricted athletes participate in risky behavior can help the clinician guide the athlete toward safe weight-loss practices.

Weight-restricted sports have created a culture that seems to imply that weight loss is a sign of mental toughness. Athletes feel a sense of belonging while "cutting weight" as a team. Many athletes want others to see them as being completely devoted to the sport, and thereby believe that being able to endure excessive or rapid weight loss shows a true devotion to one's sport. This leads to fear that coaches, athletes, and competitors view those who do not cut significant amounts of weight in weight-restricted sports as being inadequate.[63] In the eyes of the athlete, weight cutting is often directly related to discipline and status. Many athletes admit to judging athletic worth by how capable the opponent is at losing significant amounts of weight.[63] Even in the case that an athlete moves up a weight class—thereby eliminating the need to lose weight—feelings of inadequacy prior to competition due to eliminating the weight loss routine leads them to purposefully weighing more than their required competition weight.[64] This allows restoration of a weight loss routine and the feeling of inclusion in the hours leading up to competition while the rest of the team is losing weight.[63] Without excessive exercise for the purpose of losing weight prior to the weigh-in, the athlete may feel unprepared for competition. The activity associated with weight reduction has a mental effect on athletes during competition preparation.[63] The weight cutting process prior to a weigh-in gets the athlete to focus by serving as a precompetition warm up, much like a baseball player would take batting practice before a game. The outcome of the competition is somewhat out of the athlete's control, but manipulation of weight loss via food intake, fluid restriction, and exercise restores control and self-confidence.[63]

Regulating weight prior to competition provides a mental advantage by creating a sense of accomplishment.[63] Many athletes refer to the practice of weight loss as it relates to the fictional character Rocky Balboa. Similar to Rocky running up the steps at the Philadelphia Museum of Art the day before his fight, near the end of weight cutting the athlete feels an end to the tough training in preparation for competition. In combative sports, resisting hunger and thirst has been described as one of the greatest tests of an individual's willpower.[64] In addition to feeling accomplished, the athlete may experience an increase in self-confidence after a challenging period of weight cutting.[63] For example, during weigh-ins and prior to the start of competition, many athletes want to look "bigger" than opponents in the same weight class, which many believe is accomplished by competing at the lowest weight class possible. Looking larger creates a sense of power, therefore lowering the self-esteem of the opponent by not only physically intimidating them but also mentally intimidating them by flaunting the ability to endure stress and dangerous behaviors.[63]

Weight loss behavior is concerning as young athletes are idolizing college and professional athletes who practice these dangerous weight loss methods. Many athletes describe weight cutting as a way to control something before feeling out of control during competition.[63] Some athletes are using weight cutting as a way to reduce stress and anxiety,[63] but that often comes at the cost of decreased performance.[64] Understanding the culture of weight-restricted sports can assist the clinician in showing empathy and compassion. Understanding the culture of weight-restricted sports will build trust in the clinician–client relationship and assist in guiding the client in safe weight loss strategies.

Conclusion

Clients choose to reduce body weight for multiple reasons, including sport-specific goals such as weight restrictions, performance, and aesthetics. Unfortunately, many individuals tend to use dangerous weight loss strategies. Creating a health care team consisting of a registered dietitian, athletic trainer, physician, coach, and most importantly the client or athlete will benefit the weight loss process, support the safety of the client, and negate detrimental effects on athletic performance. Although education of athletes and coaches is important, the clinician should learn the culture of the sport to understand why clients gravitate toward these unhealthy behaviors and help the client build a plan for safe and successful competition.

Discussion Questions

1. Sam recently accepted an athletic training position with a NCAA Division II wrestling program. Prior to Thanksgiving break he hears the team talking about eating in excess while they are home for the holiday and how they will have to lose all the weight before their next tournament. The upperclassmen are providing methods to the freshmen for rapid weight loss that include many unsafe techniques. Although Sam has not witnessed any of these unsafe weight loss methods, what could he do in this situation?

2. Leslie is an athletic trainer for the men's and women's cross-country teams. While eating dinner with the team after a race, she hears a female runner talking to her teammate about dieting. She is counting calories and eliminating all carbohydrates from her diet. She claims that she lost 8 pounds last week and was able to shave a few seconds off her time. She is going to continue to lose weight so she can qualify for nationals. What should Leslie do in this situation?

3. You accepted a job as an athletic trainer for a collegiate cycling team. When you arrive for the first day of practice, the coach is providing each cycler with a detailed diet that will ensure they reach a weight that will maximize speed and performance. After talking with the coach, you find out she is not a registered dietitian and gets most of her information from other coaches and online cycling blogs. She mentions that no one is available on-campus to provide nutritional advice. In this situation, what is your plan to provide the cyclers with proper nutritional advice?

References

1. McArdle WD, Katch FI, Katch VL. *Sports & Exercise Nutrition.* Lippincott Williams & Wilkins; 1999.

2. Hall KD, Heymsfield SB, Kemnitz JW, Klein S, Schoeller DA, Speakman JR. Energy balance and its components: implications for body weight regulation. *Am J Clin Nutr.* 2012;95(4):989-994.

3. Gonzalez JT, Betts JA, Thompson D. Carbohydrate availability as a regulator of energy balance with exercise. *Exerc Sport Rev.* 2019:215-222.

4. Henry CJK. Basal metabolic rate studies in humans: measurement and development of new equations. Public health nutrition, 8(7a). *Public Health Nutrition.* 2005:1133-1152.

5. Thomas J. Energy balance in young athletes. *J Int Soc Sports Nutr.* 1998:160-174.

6. Blundell JE, Caudwell P, Gibbons C, et al. Role of resting metabolic rate and energy expenditure in hunger and appetite control: a new formulation. *Disease Models & Mechanisms.* 2012;5(5):608-13. doi:10.1242/dmm.009837

7. Tuner J, Markovitch D, Betts JA, Thompson D. Nonprescribed physical activity energy expenditure is maintained with structured exercise and implicates a compensatory increase in energy intake. *Am J Clin Nutr.* 2010;92(5):1009-16. doi:10.3945/ajcn.2010.29471

8. Beaulieu K, Hopkins M, Long C, Blundell J, Finlayson G. High habitual physical activity improves acute energy compensation in nonobese adults. *Med Sci Sports Exerc.* 2017;49(11):2268-2275. doi:10.1249/MSS.0000000000001368

9. Markwald RR, Melanson EL, Smith MR, et al. Impact of insufficient sleep on total daily energy expenditure on food intake, and weight gain. *Proceedings of the National Academy of Sciences of the United States of America.* 2013:5695-5700. doi:10.1073/pnas.1216951110

10. Doucet E, St-Pierre S, Almeras N, Despres JP, Boichard C, Tremblay A. Evidence for the existence of adaptive thermogenesis during weight loss. *Br J Nutr.* 2001;85(6):715-723.

11. Rosenbaum M, Hirsch J, Gallagher DA, Leibel RL. Long-term persistence of adaptive thermogenesis in subjects who have maintained a reduced body weight. *Am J Clin Nutr.* 2008;88(4):906-12. doi:10.1093/ajcn/88.4.906

12. Rosenbaum A, Leibel R. Adaptive thermogenesis in humans. *Int J Obes.* 2010:47-55.

13. Donnelly JE, Blair SN, Jakicic JM, et al. American College of Sports Medicine Position Stand. Appropriate physical activity intervention strategies for weight loss and prevention of weight regain for adults. *Med Sci Sports Exerc.* 2009;41(2):459-471.

14. Jakicic JM, Clark K, Coleman E, et al. American College of Sports Medicine position stand. Appropriate intervention strategies for weight loss and prevention of weight regain for adults. *Med Sci Sports Exerc.* 2001;33(12):2145-2156.

15. Rodriquez N, Di Marco N, Langley S. American College of Sports Medicine position stand, Nutrition and athletic performance. *Med Sci Sports Exerc.* 2009;41(3):709-31. doi:10.1249/MSS.0b013e31890eb86

16. Steen SN, Oppliger RA, Brownell KD. Metabolic effects of repeated weight loss and regain in adolescent wrestlers. *JAMA.* 1988;260(1):47-50.

17. Manore MM. Nutritional needs of the female athlete. *Clin Sports Med.* 1999:549-563.

18. Martin JT, Johnson MD. American Academy of Pediatrics Policy Statement: promotion of healthy weight-control practices in young athletes. *Pediatrics.* 2005:1557-1564.

19. Turocy PS, DePalma BF, Horswill CA, et al. National Athletic Trainers' Association position statement. Safe weight loss and maintenance practices in sport and exercise. *J Athl Train.* 2011;46(3):322-336.

20. Phillips SM. A brief review of higher dietary protein diets in weight loss: a focus on athletes. *Sports Med.* 2014:149-153.

21. Mettler S, Mitchell N, Tipton KD. Increased protein intake reduces lean body mass loss during weight loss in athletes. *Med Sci Sports Exerc.* 2010;42(2):326-337.

22. Murphy CH, Hector AJ, Phillips SM. Considerations for protein intake in managing weight loss in athletes. *Eur J Sport Sci.* 2015;15(1):21-28.

23. Maestu J, Eliakim A, Jurimae J, Valter I, Jurimae T. Anabolic and catabolic hormones and energy balance of the male bodybuilders during the preparation for the competition. *J Strength Cond Res.* 2010;24(4):1074-1081.

24. Pelly F, Burkhart S, Dunn P. Factors influencing food choice of athletes at international competition events. *Appetite.* 2018:173-178.

25. Reel J, SooHoo S, Petrie TA, Greenleaf C, Carter JE. Slimming down for sport: developing a weight pressures in sport measure for female athletes. *J Clin Sport Psychol.* 2010;4(2):99-111.

26. Cheek C, Hill K, Carlson J, Lock J, Peebles R. Weight-related coaching pressures, mental health, sleep, and quality of life in competitive university athletes. *J Adolesc Health.* 2015;56(2):88.

27. Scott C, Haycraft E, Plateau R. Teammate influences and relationship quality are associated with eating and exercise psychopathy in athletes. *Appetite.* 2019:1-10.

28. Ehrman J. *ACSM's Resource Manual for Guidelines for Exercise Testing and Prescription.* Lippincott, Williams & Wilkins; 2010.

29. Davis SE, Dwyer GB, Reed K, Bopp C, Stosic J, Shepanski M. Preliminary investigation: the impact of the NCAA wrestling weight certification program on weight cutting. *J Strength Cond Res.* 2002;16(2):305-307.

30. Franchini E, Brito C, Artioli G. Weight loss in combat sports: physiological, psychology, and performance effects. *J Int Soc Sports Nutr.* 2012;9(52).

31. Oppliger R, Case HM, Horswill CA, Landry GL, Shelter AC. ACSM Position Stand: weight loss in wrestlers. *Med Sci Sports Exerc.* 1996;28(10):135-138.

32. McMurray R, Proctor C, Wilson W. Effect of caloric deficit and dietary manipulation on aerobic and anaerobic exercise. *Int J Sports Med.* 1991:167-172.

33. Sundgot-Borgen J, Garthe I. Elite athletes in aesthetic and Olympic weight-class sports and the challenge of body weight and body composition. *J Sports Sci.* 2011:25-27.

34. Reibe DE. *Exercise prescription in ACSM's guidelines for exercise testing and prescription.* Lippincott, Williams & Wilkins; 2010:216-231.

35. Grindstaff T, Potach D. Prevention of common wrestling injuries. *Strength Cond J.* 2006;28(4):20-28.

36. Santos SLC. Pre-competitive period in olympic wrestling athletes: losing weight, a risk factor. *Journal of Scientific & Technical Research.* 2019:10532-10535.

37. Garthe I, Raastad T, Refsnes PE, Koivisto A, Sundgot-Borgen J. Effect of two different weight-loss rates on body composition and strength and power-related performance in elite athletes. *Int J Sport Nutr Exerc Metab.* 2011;21(2):97-104. doi:10.1123/ijsnem.21.2.97

38. Bryner RW, Ullrich IH, Sauers J, et al. Effects of resistance vs. aerobic training combined with an 800 caloric liquid diet on lean body mass and resting metabolic rate. *J Am Coll Nutr.* 1999;18(2):115-21. doi:10.1080/07315724.1999.10718838

39. Beyranvand R, Moradi A, Fatahi F, Mirnasouri R. Assessment and comparison of rapid weight loss methods and its complications in various weight groups of adult elite wrestlers. *J Rehab Sci Res.* 2017;4(2):41-46.

40. Cengiz A. Effects of self-selected dehydration and meaningful rehydration on anaerobic power and heart rate recovery in elite wrestlers. *J Phys Ther Sci.* 2015;27(5):1441-1444.

41. Landers DM, Arent SM, Lutz RS. Affective and cognitive performance in high school wrestlers undergoing rapid weight loss. *J Sport Exerc Psychol.* 2011;23(4):307-316.

42. Wilson G, Hawken MB, Poole I, et al. Rapid weight loss impairs simulated riding performance and strength in jockeys: implications for making-weight. *J Sports Sci.* 2014;32(4):389-391.

43. Aghaei N, Rohani H. Heart rate; blood pressure; and lactate response to sauna induced rapid weight loss in elite wrestlers. *Electronic Physician.* 2011:171.

44. Artioli GG, Franchini E, Lancha A. Weight loss in grappling combat sports: review and applied recommendations. *Revista Brasileira de Cineantropometria e Desempenho Humano.* 2006;8(2):92-101.

45. Silva JML, Gagliardo LC. Analysis of methods and strategies and weight loss in athletes of mixed martial arts during pre-competitive period. *Revista Brasileira de Nutrição e Esportiva.* 2014:74-77.

46. Coswig VS, Fukuda DH, Del Vecchio FB. Rapid weight loss elicits harmful biochemical and hormonal responses in mixed martial arts athletes. *Int J Sport Nutr Exerc Metab.* 2015;25(5):480-486.

47. Moghaddami A. Kinematic analysis of the effect of rapid weight loss by sauna on elite wrestlers' single leg takedown technique. *Evropejskij Žurnal Fiziceskoj Kul'tury i Sporta.* 2015:197-205.

48. Morales J, Ubasart C, Solana-Tramunt M, et al. Effects of rapid weight loss on balance and reaction time in elite judo athletes. *Int J Sports Physiol Perform.* 2018;1-7. doi:10.1123/ijspp.2018-0089

49. Roemmich JN, Sinning WE. Weight loss and wrestling training: effects on nutrition, growth, maturation, body composition, and strength. *J Appl Physiol (1985).* 1997;82(6):1751-9. doi:10.1152/jappl.1997.82.6.1751

50. Buford TW, Rossi SJ, Smith DB, O'Brien MS, Pickering C. The effect of a competitive wrestling season on body weight, hydration, and muscular performance in collegiate wrestlers. *J Strength Cond Res.* 2006;20(3):689-92. doi:10.1519/R-19955.1

51. Ghaemi J, Rashidlamir A, Hosseini SRA, Rahimi GRM. The effect of rapid and gradual weight loss on some hematological parameters in trained wrestlers. *International Journal of Wrestling Science,* 2014;4(2):37-41.

52. Lambert CJ, Jones B. Alternatives to rapid weight loss in US wrestling. *Int J Sports Med.* 2010;31(8):523-528. doi:10.1055/s-0030-1254177

53. Matthews JJ, Nicholas C. Extreme rapid weight loss and rapid weight gain observed in UK mixed martial arts athletes preparing for competition. *Int J Sport Nutr Exerc Metab.* 2017;27(2):122-129. doi:10.1123/ijsnem.2016-0174

54. Krentz E, Warschburger P. Sports-related correlates of disordered eating in aesthetic sports. *Psychol Sport Exerc.* 2011;12(4):375-382.

55. Reale R, Slater G, Burke LM. Individualised dietary strategies for Olympic combat sports: acute weight loss, recovery and competition nutrition. *Eur J Sports Sci.* 2017;17(6):727-740.

56. Park S, Alencar M, Sassone J, Madrigal L, Ede A. Self-reported methods of weight cutting in professional mixed-martial artists: how much are they losing and who is advising them? *J Int Soc Sports Nutr.* 2019;16(52):1-8.

57. Reale R, Slater G, Burke LM. Acute-weight-loss strategies for combat sports and applications to Olympic success. *Int J Sports Physiol Perform.* 2017;12(2):142-151. doi:10.1123/ijspp.2016-0211

58. Choma CW, Sforzo GA, Keller BA. Impact of rapid weight loss on cognitive function in collegiate wrestlers. *Med Sci Sports Exerc.* 1998;30(5):746-749. doi:10.1097/00005768-199805000-00016

59. Koral J, Dosseville F. Combination of gradual and rapid weight loss: effects on physical performance and psychological state of elicit judo athletes. *J Sports Sci.* 2009;27(2):115-20. doi:10.1080/02640410802413214

60. Fogelholm GM, et al. Gradual and rapid weight loss: effects on nutrition and performance in male athletes. *Med Sci Sports Exerc.* 1993:371-377.

61. Mendes SH, Tritto AC, Guilherme JPLF, et al. Effect of rapid weight loss on performance in combat sport male athletes: does adaptation to chronic weight cycling play a role. *Br J Sports Med.* 2013;47(18):1155-60. doi:10.1136/bjsports-2013-092689

62. Reljic D, Jost J, Dickau K, et al. Effects of pre-competitional rapid weight loss on nutrition, vitamin status and oxidative stress in elite boxers. *J Sports Sci.* 2015;33(5):437-448.

63. Pettersson S, Ekström MP, Berg CM. Practice of weight regulation among elite athletes in combat sports: a matter of mental advantage? *J Athl Train.* 2013;48(1):99-108. doi:10.4085/1062-6050-48.1.04

64. Hall C, Lane A. Effects of rapid weight loss on mood and performance among amateur boxers. *Br J Sports Med.* 2001;35(6):390-5. doi:10.1136/bjsm.35.6.390

Chapter 8

Nutrition for Injury Recovery

Kyla Cross, MS, MPH, RD, LD
Brett Singer, MS, RD, CSSD, LD

Commission on Accreditation of Athletic Training Education *2020 Standards*

This chapter addresses the following *2020 Standards for Accreditation of Professional Athletic Training Programs*:

- Standard 61: Practice in collaboration with other health care and wellness professionals.
- Standard 69: Develop a care plan for each patient. The care plan includes (but is not limited to) the following:
  - Referral when warranted
- Standard 76: Evaluate and treat a patient who has sustained a concussion or other brain injury, with consideration of established guidelines. [Implementation of a plan of care (nutrition).]
- Standard 82: Develop, implement, and supervise comprehensive programs to maximize sport performance that are safe and specific to the client's activity.

Learning Objectives

After reviewing this chapter, readers will be able to:

- Differentiate nutrition needs according to the stage of injury recovery.
- Identify common nutrition concerns regarding injury rehabilitation.
- Calculate protein needs according to the stage of injury.
- Select the appropriate supplement according to recovery needs.

Knoblauch M, ed. *Clinical Nutrition in Athletic Training* (pp 89-97).
© 2023 Taylor & Francis Group.

Introduction

Injuries are a common challenge faced by athletes of all ages and levels. From bumps, bruises, and abrasions to significant surgeries requiring lengthy rehabilitation schedules, athletes and their sports medicine support staff work together to get the athlete back on the field as soon as possible. Upon injury, the main focus of attention from the sports medicine team is directed toward injury evaluation, followed soon after by outlining a plan of care to treat that injury. An often-neglected component of injury rehabilitation is the athlete's nutrition status as well as their dietary intake in support of recovery. This chapter will discuss how nutrition can play a role in recovery, and how various stages of injury rehabilitation may alter the athlete's nutrition needs. The primary focus of this chapter will be on injuries requiring lengthier periods of time away from sport, particularly when muscle atrophy and loss of strength is a significant concern. It is important to note, however, that the amount of evidence specifically addressing nutrition and sports medicine–specific injuries is extremely limited. Instead, many of the recommendations provided within this chapter will be based on research taken from bed rest and immobilized limb studies in healthy populations. Other notable studies related to ill patients as well as recommendations related to general sports nutrition will also be utilized. To best describe the differences within nutritional needs, this chapter will be broken into 2 main parts, the immobilization phase and the rehabilitation phase as described in Tipton.[1]

Immobilization Phase

The immobilization phase of injury recovery is the period of time in which the athlete is either limited to bed rest, is non–weight bearing, or is in a cast, thereby preventing activity from occurring within the injured limb or body part. During this period of time several challenges may arise, including muscle atrophy, loss of strength, an accumulation of unwanted body fat mass, as well as a decline in insulin sensitivity.[2] There are a few simple primary nutrition objectives within the immobilization phase, which include providing adequate energy and high-quality nutrient-dense foods to support the healing process, as well as mitigating muscle atrophy and body fat accumulation. When injured and away from sport, athletes have a tendency to put nutrition in the back of their thought process, as they are often unaware of its role outside of training and competition. Through consistent education and frequent reminders from the sports medicine team, athletes can implement appropriate nutrition tactics to support the recovery process.

Over a 1% loss of leg lean mass and a 9% reduction in strength can be noted in as little as 5 days of limb immobilization.[3] When a limb is immobilized, there is a notable reduction in muscle protein synthesis (MPS). When synthesis occurs to a lesser degree than muscle protein breakdown, a negative protein balance is generated such that there is a reduction in lean mass and strength. This reduction in MPS is thought to be due to a reduced sensitivity to amino acids, often referred to as "anabolic resistance."[4] Anabolic resistance resulting in a net negative protein balance increases the likelihood of muscle atrophy as well as a loss of muscle strength and function. Recognizing this challenge, it is the goal of the dietitian and sports medicine staff to minimize the impact caused by the reduction of MPS, while avoiding any dietary behaviors that may further suppress protein synthesis.

During periods of immobilization, there is the tendency for athletes and coaches to believe energy demands are dramatically reduced and thus food intake should be minimized. While exercise-induced energy expenditure may decline, there may also be a short-term rise in resting energy expenditure as a result of the stress related to the injury and surgical procedure. Consequently, the decline in total energy needs may not be as significant as athletes perceive.

As with healthy athletes, energy needs will vary dependent upon numerous factors, as discussed in the nutrition assessment chapter of this textbook. While total energy needs may vary, it is likely best to avoid a large surplus or deficit of calories relative to total needs during the immobilization phase. Consuming too few calories will result in weight loss, a further decline in MPS, and an acceleration of muscle atrophy.[5] Consuming a substantial surplus of calories is likely to result in an accumulation of fat mass with the added risk of accelerated muscle atrophy similar to when the athlete may consume too few calories.[6]

Particularly during the first several days after a surgical procedure when appetite is reduced, consuming enough food may be quite challenging for the injured athlete due to effects from medications, nausea, exhaustion, and their ability to ambulate and access food. To meet energy demands, liquid calorie sources such as a fruit smoothies, kefir, milk, or protein shakes can be utilized. In addition to liquid calories, energy-dense foods high in fat such as avocado, nuts, or seeds may be beneficial to include if the athlete is struggling to eat enough. While lower-calorie foods such as fruits and vegetables are an important part of the diet, athletes should exercise caution. Relying too heavily on these food options, particularly when appetite is poor, may cause the athlete to feel full while still falling short of energy demands. As appetite returns, a more normalized diet is appropriate and the dependence on liquid calorie sources is likely unnecessary. With a small reduction in total energy needs, athletes will need to reduce calories, primarily in the form of carbohydrate and fat sources, while continuing to meet the high demand for protein. As will be discussed shortly, protein, which often promotes satiety, may need to be emphasized first within meals in order to ensure needs are met despite a poor appetite.

Protein

Among its many roles within the body, protein plays a significant role in the health and function of skeletal muscle. As noted previously, during times of injury and immobilization, the patient can experience anabolic resistance that suppresses the skeletal muscle response to protein feedings. To mitigate the loss of muscle mass athletes must focus on 3 main protein goals, often referenced as the 3 Ts of protein:

1. Total: Consume adequate total protein within each meal to maximize MPS.
2. Timing: Consume protein throughout the day, preferably every 3 to 5 hours.
3. Type: Consume the right types of protein, preferably high-quality leucine-rich protein sources, when possible.

In healthy adults it has been suggested that each feeding should contain approximately 0.25 to 0.4 g/kg of protein to maximally stimulate MPS.[7] However, due to anabolic resistance it is likely that a protein dose at this level will fall short of maximally stimulating MPS. As an example, in older adults over the age of 65 years where age-related anabolic resistance is believed to occur, higher intakes of protein closer to 35 to 40 g per feeding are required in order to maximally stimulate protein synthesis in comparison to typical recommendations of 20 g per feeding.[3] For this reason, recommendations have been made to consume as much as 2 to 2.5 g/kg of protein daily during the immobilization phase.[1] With these higher recommendations in total protein, injured individuals may benefit from consuming closer to 0.4 to 0.55 g/kg of protein in each feeding.[8] Consuming protein approximately every 3 hours could be a beneficial tactic for maximizing MPS throughout the day.[9] To simplify, most athletes should consume between 20 to 50 g of protein in each feeding, meaning both meals and snacks, approximately 4 to 6 times a day during immobilization.

The type of protein consumed also plays a role in the muscle protein synthesis response. Leucine, an essential amino acid, is often described as the "trigger" for MPS.[10] Leucine and the remaining essential amino acids are responsible for MPS. Leucine can be found predominantly in animal-based protein sources such as dairy, eggs, meat, and fish. Some plant-based sources including peas, soy, and black beans are also quality sources of leucine.[11]

A popular protein-based supplement often recommended during times of injury is beta-hydroxy-beta-methylbutyrate, also referred to as HMB. HMB, a leucine metabolite, has been used with some success during times of injury or bed rest. In a 10-day study in which participants were confined to bed rest, atrophy was reduced when 3 g of HMB was consumed on a daily basis.[12] In comparison to leucine, HMB is not superior for stimulating MPS[13] or in improvements of strength and lean mass.[14] It appears unlikely that HMB will provide a superior or improved response when leucine-rich, high-quality protein sources are already consumed. Thus, rather than spending significant amounts of money on HMB,

it is likely best to consume a high-quality whey protein that will provide leucine in addition to the remaining essential amino acids.

In addition to HMB and protein, there are several other potential supplements often recommended during times of immobilization. Among these are omega-3 and creatine monohydrate, as well as different vitamins and minerals. As is the case with most nutrition tactics in response to sports-related injuries, evidence remains limited. While more research is needed, omega-3 appears to be a promising option.

Omega-3

Omega-3 fatty acids are an essential polyunsaturated fatty acid (PUFA), meaning they must be obtained from the diet. There are 3 forms of omega-3, including docosahexaenoic acid (DHA), eicosapentaenoic acid (EPA), and alpha-linolenic acid (ALA). Cold water fish and marine algae are sources of EPA and DHA while plant-based sources such as walnuts and flaxseeds are sources of ALA. The 2019 International Olympic Committee recommendation is approximately 2 g total of omega-3 daily, while the Academy of Nutrition and Dietetics recommend 500 mg of EPA + DHA daily.

While omega-3 has been noted for its potential anti-inflammatory properties, there is a growing interest in its potential role within skeletal muscle and the reduction of muscle atrophy. An increase in MPS has been reported in both young and older adults.[15] Improvements have also been reported in strength[16] and lean mass[17] in older adult populations supplemented with omega-3 fatty acids. The suspected mechanism of action is that omega-3 may enhance the MPS response, particularly during times when it is suppressed (eg, during immobilization).[3] These results may be even more pronounced in women relative to men.[18]

Two to 4 weeks of supplementation are required in order to increase omega-3 composition within skeletal muscle.[19] When possible, it is likely best to supplement with omega-3 for several weeks prior to immobilization and expected muscle atrophy. A potential example could be an athlete completing a few weeks of therapy prior to surgery and supplementing during this time. A common presurgery recommendation is for patients to refrain from supplementing with omega-3. This is due to the perceived increased bleeding risk related to omega-3 supplementation. While these bleeding risks are often referenced, there does not appear to be an increased risk of bleeding when omega-3 supplementation occurs prior to surgery.[20]

In a study measuring muscle volume loss by McGlory et al, female participants were provided 5 g of omega-3 daily for 4 weeks before initiating 2 weeks of leg immobilization. Muscle volume loss was reduced in the omega-3 supplementation group in comparison to the calorie-matched placebo group.[18] These results demonstrate an improvement in myofibrillar muscle protein synthesis, thereby suggesting a potential link to omega-3 supplementation and protein synthesis, leading to a reduction in muscle atrophy.[18] Based on such findings, it is possible that supplementing with 3 to 5 g of omega-3 daily over a period of at least 2 to 4 weeks prior to and during immobilization may increase muscle protein synthesis and reduce expected muscle atrophy.

Creatine Monohydrate

Creatine monohydrate is a supplement often utilized by athletes as a result of its role in strength, power, hypertrophy, and high-intensity exercise performance. Levels of creatine within skeletal muscle may decrease by as much as 24% during immobilization, thus there is a question as to whether creatine supplementation may benefit athletes during the immobilization phase of rehabilitation.[21] Indeed, supplementation with creatine during immobilization has improved maintenance of muscle creatine. While data are limited, there have been several studies reviewing the use of creatine during immobilization and its potential role in muscle atrophy; however, results have been mixed at best. Creatine supplementation has been reported to attenuate muscle atrophy during upper extremity immobilization to a greater extent in comparison to lower extremity immobilization.[22] In addition, creatine has been used with some levels of success, in cases of cachexia and wasting.[23] While there is no strong consensus on whether creatine supplementation can improve outcomes during immobilization, creatine is recognized as one of the most significantly researched and effective supplements available. It is recognized as not only safe but potentially therapeutic in both healthy and diseased populations.[24] For these reasons, creatine monohydrate is worth strong consideration for supplementation during the immobilization phase. For those who choose to utilize creatine during the injury rehabilitation stage, there are several potential dosing protocols available. Most commonly, 20 g/day consumed in 4 separate 5 g doses for a period of 5 to 7 days is utilized as a loading phase. From there, 3 to 5 g of a single dose can be utilized on a daily basis.[25]

Vitamins and Minerals

During times of stress, such as during an illness or after an injury, athletes have the tendency to grab whatever vitamins and minerals they can find on the shelf to help shorten recovery time. This often includes antioxidants, such as high doses of vitamin C and vitamin E. Despite this common approach, there does not appear to be a need for high-dose micronutrient supplementation, including antioxidants, when individuals are within the normal limits of vitamin and mineral status.[1] Injured athletes should be encouraged to consume a wide variety of fruits and vegetables along with a complete diet, just as all athletes should, in order to meet their baseline micronutrient needs.

Other Considerations

Nutrition considerations such as energy intake, protein, and other key nutrients are typically at the forefront of any practitioner's thought process during rehabilitation. While dietitians may put together an ideal nutrition protocol to implement during immobilization, there may be other barriers, such as food access and poor appetite, preventing the athlete from adhering to the plan. Therefore, an interdisciplinary approach to identify potential barriers and provide practical solutions is necessary. This starts with consistent open dialogue between the athlete and practitioner.

Poor appetite and nausea, particularly within the first few days to weeks initially following surgery, may prevent the athlete from meeting their energy and macronutrient demands. In a recent study from Weijzen et al, participants admitted to the hospital for elective hip or knee arthroplasty were unable to consistently consume even up to 0.8 g/kg of protein per day.[26] Protein intake at this level falls as much as 3 times less than protein recommendations call for during immobilization. In addition to poor appetite, food access and the ability to prepare meals may be impaired while injured. Furthermore, injuries may prevent the athlete from driving to the grocery or efficiently walking to the kitchen to grab a snack, and some upper extremity injuries may even prevent athletes from cutting their own food.

Athletic trainers can help identify high-risk athletes by asking some simple questions:

- How hungry is the athlete on a scale of 1 to 10?
- How many feedings is the athlete having each day?
- What percentage of each meal is the athlete consuming?
- Who is handling the grocery shopping and cooking at home? Does the athlete have any additional forms of support that can help with food preparation?

If athletes report a consistently poor appetite, are frequently eating less than half of their meals, or are eating less than 3 times per day, it is unlikely they are meeting their energy demands or total protein and protein distribution recommendations. Asking the previous questions may initiate dialogue with athletes, while also finding cases where sports dietitians may contribute most to the rehabilitation process.

Summary

With bed rest or limb immobilization comes significant risk of muscle atrophy, loss of strength, and accumulation of body fat. It can be a challenging time for athletes both physically and psychologically after being removed from their sport and forced to reduce their activity levels. By taking a multidisciplinary approach, the sports medicine and performance team can assist the athlete in navigating the many challenges that come with inactivity. Maintaining energy balance through a moderate reduction in energy, carbohydrate, and fat intake can help mitigate the risk of unwanted weight loss or weight gain. Emphasizing high-quality, leucine-rich protein sources at each feeding can provide the athlete with the best chance for preservation of muscle mass. Including supplements such as omega-3 and creatine monohydrate may also help. Lastly, athletes should be encouraged to include as many nutrient-dense foods such as fruits and vegetables as possible to support the healing process.

Rehabilitation Phase

During the rehabilitation phase, the athlete will gradually transition from immobilization to a more physically active state. With changes in activity levels as well as the goals of rehabilitation, athletes should be mindful of evolving nutrition needs. The focus of nutrition will transition from preservation of muscle mass and avoiding fat mass gain (as discussed in the prior section) to supporting an individual's growing energy demands for advanced activity while assisting with muscle strength and hypertrophy.[4] While there may be some differences, in general nutrition recommendations during the rehabilitation phase will be similar to those when working with any athlete attempting to build muscle and strength.

As the athlete becomes more mobile, therapy sessions may become more labor intensive while also incorporating some return-to-play activity. As this occurs, energy demands may also begin to increase. To support these increased energy demands, athletes will need to gradually increase their intake of carbohydrates, particularly around their workout. Daily recommendations for carbohydrates and various levels of activity can be found in Chapter 10. Special attention should be paid to those athletes who may be progressing to multiple sessions of activity within a given day. Carbohydrates should be emphasized as part of the pre-exercise meal as an opportunity to provide energy, as well as post-exercise to initiate glycogen resynthesis.

During immobilization, one of the main factors driving increased protein demands is inactivity leading to anabolic resistance and a suppression of muscle protein synthesis. Once activity is increased and resistance training is incorporated into rehabilitation, muscle begins to respond more significantly to protein in comparison to the immobilization phase. During this time, protein needs decline slightly to match those of any healthy athlete. As discussed in Chapter 10, athletes can maximize their response to physical activity with 1.6 to 2.0 g/kg/day of protein. As noted previously, protein intake should be distributed throughout the day, with protein coming predominantly in the form of high-quality, leucine-rich sources. A presleep protein-based snack may also be an effective strategy for increased net protein balance and improved strength and hypertrophy.[27]

Creatine monohydrate is well known for its potential benefits with strength, hypertrophy, and high-intensity exercise performance. As discussed earlier in this chapter, there are questions regarding a potential creatine benefit during immobilization; however, it is well established that it can be beneficial in healthy athletes.[25] Despite questions regarding creatine's ability to attenuate muscle atrophy during immobilization, it has been shown that supplementation during immobilization can enhance rehabilitation after immobilization.[28] If supplementation has not been initiated during immobilization, intake can be started with a loading protocol followed by daily maintenance doses according to the recommendations described earlier in this chapter.

Summary

Once athletes reach the rehabilitation phase of injury care, their nutrition focus should begin to look similar to a standard athlete diet supporting their growing level of activity. As athletes gradually build up their level of activity, they can continue to increase calorie and carbohydrate intake. With the incorporating of resistance training back into their rehabilitation, slightly lower levels of protein intake can be appropriate. As with all athletes, a balance of lean, high-quality protein, nutrient-dense fats and carbohydrates along with plenty of fruits and vegetables will provide the athlete with the energy and nutrients required for health and the final stages of their injury recovery.

Other Potential Considerations

Collagen and Gelatin Use in Bone, Ligament, and Tendon Healing

More than 50% of all injuries in sports can be classified as sprains, strains, ruptures, or breaks of musculoskeletal tissues. Collagen is the main structural protein of the different connective tissues such as bone, cartilage, tendon, and skin. The function and strength of these tissues are also dependent on the collagen-rich matrix. Nutrition interventions that increase collagen synthesis and strengthen connective tissue can have a huge impact on injury rates in athletes.

Physiology of Collagen

Even though it remains unclear as to whether specific nutrients can positively affect soft tissue, the physiology of tendons and ligaments suggests that nutrition interventions will provide a different response compared to muscle injuries. Research is currently utilizing in vitro engineered tissues to evaluate the impact that different nutritional factors have on the collagen structural matrix and production. It is known that the limited blood flow to ligaments and tendons creates a unique predicament as these tissues get their nutrients through interstitial fluid flow.[29] Therefore, when the tendon or ligament is loaded the fluid moves out of the tissue and when it is relaxed the fluid is drawn into the tissue from the surrounding cellular environment. To ensure proper growth and healing, the nutrients required by these specialized cells must be present in the surrounding environment prior to exercise in order for the loading activity to adequately deliver these key nutrients to the cells.[30]

Vitamin C has an essential role in connective tissue healing; it regulates the structural protein collagen through hydroxylation. Hydroxylation (adding hydrogen and oxygen to amino acids) of collagen is necessary for its synthesis and production. One study found that vitamin C supplementation accelerates bone healing after fractures, increases type 1 collagen synthesis, and reduces oxidative stress parameters.[31] As a result, vitamin C has been increasingly studied in the treatment of musculoskeletal injuries in addition to other nutrients such as collagen and gelatin.

Collagen and Gelatin

Collagen and gelatin have the same nutrient profile; both are high in glycine, proline, hydroxyproline, hydroxylysine, and arginine.[32] It is thought that certain nutrition interventions increase amino acid components of collagen, and the cofactor vitamin C may improve collagen synthesis. Using a tissue-engineered ligament model, amino acids enriched in collagen added together with vitamin C improved collagen synthesis.[33] An indirect marker of collagen synthesis, P1NP, or N-terminal peptide of procollagen, can be measured via the blood. One study found that a dose of 15 g of vitamin C–enriched collagen taken 1 hour prior to exercise increased P1NP in the blood.[34] Another study found that consuming a gelatin and vitamin C–rich supplement prior to exercise increases the appearance of the amino acid components of collagen within human serum and results in greater collagen synthesis in the recovery period after exercise.[35] Further, evaluating serum samples taken before or 1 hour after feeding a placebo revealed that 5 or 15 g of vitamin C–enriched gelatin resulted in a dose-dependent increase in collagen within engineered ligaments.[35]

Recommendations

Based on the limited evidence, it is suggested that consuming approximately 15 g of gelatin or collagen with approximately 50 mg of vitamin C 1 hour prior to physical activity may improve rehabilitation for bone-, ligament-, tendon-, or cartilage-related injuries. This process can be repeated 2 to 3 times daily during injury rehabilitation. More research is required to determine the best protocol for collagen, gelatin, and vitamin C supplementation.

Nutrition and Concussion

Concussion is defined as a complex pathophysiological process affecting the brain that is induced by traumatic biomechanical forces. There are between 1.6 and 3.8 million cases of sport-related concussions each year.[36] The return to play is often reported to be within 10 days, with some athletes taking up to 20 days. Athletes often report diverse physical, cognitive, and emotional symptoms following concussive injury, and more severe symptoms after a concussion are good predictors of the recovery time.[37] Due to the large impact that concussions have on athletes, there is a tremendous interest in identifying factors that might influence the recovery time and outcomes of sport-related concussions and the role of supplements in diminishing the length of injury.[38]

Omega-3

The last decade has introduced omega-3 supplementation and its role in athletic performance and recovery. Because of this, omega-3 is considered by some researchers to be an ergogenic aid; it may improve exercise efficiency, enhance recovery, or assist in injury prevention. Omega-3s are polyunsaturated fatty acids with more than one carbon-carbon double bond in their backbone. The body is unable to produce omega-3 fatty acids, so they must be obtained through the diet or through supplementation. ALA, EPA, and DHA are the 3 types of omega-3. The body can convert ALA to EPA and DHA, but this conversion is quite inefficient; therefore, it is important to ingest separate sources of EPA and DHA. EPA has a role in inflammation and muscle protein synthesis, while DHA has a role in both brain and eye health and development. Both EPA and DHA are found in cold water fish, seafood, and algae. ALA, the most abundant omega 3 fatty acid, is primarily utilized as an energy source and building block for long-chain fatty acids and is found in chia seeds, flaxseeds, canola oil, soybeans, pumpkin seeds, perilla seed oil, walnuts, and their derivative oils.

Despite the abundance of food sources, many athletes are lacking in omega-3 consumption. Because of this insufficient omega-3 ingestion in many athletes' diets and the success of research in rodents, researchers believe the perceived benefits for athletes are the neuroprotective effects in high-impact sports as well as neurotransmission efficiency (eg, memory and reaction time).

Omega-3 Functions in the Brain

The brain itself is made up mostly of fatty acids. The most predominant (~40%) fatty acid in the brain is DHA. It is believed that omega-3 EFAs have a positive impact on the brain's metabolism and blood flow. For example, in rats, the administration of an omega-3 EPA has a favorable effect on blood flow after suffering from brain cell death.[39] Omega-3 can also decrease the toxic effects of glutamate, which is released in large amounts after traumatic brain injury (TBI), an injury that can lead to the death of brain cells around the injury site.[40] In addition, omega-3 has been found to stabilize cell membranes by inhibiting the release of arachidonic acid, a precursor to inflammatory markers that can reduce the inflammatory response in the brain.[41]

Athletes and Omega-3

Research with athletes has been based on the omega-3 index, a measure that sums EPA and DHA as a percentage of total erythrocyte fatty acids in red blood cells. The omega-3 index has become a widely used measure for several reasons including:

- It correlates with EPA and DHA content in a variety of tissues (not just red blood cells).
- Results are not altered in the fed state and act like a hemoglobin A1C.
- Similar to hemoglobin A1C, the relationship between omega-3 index and cardiovascular risk does not change with a daily dose but rather over the course of time.

Each of these characteristics make the omega-3 index an effective measure of omega-3 status. The range of the omega-3 index is associated with cardiovascular risk and all-cause mortality such that those with a measure between 0% to 4% are associated with the highest risk of cardiovascular disease and poor status, those between 4% and 8% are at moderate risk, and those >8% are in the optimal range.[42]

Research in most athletes has shown that none are in the optimal range of the omega-3 index. Even though athletes are perceived as "healthier," many struggle to eat a variety of foods, especially those high in omega-3. Wilson and Madrigal in 2016 looked at athletes from a major university and found that their average omega-3 index was 4.79%.[43] Likewise, Anzalone et al in 2019 found that the average omega-3 index across 4 different Division I college football programs was approximately 4.4%. About 34% of these athletes were considered high risk and 66% were considered moderate risk for a cardiovascular incident.[42]

Recognizing the potential importance of omega-3 status, and that so many athletes are falling short of the recommended amounts, researchers are beginning to look into the potential benefits of omega-3 supplementation. Amen et al in 2011 looked at 30 retired NFL players who had signs of brain damage and cognitive impairment. They received 5.6 g of fish oil per day, and after 6 months it was found that they had an increase in cerebral blood flow and an increase in cognitive function.[44] Oliver et al in 2016 performed a 6-month intervention of 81 NCAA Division I football players who were given 2, 4, or 6 g per day of DHA. Afterward, researchers found a decrease of serum Nf-L, a measure of axonal injury and measurement of TBI.[45] In addition, Guzmán et al supplemented 24 elite female soccer players with 3.5 g/day of DHA and later reported that they had an increase in neuromotor function, an increase in reaction time, and increased efficiency in various soccer skills.[46] The general conclusion in most research is that most athletes have poor omega-3 status, so addressing this poor status in sports that have a majority of head impacts (ie, football, soccer) will be crucial for moving forward with creating omega-3 recommendations for athletes.

Creatine Monohydrate

In addition to omega-3, creatine has also been researched in regard to its neuroprotective effects on the brain in TBI. Creatine monohydrate is a naturally occurring nitrogenous organic acid found primarily in skeletal muscle, as well as in the brain. The neuroprotective effect of creatine may result from inhibition of the mitochondrial permeability transition pore as a result of structural and functional interactions between creatine kinase and the mitochondrial adenine nucleotide translocator not allowing oxidative stress byproducts to enter the cell.[47] Simply, creatine protects against TBI through mitochondrial bioenergetics and preservation of adenosine triphosphate levels. In children with TBIs, supplementation of creatine (0.4 g/kg/day) for 6 months showed improvements in headaches, dizziness, and fatigue scales[48] and in clinical indices.[49] However, most studies evaluating creatine and its neuroprotective effects against injury have been conducted in animals with ischemia and stroke.[50] Despite evidence of a neuroprotective effect in some studies, no research has been done directly on concussion and creatine monohydrate supplementation.

Athletic Trainer Role

Despite the promising research on omega-3 and creatine monohydrate, the connection between these nutrients and concussions is still in infancy stages. At this time, it is unrealistic to provide specific recommendations regarding dosage or timing for either supplementation in regard to the treatment or prevention of concussion. As an athletic trainer, continuing to follow return-to-play protocols, knowing the injury protocol at each institution, and communication with a dietitian and physician are crucial in determining the best plan of care for an athlete following a concussion.

Conclusion

Nutrition is a piece of the rehabilitation puzzle that often goes overlooked. Sports dietitians and athletic trainers can work together to ensure athletes are fueling appropriately throughout the different stages of rehabilitation. It is important to consider where the athlete is at in terms of their rehabilitation and what their goals are at that time. Open dialogue between all members of the sports medicine and performance staff can ensure each opportunity for success is incorporated, and nutrition can be a key variable in that success.

Discussion Questions

1. A collegiate athlete had ACL reconstruction less than 1 week ago. He currently lives in an off-campus apartment alone and his family lives across the country. What concerns do you have about this athlete's situation, and what questions could you ask to identify potential opportunities to improve upon the athlete's diet?

2. A high school athlete is in the latter stages of his rehabilitation and is performing light physical activity during school, along with a more intense rehabilitation session after school. You have noticed that he is not progressing as quickly as you would expect, and he always appears to be fatigued during the afternoon rehabilitation session. What potential nutrition tools could be utilized to ensure adequate energy is available for his afternoon therapy session?

References

1. Tipton KD. Nutritional support for exercise-induced injuries. *Sports Med.* 2015;45(1):93-104.

2. Tipton KD. *Nutritional support for injuries requiring reduced activity.* Gatorade Sports Science Institute; 2017.

3. Wall BT, Morton, JP, Loon LJCV. Strategies to maintain skeletal muscle mass in the injured athlete: nutritional considerations and exercise mimetics. *Eur J Sport Sci.* 2014;15(1):53-62.

4. Tipton KD. Nutrition for acute exercise-induced injuries. *Ann Nutr Metab.* 2010;57(Suppl.2):43-53.

5. Biolo G, Ciocchi B, Stulle M, et al. Calorie restriction accelerates the catabolism of lean body mass during 2 wk of bed rest. *Am J Clin Nutr.* 2007;86(2):366-372.

6. Biolo G, Agostini F, Simunic B, et al. Positive energy balance is associated with accelerated muscle atrophy and increased erythrocyte glutathione turnover during 5 wk of bed rest. *Am J Clin Nutr.* 2008;88(4):950-958.

7. Morton RW, McGlory C, Phillips SM. Nutritional interventions to augment resistance training-induced skeletal muscle hypertrophy. *Front Physiol.* 2015;6:245.

8. Schoenfield BJ, Aragon AA. How much protein can the body use in a single meal for muscle-building? Implications for daily protein distribution. *J Int Soc Sports Nutr.* 2018;15(1):1-6.

9. Areta JL, Burke LM, Ross ML, et al. Timing and distribution of protein ingestion during prolonged recovery from resistance exercise alters myofibrillar protein synthesis. *J Physiol.* 2013;591(1):2319-2331.

10. Breen L, Churchward-Venne TA. Leucine: a nutrient "trigger" for muscle anabolism, but what more? *J Physiol.* 2012;590(9):2065-2066.

11. Vliet SV, Burd NA, Loon LJCV. The skeletal muscle anabolic response to plant- versus animal-based protein consumption. *J Nutr.* 2015;145(9):1981-1991.

12. Deutz NE, Pereira SL, Hays NP, et al. Effect metabolite β-hydroxy-β-methylbutyrate (HMB) on lean body mass during 10 days of bed rest in older adults. *Clin Nutr.* 2013;32(5):704-712.

13. Wilkinson DJ, Hossain T, Hill DS, et al. Effects of leucine and its metabolite β-hydroxy-β-methylbutyrate on human skeletal muscle protein metabolism. *J Physiol.* 2013;591(11):2911-2923.

14. Jakubowski JS, Wong EPT, Nunes EA, et al. Equivalent hypertrophy and strength gains in β-hydroxy-β-methylbutyrate- or leucine-supplemented men. *Med Sci Sports Exerc.* 2019;51(1):65-74.

15. Smith GI, Atherton P, Reeds DN, et al. Omega-3 polyunsaturated fatty acids augment the muscle protein anabolic response to hyperinsulinaemia-hyperaminoacidaemia in healthy young and middle-aged men and women. *Clin Sci (Lond).* 2011;121(6):267-278. doi:10.1042/CS20100597

16. Rodacki CL, Rodacki AL, Pereira G, et al. Fish-oil supplementation enhances the effects of strength training in elderly women. *Am J Clin Nutr.* 2012;95(2):428-436.

17. Smith GI, Julliand S, Reeds DN, Sinacore DR, Klein S, Mittendorfer B. Fish oil-derived n-3 PUFA therapy increases muscle mass and function in healthy older adults. *Am J Clin Nutr.* 2015;102(1):115-122.

18. McGlory C, Gorissen SH, Kamal M, et al. Omega-3 fatty acid supplementation attenuates skeletal muscle disuse atrophy during two weeks of unilateral leg immobilization in healthy young women. *FASEB J.* 2019;33(3):4568-4597.

19. McGlory C, Wardle SL, Macnaughton LS, et al. Fish oil supplementation suppresses resistance exercise and feeding-induced increases in anabolic signaling without affecting myofibrillar protein synthesis in young men. *Physiol Rep.* 2016;4(6):12715.

20. Harris WS. Expert opinion: omega-3 fatty acids and bleeding—cause for concern? *Am J Cardiol.* 2007;99(6):44-46.

21. Rawson ES, Miles MP, Larson-Meyer DE. Dietary supplements for health, adaptation and recovery in athletes. *Int J Sport Nutr Exerc Metabol.* 2018;28(2):188-199.

22. Slater G, Pyne D, Tipton K. Immunity, infective illness and injury. In: *Clinical Sports Nutrition.* 5th ed. McGraw Hill Education; 2015:730-751.

23. Sakkas GK, Schambelan M, Mulligan K. Can the use of creatine supplementation attenuate muscle loss in cachexia and wasting? *Curr Opin Clin Nutr Metab Care.* 2009;12(6):623-627.

24. Kreider RB, Kalman DS, Antonio J, et al. International Society of Sports Nutrition position stand: safety and efficacy of creatine supplementation in exercise, sport and medicine. *J Int Soc Sports Nutr.* 2017;14(1):18.

25. Maughan RJ, Burke LM, Dvorak J, et al. IOC consensus statement: dietary supplements and the high-performance athlete. *Br J Sports Med.* 2018;52(7):439-455.

26. Weijzen MEG, Kouw IWK, Verschuren AAJ, et al. Protein intake falls below 0.6 g•kg-1•d-1 in healthy, older patients admitted for elective hip or knee arthroplasty. *J Nutr Health Aging.* 2019;23(3):299-305.

27. Snijders T, ResPT, Smeets JSJ, et al. Protein ingestion before sleep increases muscle mass and strength gains during prolonged resistance-type exercise training in healthy young men. *J Nutr.* 2015;145(6):1178-1184.

28. Hespel P, Eijnde BO, Van Leemputte M, et al. Oral creatine supplementation facilitates the rehabilitation of disuse atrophy and alters the expression of muscle myogenic factors in humans. *J Physiol.* 2001;536(2):625-633.

29. Benjamin M, Toumi H, Ralphs JR, Bydder G, Best TM, Milz S. Where tendons and ligaments meet bone: attachment sites ('entheses') in relation to exercise and/or mechanical load. *J Anat.* 2006;208(4):471-490.

30. Baar K. Training and nutrition to prevent soft tissue injuries and accelerate return to play. *Sports Science Exchange.* 2015;28(142):1-6.

31. DePhillipo NN, Aman ZS, Kennedy MI, Begley JP, Moatshe G, LaPrade RF. Efficacy of vitamin C supplementation on collagen synthesis and oxidative stress after musculoskeletal injuries: a systematic review. *Orthop J Sports Med.* 2018;6(10):2325967118804544.

32. Eastoe JE. The amino acid composition of mammalian collagen and gelatin. *Biochem J.* 1955;61(4):589.

33. Paxton JZ, Grocer LM, Baar K. Engineering an in vitro model of a functional ligament from bone to bone. *Tissue Engineering Part A.* 2010;16(11):3515-3525.

34. Lis DM, Baar K. Effects of different vitamin-C enriched collagen derivatives on collagen synthesis. *Int J Sport Nutr Exerc Metabol.* 2019;29(5):526-531.

35. Shaw G, Lee-Barthel A, Ross ML, Wang B, Baar K. Vitamin C-enriched gelatin supplementation before intermittent activity augments collagen synthesis. *Am J Clin Nutr.* 2017;105(1):136-143.

36. Maroon JC, Bost, J. Concussion management at the NFL, college, high school, and youth sports levels. *Clin Neurosurg.* 2011;58(suppl 1): 51-56.

37. Iverson GL, Gardner AJ, Terry DP, et al. Predictors of clinical recovery from concussion: a systematic review. *Br J Sports Med.* 2017;51(12):941-948. doi:10.1136/bjsports-2017-097729

38. Shim J, Smith DH, Van Lunen BL. On-field signs and symptoms associated with recovery duration after concussion in high school and college athletes: a critically appraised topic. *J Sport Rehabil.* 2015;24(1):72-76.

39. Wu A, Ying Z, Gomez-Pinilla F. Dietary omega-3 fatty acids normalize BDNF levels, reduce oxidative damage, and counteract learning disability after traumatic brain injury in rats. *J Neurotrauma.* 2004;21(10):1457-1467.

40. Mills JD, Hadley K, Bailes JE. Dietary supplementation with the omega-3 fatty acid docosahexaenoic acid in traumatic brain injury. *Neurosurgery.* 2011; 88(2):474-478.

41. Harper M, Thom E, Klebanoff MA, et al. Omega-3 fatty acid supplementation to prevent recurrent preterm birth: a randomized controlled trial. *Obstet Gynecol.* 2010;115(2 Pt 1):234-242. doi:10.1097/AOG.0b013e3181cbd60e

42. Anzalone A, Carbuhn A, Jones L, et al. The omega-3 index in National Collegiate Athletic Association Division I collegiate football athletes. *J Athl Train.* 2019;54(1):7-11. doi:10.4085/1062-6050-387-18

43. Wilson, PB, Madrigal LA. Associations among omega-3 fatty acid status, anxiety and mental toughness in female collegiate athletes. *J Am Coll Nutr.* 2017;36(8):602-607.

44. Amen DG, Wu JC, Taylor D, Willeumier K. Reversing brain damage in former NFL players: implications for traumatic brain injury and substance abuse rehabilitation. *J Psychoactive Drugs.* 2011;43(1):1-5.

45. Oliver JM, Jones MT, Kirk KM, et al. Effect of docosahexaenoic acid on biomarker of head trauma in American football. *Med Sci Sport Exerc.* 2016;48(6):974-982.

46. Guzmán JF, Esteve H, Pablos C, Pablos A, Blasco C, Villegas JA. DHA-rich fish oil improves complex reaction time in female elite soccer players. *J Sports Sci Med.* 2011;10(2):301-305.

47. Klivenyi P, Ferrante R, Matthews R, et al. Neuroprotective effects of creatine in a transgenic animal model of amyotrophic lateral sclerosis. *Nat Med.* 1999;5(3):347-350.

48. Sakellaris G, Nasis G, Kotsiou M, Tamiolaki M, Charissis G, Evangeliou A. Prevention of traumatic headache, dizziness and fatigue with creatine administration. A pilot study. *Acta Paediatr.* 2008;97(1):31-34. doi:10.1111/j.1651-2227.2007.00529

49. Sakellaris G, Kotsiou M, Tamiolaki M, et al. Prevention of complications related to traumatic brain injury in children and adolescents with creatine administration. An open label randomised pilot study. *J Trauma.* 2006;61:322-329.

50. Sullivan PG, Geiger JD, Mattson MP, et al. Dietary supplement creatine protects against traumatic brain injury. *Ann Neurol.* 2000;48(5):723-729.

Chapter 9

Nutrition for the Newly Active

Cathy Tillery, MS, RD, CSSD, LD

Commission on Accreditation of Athletic Training Education *2020 Standards*

This chapter addresses the following *2020 Standards for Accreditation of Professional Athletic Training Programs*:

- Standard 55: Students must gain foundational knowledge in statistics, research design, epidemiology, pathophysiology, biomechanics and pathomechanics, exercise physiology, nutrition, human anatomy, pharmacology, public health, and health care delivery and payor systems.

- Standard 58: Incorporate patient education and self-care programs to engage patients and their families and friends to participate in their care and recovery.

- Standard 61: Practice in collaboration with other health care and wellness professionals.

- Standard 69: Develop a care plan for each patient. The care plan includes (but is not limited to) the following:
  - Assessment of the patient on an ongoing basis and adjustment of care accordingly
  - Consideration of the patient's goals and level of function in treatment decisions
  - Referral when warranted

- Standard 77: Identify, refer, and give support to patients with behavioral health conditions. Work with other health care professionals to monitor these patients' treatment, compliance, progress, and readiness to participate.

- Standard 83: Educate and make recommendations to clients/patients on fluids and nutrients to ingest prior to activity, during activity, and during recovery for a variety of activities and environmental conditions.

Knoblauch M, ed. *Clinical Nutrition in Athletic Training* (pp 99-109).

Introduction

Starting a new exercise routine can be daunting. For any health professional, working with an individual who has decided to embark on a new exercise journey for the first time requires navigating many myths and misconceptions in the muddied waters of nutrition. For these individuals, views on nutrition have often been shaped by a myriad of sources such as friends, teammates, books, or the internet. While some of the information may be helpful and accurate, the information may be biased, without scientific facts, or possibly harmful. Many times individuals fall short of seeking counsel from professionals for expert advice, instead relying on friends and family or the internet as the expert. With the immense amount of information at their fingertips, decisions about what to eat, how to eat, and when to eat can often be decided upon based on popular fad diets, professional endorsements, and the marketing push of multimillion-dollar companies. This leaves consumers with conflicting advice that is often not backed by scientific research, in turn leading to risky and dangerous diet practices. As an athletic training professional, it is essential to provide accurate knowledge as it relates to health and performance in this group of newly active individuals.

The goal of this chapter is to provide the most up-to-date, evidence-based nutritional guidelines that the athletic training professional can use to ensure their clients receive nutritional recommendations that are consistent and accurate across the medical, sports and fitness, and nutrition disciplines. Newly active individuals exposed to consistent nutrition messages will be better able to navigate and succeed in the journey to achieve a more active and healthier lifestyle. General nutrition guidelines for macronutrients (eg, carbohydrates, proteins, fats) and micronutrients (eg, vitamins, minerals) will be addressed along with popular myths, misconceptions, and often poor nutrition practices inherent to many newly active individuals in order to guide them toward a better understanding of nutrition for a newly active lifestyle.

Defining the Newly Active Individual

The newly active individual comes from an incredibly diverse group and from many walks of life. In this chapter, the newly active will be defined as any individual who is initiating a new exercise regimen, whether never having exercised before or after a season of being sedentary. Young or old, healthy or not, these individuals come with set goals in mind and frequently begin their journey without help, ultimately failing before seeking the aid of an athletic training professional for motivation, accountability, and knowledge.

Food Perceptions

All individuals have a perception about food. Some eat to live, while others live to eat. Choices in food are not solely based on knowledge but on cost, emotions, and time. In this high-tech, on-the-go world, most individuals are struggling to get through the day and rarely think about when or where their next meal is coming from. Surveys completed by the US Food and Drug Administration, US Department of Agriculture (USDA), the Food Marketing Institute (FMI), and the Academy of Nutrition and Dietetics show Americans have a mixed amount of knowledge about food and nutrition and how it relates to disease and health.[1] And despite knowledge, food choices can be dependent on several factors such as attitudes about choosing healthy foods, taste/flavor of healthy foods versus unhealthy foods, and time in which it takes to prepare healthy meals. These attitudes and perceptions are often key components in shaping an individual's diet. The perceived benefit of eating healthy as it relates to cost, time, and palatability of foods will guide the choice between healthy options and unhealthy foods regardless of nutrition knowledge in relation to health and disease.[1] Therefore, the athletic trainer should be mindful of the attitudes and perceptions newly active individuals bring to the "table" in order to help guide them in making better food choices to support their healthier lifestyle.

Food as Fuel

The saying "You are what you eat" is a mantra best used for an individual navigating the waters of a healthy lifestyle for the first time. The Academy of Nutrition and Dietetics along with the Dietitians of Canada and the American College of Sports Medicine recognize energy intake as the cornerstone of the foundation of optimal nutrition. Energy, in terms of food, fuels optimal body functions and allows the body to work properly. Fuel provides the necessary macronutrients (eg, carbohydrates, proteins, fats) along with micronutrients (eg, vitamins, minerals) the body needs to fuel itself—not only for daily activity but also for physical activity.[2]

For the newly active population, the general "rule of thumb" is to focus on a well-balanced diet rich in complex carbohydrates, lean proteins, low fat dairy, and fresh fruits and vegetables. The National Academy of Medicine states in order for individuals to meet daily energy needs, including macronutrients and micronutrients, and also minimizing risk for chronic disease, adults should consume "45% to 65% calories from carbohydrates, 20% to 35% calories from fat, and 10% to 35% from protein."[3] Total calories consumed to meet energy requirements for individuals is based on height, weight, gender, and—perhaps most importantly—activity levels. In general, a well-balanced diet is the cornerstone for the newly active individual. To better illustrate these nutritional intake recommendations, there are several graphic representations of a healthy diet that can be used in suggesting nutrition information. MyPlate at www.choosemyplate.gov or a more detailed version at www.hsph.harvard.edu/nutritionsource/healthy-eating-plate can easily be accessed (Figure 9-1).

In order to properly understand the energy needs and requirements for an individual embarking on an activity-based lifestyle for the first time, it is imperative for the athletic training professional to understand exercise and nutritional goals of the client. Seasoned and elite athletes look to nutrition to achieve optimal performance while nonathletes or newly active individuals typically look to nutrition to achieve optimal health.[4] Proper nutrition can certainly enhance performance; however, for the newly active individual, balanced dietary habits with a solid foundation of proper nutrition can be utilized to improve health and potentially prevent or treat a chronic disease. Proper energy intake and balance are the core concepts for the newly active.

Carbohydrates

Carbohydrates are essential to a healthy diet, but are often at the forefront of controversy when it comes to nutritional habits in the newly active individual. In a world of low-carbohydrate diets such as Paleo, Whole 30, Atkins, and Ketogenic, carbohydrates seem to have become the figurative "enemy" among nutrients. Individuals are opting to forego

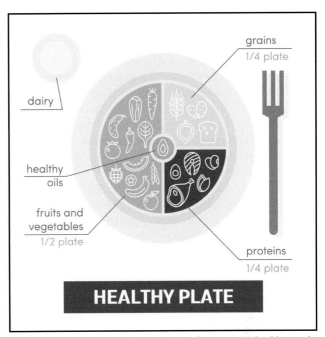

Figure 9-1. An example of a balanced plate for creating a healthy meal. (marina_ua/Shutterstock.com.)

needed fuel for the body by following these low-carbohydrate diets, choosing instead protein and fat and often leaving individuals who undertake these diets feeling tired and fatigued. With good intentions, individuals who take part in these diets cast off carbohydrates with no thought to the central role this macronutrient plays in the body. Carbohydrates supply essential substrates that fuel the body to perform daily tasks and are also imperative for brain function.[5] The body stores needed carbohydrates in the form of glycogen in muscles and liver and, whether an individual is new to exercise or highly trained, energy needs of muscles demand these stored carbohydrates be used as the predominant source of fuel for moderate-intensity exercises.[6] Individuals who opt to substantially decrease their carbohydrate intake in an effort to lose weight impede performance and thereby their ability to reach overall health goals. Research shows that a low-carbohydrate diet will in fact produce weight loss over the short term; however, long-term weight loss cannot be sustained.[7] In addition, research has shown that a diet high in fat and low in carbohydrates may not equate to better exercise efficiency and therefore may not aid in weight loss and can impair performance due to the reduced exercise efficiency, thereby reducing overall performance and calories burned.[8] Because carbohydrates are the predominant fuel during exercise, newly active individuals should be encouraged to consume complex carbohydrates such as whole wheat pasta, brown rice, or starchy vegetables like sweet potatoes. Allowing individuals to understand the need for carbohydrates as fuel to the newly exercising muscles allows for better performance and overall increased energy expenditure.

Protein

With the rise in popularity of high-protein diets, protein has become the cornerstone of many diets in the newly active population. In an attempt to lose weight, gain muscle, or improve overall health, individuals are looking to proteins as a main energy source. High-quality proteins are essential to the body to aid in protein synthesis and are needed for muscle recovery and repair after exercise. A diet that excludes or severely restricts a whole macronutrient group such as carbohydrates hinders the job of proteins in building and repairing muscle, particularly when protein is being relied upon for energy needs.[2] In addition, when previously sedentary individuals become active, severely limiting carbohydrate intake leads to fatigue and poor exercise performance.[8] Still, it is worth noting that protein needs vary per individual and are dependent upon type and intensity of exercise and the quality of protein being consumed.[9] It is generally recognized that healthy sedentary adults, or those adults initiating exercise for the first time, should consume no more than 0.8 to 0.9 g of protein/kg/body weight per day or no more than 10% to 35% of calories from protein to meet daily protein requirements.[3] In contrast, protein needs of athletes can reach the upper limits of 2 g of protein/kg/body weight per day.[9] Because the newly active individual is not expected to be exercising to the degree of a seasoned or elite athlete, the higher protein intake recommendations for athletes is not advised. All individuals should be encouraged to consume high-quality lean proteins. Good sources of lean protein are chicken, turkey, beef, pork, or fish. For vegetarians, opt for dried beans, tofu, or low-fat dairy. If individuals opt for convenience, protein supplements, with quality protein sources from whey and casein, are suggested.[10]

Fat

Fat is an essential macronutrient in all diets, facilitating the absorption of fat-soluble vitamins, providing energy, and serving as a vital component of cell membranes. Fats, in the form of free fatty acids, fuel muscle contractions during light to moderate exercise intensities and during long-duration exercises.[2] Whether an individual is newly active, sedentary, or an elite athlete, the *Dietary Guidelines for Americans* for fat remain the same. Individuals should consume 20% to 25% of total calorie intake from fat, with no more than 10% of their total caloric intake consisting of saturated fats.[3] Clients should be encouraged to choose lean proteins, low-fat dairy, and fresh fruits and vegetables to help them stay within the target guidelines and contribute to the consumption of a balanced diet.

Micronutrients (Vitamins and Minerals)

When it comes to vitamins and minerals for the newly active, individuals need only to meet the USDA recommended daily allowance. Exceeding the RDA is not advised and can even be contraindicated, especially for fat-soluble vitamins (vitamins A, D, E, and K) or minerals such as iron.[11] Encouraging a diet that emphasizes fresh fruits and vegetables and a colorful plate helps individuals get the nutrients the body needs without expensive supplements. However, one exception is the active older adult population. Older adults spend less time outside, and whether due to the lack of sunlight exposure or the decrease in the skin's availability to synthesize vitamin D, levels can be suboptimal and result in a decrease in physical performance and therefore may need additional supplementation.[11] For all individuals beginning a new exercise regimen, a diet rich in fresh fruits and vegetables is optimal to provide them with vitamins and minerals.

Hydration

In the human body, up to 60% of body weight is water. A delicate balance is maintained between total body water and hydration status and any deviation from this normal range, even at levels as little as 1% to 3%, can compromise health and organ function as well as decrease exercise performance.[12] For the purposes of the newly active individual, the athletic training professional is on the front line in helping individuals become more aware of beverage intake, relying on water as a primary hydration medium. The newly active person's exercise endeavors typically do not reach the intensity and duration that more seasoned and professional athletes perform at and therefore require a less structure hydration plan. (See Chapter 5 for a complete and comprehensive guide to hydration and fluid intake.) The athletic training professional should encourage individuals to focus on fluid intake throughout the day, keeping a water bottle accessible at all times and drinking even before feeling thirsty. Adding fresh fruits, vegetables, or herbs such as blackberries, cucumber, and mint can tremendously improve flavor and palatability to plain water—helping individuals increase daily consumption. By encouraging individuals to focus on hydration each day, the detrimental effects of dehydration can be avoided.

Sports Performance Beverages

Sports and electrolyte replacement beverages have become the preferred choice in locker rooms and conference rooms across the nation. From Little League fields to executive meeting rooms, consumers tend to believe the hype associated with sports drinks specific to rehydration and fueling of active muscles. Sports performance beverage companies make billions of dollars each year using professional athletes

Sidebar 9-1

Sports performance beverages do have a place in the diet for the newly active individual who is participating in athletic endeavors lasting greater than 1 hour, such as those undertaking their first marathon. For an athletic event lasting greater than 1 hour, consuming 30 to 60 g of carbohydrates per hour is recommended and can be easily obtained in a 20-ounce sports beverage that contains ~38 g of carbohydrates.

Sidebar 9-2

Recently, there has been an increase in popularity of athletic events that promote alcohol and reward its participants with beer or wine at the finish line. With races with names such as Run the Vineyards Wines and Vines, Lose Your Resolution Beer Run, or Fueled by Wine half marathon, the newly active or the "weekend warrior" is encouraged to "drink up" after races. The attractive appeal to these races entices participants to "throw caution to the wind" and engage in drinking after the event to celebrate their victory of crossing the finish line. However, studies show alcohol consumption after an event negatively impacts muscle damage recovery by impairing protein synthesis, and leads to negative gains in the area of resistance training.[13] The newly active individuals should be cautioned about the effects of postrace alcohol consumption and whether or not the practice fits into their overall health goals.

to endorse products promising better performance. Water is perceived to no longer be sufficient to achieve top-level sports performance and appears incapable of adequately hydrating even the "average Joe." To those individuals aware of the latest sports beverage marketing tactics, water must now have additional electrolytes and carbohydrates to fuel any and all exercise. But for the common exerciser or the newly active individual, sports performance drinks serve only to add additional calories. In fact, the position stance of the Academy of Nutrition and Dietetics, Dietitians of Canada, and the American College of Sports Medicine is that carbohydrates are not needed for activities lasting less than 45 minutes, and only small or minimal amounts of carbohydrates are needed for those individual participating in activities 45 to 75 minutes in length.[2] Because most individuals who are beginning to participate in an active lifestyle or sports activity fit into these 2 exercise-duration categories, additional carbohydrate consumption in the form of sports beverages is not warranted (Sidebar 9-1).

Alcohol

Alcohol intake is a considerable factor when it comes to the newly active individual. For any athletic trainer who is working with an individual who is transitioning from a sedentary lifestyle, alcohol consumption should be addressed. Surprisingly, research shows individuals who participate in regular activity consume alcohol at higher rates than sedentary individuals.[13] The consumption of alcohol in excess can lead to detrimental consequences for the newly active individual and has deleterious effects on an individual's overall health and athletic performance. Alcohol can affect muscle recovery, promote dehydration, and lead to poor and uncontrolled food choices as alcohol lowers inhibitions. The athletic trainer has an important role in helping individuals make smarter and healthier choices when it comes to alcohol intake and exercising. By highlighting the impact alcohol can have on exercise recovery, excessive calorie intake, and the potential to hinder the achievement of health and wellness goals, athletic trainers can help individuals navigate alcohol intake and its place in their newly active lifestyle (Sidebar 9-2).

Myths and Misconceptions

In consideration of the diet recommendations for the newly active individual, it is imperative for athletic trainers to be able to incorporate, understand, and process the thoughts and attitudes that clients often bring to the table. Will taste, cost, and convenience inhibit lifestyle change and diet modification, or is nutrition knowledge enough to promote healthy nutrition choices? When it comes to macronutrients and micronutrients, do individuals understand nutritional guidelines set forth by the USDA or will they rely on current trends found on the internet to make diet choices? The physical, emotional, and psychological reasons behind food choices and behaviors are vast and often difficult to change. The key for the athletic training professional is to work with individuals to identify obstacles and to develop strategies to improve the likelihood of behavior change in order to achieve optimal health.

Foundational Nutrition

The idea of solid foundational nutrition is often confused in the newly active individual. When an individual embarks on a new journey to become active nutrition comes to the forefront, with greater attention given to the questions "What should I be eating?", "How should I be eating?", and "When should I be eating?" Often the newly active individual ignores the need to stand fast on solid foundational nutrition and general healthy nutrition guidelines and forges ahead to sport-specific nutrition guidelines. Relying on anecdotal information found on Facebook groups, message boards, or social media that have no scientific backing, individuals find themselves embarking on nutritional strategies utilized by professional athletes instead of the recreational or newly active. Suddenly, a teenage football player tries to maintain the diet of a 350-pound lineman from the Dallas Cowboys that, based on metabolism and energy demand differences between the 2 individuals, will almost assuredly result in unwanted weight gain for the newly active individual. Similarly, a newbie to running who sets out to mimic the training diet of a 2-hour marathoner may trigger gastric issues from the improper use of energy gels and sports drinks. Or the newly active individual seeking weight loss begins a "cleanse" and suffers fatigue and headaches from inadequate energy intake and caffeine withdrawal. These are just a few examples of common mishaps seen with the newly active. As an athletic training professional, guiding individuals to start with a foundation in good nutrition is paramount. Steering individuals back to the basics of consuming a nutrient-rich diet found in whole foods and eating minimally processed foods is the backbone and cornerstone of foundational nutrition.

Popular Nutrition Practices

There are a multitude of diet and nutrition practices gaining popularity and momentum around the country. For the newly active individual, these practices have a certain appeal as individuals try to meet health and wellness goals. The list of popular diets is exhaustive, and a complete and comprehensive review can be found in Chapter 13. But for the purpose of this chapter, gluten-free diets, organic foods, and intermittent fasting will be the focus as they are relevant to the diet practices of the newly active individual. The role of the athletic training professional is to provide clients information and education around these nutrition topics while emphasizing a well-balanced diet rich in complex carbohydrates, lean proteins, fresh fruits and vegetables, and low-fat dairy.

Gluten-Free Diet

The number of individuals going "gluten-free" has increased tremendously over the last few years due to celebrity endorsements and purported health claims. In 2013 a study found "65% of American adults think gluten-free foods are healthier, and 27% choose gluten-free products to aid in weight loss."[14] The gluten-free diet has been heralded as a panacea for weight loss, improved athletic performance, and medical management of conditions such as chronic fatigue, diabetes, or gastrointestinal issues.[15] For the approximately 1% of the population that has celiac disease, the gluten-free diet is a true therapeutic diet and absolute necessity. However, for the newly active individual looking to improve optimal health, the gluten-free diet often provides no benefits other than eliminating poor food choices.[14] When faced with clients who are inquiring about beginning a gluten-free

diet, educating individuals on gluten-free products and suggesting gluten-free modifications such as gluten-free breads and grains is appropriate, along with emphasizing a well-balanced diet filled with fruits and vegetables and lean proteins. A referral to a gastroenterologist and a gastrointestinal specialist dietitian is warranted if an individual exhibits a true gluten allergy or if a sensitivity with symptoms of gastrointestinal upset occurs after gluten-free modification.

Organic Foods

Organic foods, just like "gluten-free," have become somewhat of an obsession in the American diet. Strict and comprehensive guidelines have been established by the USDA for organic labeling for produce, meat, and processed foods. In general, foods that meet the USDA organic standards "prohibit food from containing artificial preservatives, colors, or flavors."[16] Today, organic-based diets have become a multibillion-dollar food industry. Eating "organic" is considered by consumers to be the figurative "Ferrari" of diet options. As with gluten-free products, a food that is labeled as organic is not always nutritionally superior. In providing recommendations to the newly active, education geared toward balanced, healthy eating is the key—and an understanding of organic food options should be a part of this education. If a person desires to consume predominantly organic-type foods, encourage healthy choices such as fresh fruits and vegetables as well as organically raised antibiotic- and hormone-free meats and dairy. A pantry full of organic snack foods such as organic pretzels, snack crackers, or cookies will not make for a healthy diet. To be clear, an organic Oreo (Mondelez International) is still an Oreo! These "organic" snack foods could still have a high sodium content, sugar content, or be a highly processed food, which would counter any benefit of eating organic (Sidebar 9-3).

Intermittent Fasting

Fasting in its many different forms has been around almost since the creation of humans. Historically seen in the setting of religion, fasting has now been propelled to the forefront of diet practices due to celebrity endorsements and the attention of the mainstream media. The term "fasting" can encompass a variety of fasts: from a complete withholding of food to the more popular intermittent fast, which also has its own subset of varieties. For the purpose of this chapter, the term "intermittent fasting" will be defined as caloric intake restriction over a designated period of the day, followed by an ad libitum caloric intake for the remainder of the day. Most popular among the newly active population is the 16/8 intermittent fast, in which individuals remain in a 16-hour state of fast and allow for 8 hours of ad libitum eating during the remainder of the day (ie, fasting from 8 pm to noon, ad libitum eating noon to 8 pm).[17] Why are newly active individuals drawn to fasting? There are a multitude of reasons behind the

Sidebar 9-3

A family client of mine asked me to come to their house to help them clean out their pantry in light of the new meal plan I had designed for them. They had had 1 month to work with the plan, grocery shop, and make diet changes. When I arrived at their house, I dove right into the pantry. I pulled out 3 boxes of organic snack crackers, 3 bags of organic chips, 1 sleeve of organic cookies, 5 boxes of organic (refined white flour) mac and cheese, 2 boxes of organic cereal, and 6 packages of ramen noodles (non-organic). What remained in their pantry were less-processed foods such as whole grain pastas, rice, dried legumes, rolled and steel cut oats, among other products. I emphasized replacing snack foods, such as the organic cookies and chips, with fresh fruits and vegetables, low-fat yogurt and low-fat cheeses, and hummus. The pantry looked quite bare as I left, but it was full of whole grain products that would provide a solid source of fuel for their active lifestyle.

Sidebar 9-4

A pantry stocked full of healthy foods and snacks is the first line of defense against poor food choices. When faced with preparing a healthy snack and grabbing a bag of chips, convenience wins every single time. Encouraging clients to have handy "grab and go" snacks is essential to healthy eating. Stocking the refrigerator with low-fat yogurt, low-fat cheeses in individual servings, and precut fruits and vegetables makes healthy snacking easy and convenient. When it comes to the pantry, individual servings of nuts, trail mix, granola bars, and/or dried fruits help eliminate the urge to grab junk food when hunger cravings abound.

choice to fast; however, within this population the desire for weight loss and improved health is pervasive. For the athletic training professional working with the newly active individual practicing intermittent fasting, emphasis should remain on the individual consuming a well-balanced diet that is rich in complex carbohydrates, lean proteins, an array of fruits and vegetables, and low-fat dairy, whether this occurs over a 24-hour period of time or an 8-hour period of time.

Nutritional Pitfalls of the Newly Active Individual

Despite being armed with up-to-date, scientific-based nutrition knowledge, the newly actively athlete can fail at their efforts to make significant diet changes due to improper preparation and organization. Whether from inappropriate meal timing, poor meal planning and preparation, or improper fueling for performance, these pitfalls can wreak havoc on the newly active individual. The athletic training professional has a fundamental role in helping individuals organize their nutrition plans in order to bring about change and maintain long-term healthy eating goals.

Planning and Organizing

For the newly active individual, poor planning and organization can quickly defeat even the most well-laid-out plans to eat nutritionally for optimal health. Unlike most elite athletes who have personalized plans, private chefs, and refrigerators and pantries stocked with healthy foods to fuel performance, most newly active individuals have limited time due to constraints of work and family life. Said simply, work–life balance often gets in the way of preparing and organizing meals to promote healthy choices. For the average individual, kitchens often lack healthy snack options with pantry shelves lined with highly processed junk foods and refrigerators full of sodas and "take out" while lacking in fresh whole foods. Providing individuals with practical tips for meal prep and organizing is the first step to helping individuals eat healthy for their new active lifestyle (Sidebar 9-4).

Menus and Meal Planning

For a multitude of individuals, the road to fueling properly for their new active lifestyle is met with roadblocks and potholes due to improper menu planning. In today's fast-paced, on-the-go lifestyle, eating healthy is difficult. When met with the question of "What's for dinner?", individuals without a plan often succumb to convenience. Drive thrus, take out, and meal delivery services dominate the landscape of dinner options and further prevent individuals from achieving optimal success when it comes to healthy eating. However, individuals can improve the likelihood of eating healthy meals by creating menus, making a grocery list, and food shopping each week. Those who have planned menus, know precisely what is for dinner, and have prepared all the ingredients are better equipped to succeed in reaching health and wellness goals. It is no secret, planning, shopping, and preparing takes time and effort, but having minimally processed homemade meals provides the fuel that an active individual needs to succeed in achieving optimal health (Sidebar 9-5).

Sidebar 9-5

Creating weekly menus can seem daunting to the newly active individual. Most individuals feel like time and cost inhibit the likelihood of preparing freshly made meals at home. The internet is a useful tool for menu planning. Apps and sites such as Pinterest can make menu planning simple and easy while adding variety. Using the USDA's MyPlate (www.choosemyplate.gov) provides a solid foundation and ensures each meal has a lean protein, a complex carbohydrate, and ample fresh fruits and vegetables. Not every individual will prepare gourmet or 5-star cuisine like Gordon Ramsay or Martha Stewart, however, choosing to prepare healthy homemade meals can be both rewarding and effective in achieving health goals.

Sidebar 9-6

A 47-year-old female client contacted me to help her prepare for a 3-day "walk for a cause" event. The event would cover 15 to 22 miles per day over a 3-day time period. Her training consisted of 4 days of walking per week, starting with 1-mile walks and then increasing to a goal of a single, long-training walk of 15 miles each week. Her goal was to achieve a healthier lifestyle and lose weight. At her initial consultation, she weighed 165 pounds with her estimated needs to be ~1400 to 1600 kcals/day on nontraining days and ~1900 to 2400 kcals on training days. She was given a meal plan and educated on a well-balanced diet for exercise and weight loss. At her follow-up appointment, 3 months later, she had gained 10 pounds. After a careful review of her diet log, it was apparent she was deviating from her original meal plan and consuming ~2500 calories on training days. In discussion, she held to the belief, "I can reward myself with extra food because I'm exercising"—often eating out and consuming desserts on training days. Through our discussion, she quickly realized that exercise doesn't equate to eating "whatever!" After reinforcing calorie intake and calorie goals, with emphasis on a balanced diet that incorporated an occasional "treat meal" or dessert indulgence, she began to lose weight and reported an improvement in her training.

Meal Timing

Meal timing is an essential aspect of the newly active individual's daily nutritional intake. Questions begin to arise when it comes to timing of food, with many struggling with the answers for "Should I eat breakfast?" "How late is too late to eat?" or "What should I eat before and after an event?" Also, do the answers to these questions differ for the newly active individual as compared to a conditioned athlete? As with any individual, whether it is a professional athlete or an individual starting to exercise for the first time, nutrient timing is going to be individualized based on time of activity, intensity, and duration. Just like no 2 individuals are alike, no 2 nutrition plans are alike. Impressing upon individuals to consume a healthy well-balanced diet that includes meals and snacks is the first line of defense in preparing to engage in an active lifestyle. For individuals seeking personalized meal plans to develop timing of meals and snacks for daily activity and exercise, a referral to a registered dietitian is warranted.

Improper Fueling for Performance

As stated from the beginning, the newly active individual comes from an incredibly diverse group and from many walks of life, bringing nutritional biases, beliefs, and habits to the table on their journey to seek an active lifestyle. Athletic trainers have a unique opportunity as the front-line expert to guide individuals to avoid pitfalls from improper fueling for sports performance, whether it be overindulging, using improper fueling techniques, or trying new practices on race day. Steering the newly active individual back to basic solid nutrition practices of consuming a well-balanced diet rich in complex carbohydrates, lean proteins, low-fat dairy, and fresh fruits and vegetables will bring success in every endeavor.

Food as a Reward

Indulging in excess caloric intake, or "bingeing," is another practice often seen in the newly active person. Perhaps unfortunately, the concept of food as a reward for exercise is pervasive. "I deserve it" often predominates an individual's mindset, and energy expended through exercise is often overcompensated with a high-calorie meal postexercise. This use of food as a reward for training is especially true for those whose endeavors involve a first-time training for events such as a marathon, triathlon or multiple-day events. For the newly active individual, a balanced diet consisting of whole grain carbohydrates, lean proteins, low-fat dairy foods, and a variety of fruits and vegetables is the cornerstone to achieving a healthy lifestyle (Sidebar 9-6).

Race Day Mistakes

It is not uncommon for the newly active individual to adhere to strict and rigid exercise and diet regimens for months, only to the watch their hard work "go down in flames" on race day. Whether due to trying out new foods, tackling race day nerves and jitters, or experimenting with new nutritional strategies, individuals can sabotage months

Sidebar 9-7

The timeless practice of carbohydrate loading before an endurance event is recognized across many generations. In a study published by Bergström et al. in 1967, they discussed the idea of carbohydrate loading, stating "The muscle glycogen concentration in man can be considerably increased by first emptying the glycogen stores through hard work, and then giving a carbohydrate rich diet."[18] Over the past 50 years, research in the area of carbohydrate loading and carbohydrate intake before competition has been widely studied and established; however, the training and nutritional complexities involved in carbohydrate loading is highly unlikely to be properly performed and accomplished in the newly active population and therefore is not recommended.

Sidebar 9-8

A 35-year-old male, former Division I collegiate athlete, signed up to run his first ever 10K race. Having been an athlete in his teens and early 20s he had a framework of nutrition knowledge. The night before his race, he attempted to "carbohydrate load" by consuming a large Italian dinner at a local eating establishment, overindulging on pasta and bread. On race morning, he awoke feeling "bloated" and "heavy" and unable to consume breakfast. After completing the race, he reported he was only able to run a portion of the race and was forced to walk the remaining distance due to GI distress during the race. This simple diet mistake of making a poor diet choice the night before his race ruined his race opportunity, thereby ruining his chance to see what his training gained him. As a result, he will have to enter another race and continue to train at a race-training pace to see what he is capable of running in a 10K race in when fueled appropriately.

of training with improper race day fueling. Athletic trainers must stress the importance of diet consistency with the solid stance, "Nothing new is ever tried on race day, EVER!" To prevent suboptimal performance or, even worse, having to pay for and enter a new race because of poor choices, individuals should adhere to eating practices they have used during training (Sidebars 9-7 through 9-9).

Special Populations

Numerous individuals move from a sedentary to active lifestyle as a result of a health concern or crisis. Whether it is cardiovascular disease, diabetes, cancer, or obesity, athletic trainers will encounter individuals with special needs both physically and nutritionally. Understanding those needs and considerations is pivotal, as what is advisable for one individual or population group may possibly be inadvisable or unsafe for another. Additionally, assessing and providing nutritional advice for these special populations may well be outside the scope of practice of an athletic trainer, and a referral to a clinical or sports dietitian is warranted. Encouraging a balanced diet rich in complex carbohydrates, fresh fruits and vegetables, lean proteins, low-fat dairy, and low fats is the goal. Specific recommendations should be avoided and left to a registered dietitian who specializes in these areas (Sidebar 9-10).

Tweens and Teens

The final consideration is the ever-increasing "tween" and teenage newly active population. According to *Cambridge Dictionary*, tweens are defined as a young person between the ages of approximately 8 to 12 years old. Despite the size of some teenagers, kids in the prepuberty and puberty development stages should not be considered as "little adults." The

Sidebar 9-9

A 41-year-old male client met with me to help him clean up his diet and provide a nutrition training regimen to coincide with his goal of completing his first triathlon. During the training phase, he had issues with calf cramping during the later portion of his cycling and into his run. We adjusted his sodium and potassium intake, working with food sources and electrolyte replacements during longer training sessions. Training sessions were going great; however, on race day, all went well until the run portion where he experienced severe leg cramps. After a careful review of his diet intake and his fluid intake on race day it was evident that he deviated from the diet and hydration plan he had been following during his training. Due to nerves and his fear of becoming dehydrated, he overhydrated and veered from his nutritional plan that was working. This simple deviation in his diet caused deleterious effects on his expected outcome, leading him to enter and train again for another race.

individualized needs of tweens and teens change depending on the stage of puberty and development. Prior to puberty, nutritional needs and requirements for boys and girls are the same, but once puberty is reached, an individual's physical maturity, physical activity level, and the nutrition and exercise goals must be taken into consideration.[19]

Sidebar 9-10

Special populations can be a challenge to the athletic trainer when addressing the nutritional needs of these individuals and giving appropriate nutritional advice and guidance. Such populations who warrant a referral to a dietitian include, but are not limited to, those with eating disorders, pregnancy, new onset diabetes, cancer, undergoing chemotherapy or radiation, or those who have experienced a recent heart attack or stroke. Individuals in these categories may require specialized diet intervention outside the scope of practice and knowledge of the athletic training professional. Providing clients with an interdisciplinary approach to their training by incorporating a dietitian can improve client outcomes and elevate your level of professionalism as seen by both your client and other disciplines.

It cannot be stated enough, habits that begin in adolescence can be carried over to adulthood and helping the tween and teen establish a well-balanced eating plan is of utmost importance in this age group. During this time, tweens and teens need enough nutrients to support adequate growth, tissue maintenance, and tissue repair to perform both physically and mentally, but not in excess, which could lead to childhood obesity. The consequences of poor eating habits among tweens and teens can lead to health concerns such as high blood pressure, type 2 diabetes, or gastric reflux. In addition, kids with obesity have a greater propensity of being adults with obesity with an increased likelihood of developing heart disease, diabetes, or cancer as adults.[20] Though tweens and teens may not see or understand the benefit of eating healthy to prevent disease, they feel deeply the social stigma of being overweight with many dealing with body image issues or even eating disorder behaviors. The main goal for the athletic training professional is to provide basic nutrition advice and guidance, while answering the questions "What are carbohydrates, proteins, and fats?" and "What are the best sources to obtain them?" The aim is to help young adolescents grow, provide fuel for the exercising muscles, and achieve overall sound healthy eating habits. Athletic training professionals should emphasize the importance of a healthy and balanced diet with good sources of complex carbohydrates, lean proteins, low-fat dairy, and lots of fruits and vegetables.

The job of the athletic training professional is to encourage their newly active clients toward optimal health and a new, active lifestyle. Although they are not expected to provide one-on-one nutrition counseling, the athletic training professional is on the figurative "front line," specific to an athlete's, patient's, or client's nutritional concerns and diet choices. Guiding each individual to consume a well-balanced and well-rounded nutrition plan is vital. Encouraging eating at home by preparing fresh foods, loading plates with fruits and vegetables, cutting down on highly processed foods, and avoiding fast foods goes a long way in preventing disease and can help establish habits that can last a lifetime.

Conclusion

Newly active individuals are a unique population who, given their newfound interest in physical activity, crave nutritional advice. Because this group may have limited nutritional knowledge, it is vital for athletic trainers to stress the importance of a well-rounded nutrition plan. It is equally important to stress to this population that there is no magic pill nor magic diet that will make weight loss or achieving fitness goals easier. As with a well-rounded exercise plan, diet and nutritional success takes consistency, planning, hard work, and the desire to improve. Making healthy choices as well as planning and preparing in advance is a must. Emphasis should always be focused toward moderation and healthy eating, consuming whole grains, lean proteins, fresh fruits and vegetables, and low-fat dairy. Emphasize to all newly active individuals that no one is perfect; equally, no diet will ever be perfect—moderation is the goal. Athletic trainers should also be able to recognize when a higher level of nutritional guidance is needed; in such cases the athletic trainer should refer the newly active individual to a registered dietitian. Working closely with the client and a nutrition professional promotes a lifetime of optimal health and success for the newly active individual.

Discussion Questions

1. When making nutrition recommendations to the newly active individual, would sport-specific guidelines be addressed as a first round of discussion or would general nutrition practices and guidelines be the starting point for discussion? Why?
2. How might a newly active individual be advised to change their eating behaviors or patterns when training for their first athletic event/race when their goal is weight loss? Why?

References

1. Guthrie JF, Derby BM, Levy AS. What people know and do not know about nutrition. In: *What People Know.* USDA/ERS; 2019:243-274.

2. Thomas DT, Erdman KA, Burke LM. Position of the Academy of Nutrition and Dietetics, Dietitians of Canada, and the American College of Sports Medicine: nutrition and athletic performance [published correction appears in *J Acad Nutr Diet.* 2017;117(1):146]. *J Acad Nutr Diet.* 2016;116(3):501-528.

3. Institute of Medicine. *Dietary Reference Intakes for Energy, Carbohydrate, Fiber, Fat, Fatty Acids, Cholesterol, Protein, and Amino Acids.* The National Academies Press; 2005.

4. Braun, B, Miller BF. Nutrition, physical activity, and health. In: Maughan RJ, ed. *Sports Nutrition.* Wiley Blackwell; 2014:455-465.

5. Burke, LM. Carbohydrate needs of athletes in training. In: Maughan RJ, ed. *Sports Nutrition.* Wiley Blackwell; 2014:102-112.

6. Coleman, EJ. Carbohydrate and exercise. In: Rosenbloom CA, ed. *Sports Nutrition: A Practice Manual for Professionals.* Academy of Nutrition and Dietetics; 2012:16-35.

7. Noble CA, Kushner RF. An update on low-carbohydrate, high-protein diets. *Curr Opin Gastroenterol.* 2006;22(2):153-159.

8. Burke LM, Ross ML, Garvican-Lewis LA, et al. Low carbohydrate, high fat diet impairs exercise economy and negates the performance benefit from intensified training in elite race walkers. *J Physiol.* 2017;595(9):2785-2807.

9. Phillips, SM. Defining optimum protein intakes for athletes. In: Maughan RJ, ed. *Sports Nutrition.* Wiley Blackwell; 2014:136-146.

10. Jäger R, Kerksick CM, Campbell BI, et al. International Society of Sports Nutrition position stand: protein and exercise. *J Int Soc Sports Nutr.* 2017;14:20.

11. Volpe SL, Bland E. Vitamins, minerals, and exercise. In: Rosenbloom CA, ed. *Sports Nutrition A Practice Manual for Professionals.* Academy of Nutrition and Dietetics; 2012:75-105.

12. McDermott BP, Anderson SA, Armstrong LE, et al. National Athletic Trainers' Association position statement: fluid replacement for the physically active. *J Athl Train.* 2017;52(9):877-895.

13. Duplanty AA, Budnar RG, Luk HY, et al. Effect of acute alcohol ingestion on resistance exercise-induced mTORC1 signaling in human muscle. *J Strength Cond Res.* 2017;31(1):54-61.

14. Jones AL. The gluten-free diet: fad or necessity? *Diabetes Spectr.* 2017;30(2):118-123.

15. Johanson L. The gluten-free frenzy: fad or fitting? *Medsurg Nurs.* 2015;24(4):213-217.

16. McEvoy M. Organic 101: what is the USDA organic label mean. United States Department of Agriculture. Published March 13, 2019. Accessed April 13, 2019.

17. Levy E, Chu T. Intermittent fasting and its effects on athletic performance: a review. *Curr Sports Med Rep.* 2019;18(7):266-269.

18. Bergström J, Hermansen L, Hultman E, Saltin B. Diet, muscle glycogen and physical performance. *Acta Physiol Scand.* 1967;71(2):140-150.

19. Hoch AZ, Goossen K, Kretschmer T. Nutritional requirements of the child and teenage athlete. *Phys Med Rehabil Clin N Am.* 2008;19:373-398.

20. Centers for Disease Control and Prevention. Childhood obesity causes and consequences. Published December 15, 2016. Accessed April 8, 2020.

Chapter 10

Activity-Based Nutrition

Melissa Brown, PhD, RD, CSSD, LD

Commission on Accreditation of Athletic Training Education *2020 Standards*

This chapter addresses the following *2020 Standards for Accreditation of Professional Athletic Training Programs*:

- Standard 62: Provide athletic training services in a manner that uses evidence to inform practice.
- Standard 82: Develop, implement, and supervise comprehensive programs to maximize sport performance that are safe and specific to the client's activity.
- Standard 83: Educate and make recommendations to clients/patients on fluids and nutrients to ingest prior to activity, during activity, and during recovery for a variety of activities and environmental conditions.

Learning Objectives

After reviewing this chapter, readers will be able to:

- Explain the importance of understanding the energy systems in use for specific types of activity in order to appropriately select nutrition strategies to optimize performance.
- Identify the optimal nutrition strategies for fueling athletes before, during, and after training and competition based on the type of activity and individual needs.
- Describe the common pitfalls, dietary deficiencies, and limitations observed in athletes from each type of activity.

Knoblauch M, ed. *Clinical Nutrition in Athletic Training* (pp 111-120).
© 2023 Taylor & Francis Group.

Introduction

The field of sports nutrition has evolved into a complex specialty area with sports dietitians as the recognized experts in the field. However, the field is still growing and sports dietitians are not always readily available for athletes, and active individuals have even less access typically. As the member of the sports medicine team that typically has the most frequent contact with the athletes, the responsibility of providing knowledge in all areas, including nutrition, often falls to the athletic trainer. Athletic trainers are often expected to provide basic evidence-based nutrition and fluid recommendations to clients based on specific activities, despite relatively little focused training in nutrition. Therefore, it is critical for athletic trainers to have a basic understanding of the energy systems in use during different types of activity. This basic understanding will allow athletic trainers to recommend appropriate nutritional strategies to help individuals optimize performance. Each individual has their own unique nutrient needs, and these needs may change on a daily basis depending on the type of activity that is planned. For example, the same individual may engage in strength training exercises on certain days and endurance exercises on other days; consequently, the nutrition recommendations must match the energy usage of the specific activity type. The most successful training programs include a well-designed, intentional meal plan that meets energy and nutrient needs with strategic timing built into that plan. In this chapter, the reader will learn how to apply activity-based nutrition strategies to help clients achieve peak performance in conjunction with an individual's nutrient needs for overall health. This chapter will also cover potential pitfalls, nutrient deficiencies, and limitations that common athletes and active adults experience and how to address them. A specific section is included at the end of the chapter that addresses active individuals who are considered separate from athletes. The information in this chapter will help athletic trainers achieve the professional standards for the CAATE listed in the beginning of this chapter.[1]

Common Pitfalls, Nutrient Deficiencies, and Limitations

Throughout this chapter the reader will gain an understanding of some of the more common pitfalls, nutrient deficiencies, and limitations that athletes and active adults experience. The information provided will hopefully help athletic trainers to address these in advance and prevent them whenever possible. Some of the more common nutrient deficiencies affecting performance are inadequate carbohydrate, electrolyte, and fluid intake, as well as inadequate overall energy intake. Frequently skipping meals and scheduled snacks easily leads to athletes failing to meet their energy and nutrient needs. Inadequate intake of carbohydrates, fluids, and electrolytes can result in poor performance related to (among other things) fatigue, dehydration, headaches, nausea, vomiting, and cramping. Two of the biggest limitations for athletes is a lack of nutrition knowledge and finding a credible source of nutrition information. It can be difficult to sift through all the nutrition information that is available on the internet and from various sources and knowing which is based on scientific evidence and which is just a fad or misinformation. Furthermore, athletes often have very busy schedules and feel they do not have enough time to meal plan properly to ensure adequate fueling and hydration. In addition, upon completion of a workout or athletic event, many athletes do not have an appetite and do not want to eat anything. They may instead prefer to enjoy an alcoholic beverage after a training session or competition as part of a social activity. However, most of these athletes are unaware of the effects of alcohol on performance and the training-based recovery process. Lastly, there are pitfalls for active adults as well, such as a general lack of knowledge on what a healthy eating plan should include to sustain an active lifestyle.

Nutrition Strategies for Specific Types of Activity

Metabolic requirements differ based on the type of activity, and these metabolic requirements subsequently dictate the optimal fueling strategy. The fueling strategy will be based on whether the activity involves high intensity with short-duration movements, continuous movements of lower intensity for long stretches of time, or a combination of the 2 utilizing aspects of power, speed, and endurance (Table 10-1). These different types of activity can be categorized generally as power sports, endurance sports, and team sports, respectively. Different muscle types and energy systems will be involved based on the type of activity. Calculating macronutrient needs to meet the training needs starts with determining the carbohydrate and protein needs for the athlete, and then the remaining calories are allotted to fat based on the Acceptable Macronutrient Distribution Ranges (AMDR; 20% to 35% of total energy from fat), which are part of the Dietary Reference Intakes developed by the National Academies of Sciences, Engineering, and Medicine.[2-4] Fat intake can be adjusted to promote weight loss, weight gain, or to improve physique. Caution should be taken when restricting to very low levels (<20% of total energy from fat), as this may result in an inadequate intake of essential fatty acids and fat-soluble vitamins.[2-4] The macronutrients, and protein in particular, should be spaced equally throughout the day as 4 to 6 small meals and snacks to reap the most benefits. General fluid requirements vary widely and should be individualized based on losses.[2] Table 10-1 provides guidance on how to determine fluid needs for each athlete, as well as general guidelines for key minerals and electrolytes. The following sections will discuss the overall activity-based nutrition recommendations for athletes based on the type of activity, with specific regards to carbohydrate and protein needs.

Table 10-1

Overall Activity-Based Nutrition Recommendations

NUTRIENT	TYPE OF ACTIVITY/ TRAINING	RECOMMENDED INTAKE[2]	EXAMPLE OF DAILY RECOMMENDATION
Carbohydrate	Low-intensity exercise or skill-based drills	3 to 5 g/kg/day	A 71-kg (156-pound) athlete would need 213 to 355 g/day.
	Moderate-intensity exercise, ~60 minutes/day	5 to 7 g/kg/day	A 71-kg (156-pound) athlete would need 355 to 497 g/day.
	High-intensity endurance exercise, ~1 to 3 hours/day	6 to 10 g/kg/day	A 71-kg (156-pound) athlete would need 426 to 710 g/day.
	Very high-intensity exercise, ~4 to 5 hours/day	8 to 12 g/kg/day	A 71-kg (156-pound) athlete would need 568 to 852 g/day.
Protein	Endurance	1.2 to 1.4 g/kg/day	A 71-kg (156-pound) athlete would need 85 to 99 g/day.
	Resistance/strength-based	1.6 to 2.0 g/kg/day	A 71-kg (156-pound) athlete would need 114 to 142 g/day.
Fat	Typically, the carbohydrate and protein amounts are calculated first and then the remainder of the calories are allotted to fat based on the AMDR of 20% to 35% of energy from total fat, <10% from saturated fat, and <1% from *trans* fat.[5] Fat can be adjusted to promote weight loss, weight gain, or improve physique. Caution should be taken when restricting to very low levels, as this may result in an inadequate intake of essential fatty acids and fat-soluble vitamins.[3,4]		

Fluid/electrolytes (Requirements vary widely and should be individualized based on losses.)	*Fluid*[4]	*Mineral/Electrolyte Recommended Intake*[4]	
	• Males: ~3.7 L/day	Sodium	1500 mg/d
	• Females: ~2.7 L/day	Chloride	1500 mg/d
	(or divide body weight in pounds by 2 for fluid ounces required/day)	Potassium	4700 mg/d
		Magnesium	240 to 420 mg/d
	Ensure enough fluid to urinate every 2 to 4 hours each day.	Calcium	1000 to 1300 mg/d

High-Intensity, Short-Duration Activity

High-intensity, short-duration activities are often referred to as power sports and are those that involve near maximal effort and are no longer than a few minutes in duration. Activities that are most often considered to be high intensity and short duration are activities involving sprints (very high intensity), middle-distance events such as running or rowing, or field events such as throwing or jumping. The higher the intensity of the activity, the more reliant the body is on the anaerobic energy system and the breakdown of glycogen into glucose for fuel. Diets that are high in carbohydrates contribute to glycogen stores; however, power sport athletes often focus primarily on their protein intake without regard to adequate carbohydrate intake (Sidebar 10-1). The heavy focus on protein is usually due to the desire to gain as much muscle mass as possible without losing speed. While protein intake is important, without adequate carbohydrates the athlete will not have the necessary glycogen stores to supply glucose for fuel and perform their activity at the highest level. One bout of short-duration activity will not deplete one's glycogen stores, but most athletes are not performing a single bout of activity. Rather, bouts are usually repeated over a defined time period and/or involve other activities and events throughout the day as well. Glycogen depletion becomes a concern in these situations. The overall nutrition recommendations for high-intensity, short-duration activity is 5 to 7 g/kg/day carbohydrate to ensure adequate glycogen stores and 1.6 to 2 g/kg/day protein to support muscle mass.[2]

Endurance Activity and Potential Uses for Carbohydrate Loading

Endurance activities include a wide array of different events such as cross country ski races, half marathons/marathons, and Olympic distance triathlons. While the

Sidebar 10-1

Pitfall #1: Inadequate carbohydrate intake related to misinformation on performance related nutrient needs. A male collegiate freshman sprinter was feeling extreme fatigue and heavy legs, and could not finish his sprint workouts. After analyzing his dietary intake, it was revealed that this sprinter was consuming a very low carbohydrate diet. When asked for the reason for this, he stated that it was because his high school biology teacher told him that protein was the main source of energy for him; therefore, he should limit carbohydrates and consume mainly protein for energy. Once the physiologic need for carbohydrates was explained to the athlete and the misinformation had been corrected, carbohydrates were introduced back into his diet, his fatigue resolved, and he started achieving personal bests again.

Sidebar 10-2

Pitfall #2: Lack of proper planning to ensure adequate energy and fluid intake to sustain long duration activities. A competitive, amateur female endurance runner was experiencing extreme fatigue and severe headaches after long training runs of >10 miles while preparing for her first marathon. She was eating very little before a run, consuming minimal fluid during the run, and zero electrolytes or fuel during the run. Further, she is a mother of 4 and works full-time; therefore, once the long training runs were completed, she did not refuel and rehydrate because she felt she did not have time. This athlete needed to learn some strategies to plan ahead and simplify the process through the use of meal-delivery services. A back-up option was also provided that included taking 1 day a week to cook several meals at a time and have them ready for use throughout the week. In addition, she was educated on how to prepare for early morning runs the night before. She learned how to prepare something simple like overnight oats for a quick easy breakfast and also how to prepare fuel and hydration packs with fruit, sports gels, and sports drinks on Saturday nights before her early Sunday runs (the longest run of her week) and prepare a recovery smoothie for right after her run. She was also provided with a plan to fuel and hydrate every couple of miles during the marathon. Once a proper fuel and hydration plan was put into place, her training runs improved and she achieved a personal best in the New York City marathon.

high-intensity, short-duration sports rely most heavily on the anaerobic energy systems, endurance activity requires the aerobic energy systems. Glucose is typically the predominant substrate in use during aerobic activity, but as the duration of the activity increases so does the ability to utilize fat as an energy source. Intensity of the activity also impacts the fuel substrate.

- Low-intensity exercise, or skill-based drills, requires 3 to 5 g/kg/day of carbohydrates.
- Moderate-intensity exercise (~60 minutes/day) requires 5 to 7 g/kg/day of carbohydrates.
- High-intensity endurance exercise (~1 to 3 hours/day) requires 6 to 10 g/kg/day of carbohydrates.
- Very high–intensity exercise (~4 to 5 hours/day) requires 8 to 12 g/kg/day of carbohydrates (Sidebar 10-2).[2]

These carbohydrate amounts should be accompanied by 1.2 to 1.4 g/kg/day of protein.[2] Carbohydrate loading may be of benefit to athletes involved in events that last ≥90 minutes.[2] Carbohydrate loading is the practice of consuming a high amount of carbohydrates in the time leading up to an event, at the same time that the training load decreases. This practice can lead to maximizing the glycogen stores and help to prevent early fatigue during the event or competition. A typical carbohydrate-loading protocol would be 10 to 12 g/kg/day of carbohydrates in the 2 days prior to the event or competition paired with rest days without any activity.[2] The athlete would then resume normal carbohydrate intake on the day of the event or competition in line with their activity.

Intermittent, High-Intensity Activity Utilizing Aspects of Power, Speed, and Endurance

Some activities cannot be categorized as just power or just endurance but instead are a combination of the two. This is most often the case with team sports such as soccer, basketball, tennis, and ice hockey (Sidebar 10-3). The recommended level for intake of carbohydrate and protein for athletes involved in team sports typically falls somewhere in the middle between pure power sports and pure endurance sports, and will depend on many factors such as the duration of the activity. Most team sports will have a duration somewhere between 1 to 3 hours in length and therefore 6 to 10 g/kg/day of carbohydrate would be appropriate along with 1.2 to 1.4 g/kg/day of protein.[2]

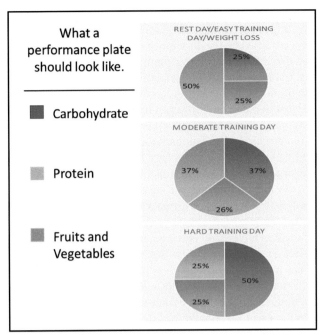

Figure 10-1. Overall guidelines for training day. Performance nutrition.

Nutrient and Fluid Timing Related to Activity and Individual Needs

The days of only paying attention to nutrition on competition days or game days are in the past. Successful athletes now apply a more modern approach to nutrition, in which the energy and nutrient intake is matched to the usage on a daily basis to maximize performance and overall health. Training cycles have long been a staple for the competitive athlete but it is only more recently that nutrition-specific cycles, or periodized nutrition,[5,6] have been adopted and put into practice. The concept of periodized nutrition is based on the technique of pairing nutrition and fluid intake to an athlete's training load on any given day to meet specific performance, body composition, and overall health-related goals.[5,6] For example, these goals may include a desire to improve speed, strength, and endurance or increase lean body mass all while helping to prevent nutrient deficiencies, injury, and illness.

Training Days Versus Competition Days Versus Rest Days

In general, energy and nutrients should be distributed throughout the day rather than consumed all in one sitting.[2,3,5,6] This concept applies to all individuals and not just athletes, but for athletes in particular, this distribution of nutrients takes on even greater significance. The total amount

of energy and nutrients needed, and how they will be distributed throughout the day, will differ based on whether it is a rest day; a light, moderate, or heavy training day; or whether it is a competition day (Figure 10-1). Meals, or the performance plate, on rest days or light training days should consist of half of the plate from fruits and vegetables (50%), and the other half of the plate divided between complex carbohydrates (25%) and lean protein (25%).[2,3,5,6] As the athlete moves through training cycles and increases intensity and duration, complex carbohydrates will increase to support the energy needs. The performance plate on a moderate training day should reflect an increase in complex carbohydrates to ~37% of the plate with the remainder consisting of fruits and vegetables (~37%) and lean protein (~26%).[2,3,5,6] For a hard training day or game day, the performance plate should reflect half of the plate from complex carbohydrates (50%) with the remainder split between fruits and vegetables (25%) and lean protein (25%).[2,3,5,6] It is also noteworthy to point out that the rest day performance plate can also be recommended for athletes who are trying to lose weight, regardless of whether it is a rest day or not. However, caution should be taken when recommending weight loss for any athlete during an intense training cycle or while in-season to prevent detrimental effects on overall health and performance. Nutrient needs also vary based on whether an athlete is in-season, pre-season, or off-season. Typically athletes who are either in-season or in pre-season will have higher overall energy and nutrient needs than those in the off-season.

The nutrition plan for training days should be developed to provide support for the necessary physiologic adaptations that are needed to continue to improve athletic performance.[5,6] This is in contrast to competition day nutrition strategies that are more focused on providing the right combination of energy, nutrients, and fluid and the right timing for peak performance.[5,6] Nutrition strategies for training days are based on the duration, intensity, and type of activity and decisions regarding nutrition can either support or hinder training effects. Some training days may be more taxing on the body and longer in duration than a game day or competition day, and this must be taken into account when developing the nutrition plan. The nutrition plan for competition day focuses on familiar foods that the athlete tolerates and will provide enough energy for the singular event that day or for multiple events. Athletes should be advised to test out any fueling strategies during training rather than implement something new on a competition day to avoid any unknown or unexpected negative effects.

When it comes to nutrition, it is not a "one-size-fits-all" mantra. Furthermore, there is not one particular set of nutrient guidelines that applies to an individual. An effective nutrition plan will be dynamic and will change to match the training. An athlete may change nutrition strategies for one specific event such as the practice of carbohydrate loading prior to a marathon or increasing protein intake when trying to lose body fat while simultaneously maintaining lean body mass. These particular changes are intended to be temporary and not reflective of what the individual would typically be following for a nutrition plan.

Carbohydrate Intake Before, During, and After Activity

Prior to any training session or competition, an athlete should focus on "topping" off their glycogen stores in order to ensure adequate energy will be available to fuel the activity (Table 10-2). Athletes should select fueling options that are "tried and true," meaning that the athlete has tested them out during training to determine how their body will react. The carbohydrates should be easy to digest; they should be familiar foods that will not upset the stomach of the athlete or lead to any gastrointestinal distress. Specific recommendations for quantity is for athletes to consume the largest amount of carbohydrates (combination of complex and simple carbohydrates) about 2 to 4 hours prior to the activity and then to decrease the quantity the closer they get to the start of the activity. For instance, a general guideline would be to match the grams of carbohydrate to the number of hours preceding the activity such as[2,3]:

- 4 g of carbohydrates per kg of body weight consumed 4 hours before

- 3 g of carbohydrates per kg of body weight consumed 3 hours before

- 2 g of carbohydrates per kg of body weight consumed 2 hours before

- No more than 1 g of carbohydrate per kg of body weight consumed 1 hour before

This is to ensure adequate digestion prior to the start of the event.[2,3] Carbohydrate intake during activity will vary based on the length of time of the activity and the intensity.[2] For activity lasting less than 30 minutes, carbohydrate intake is typically not necessary. For high-intensity exercise lasting from 30 to 75 minutes, a small amount of carbohydrates may be beneficial. For endurance and intermittent high-intensity activities lasting from 1 to 2 hours, consumption of ~30 g/hour will help to sustain blood glucose levels and prolong the time to glycogen depletion. That amount will increase to ~60 g/hour and ~90 g/hour, if the endurance activity lasts from 2 to 3 hours and more than 2.5 hours, respectively. Since there is a maximum amount of glucose that can be absorbed per minute and per hour (~1 g/minute or ~60 g/hour), longer-duration activities may require utilizing additional sources of energy simultaneously, such as fructose rather than just glucose.[2,3] If both glucose and fructose are consumed, the grams of carbohydrate absorbed per minute increases to ~1.8 g/minute or 108 g/hour by utilizing multiple transporters in the intestinal tract.[2,3]

Carbohydrate consumption is equally important after the activity concludes. A typical guideline for athletes to follow after glycogen-depleting activity is to consume 1 to 1.2 g of carbohydrates per kilogram of body weight every hour for the next 4 hours.[2,3] This is most crucial when the athlete has another training session or competition within 8 hours of the first. Since many athletes have a poor appetite immediately after an intense training session or competition, liquid options may be best for those who experience poor appetite after exercise.

Protein Intake Before, During, and After Activity

Less of an emphasis is placed on protein consumption before and during exercise for most athletes. A general guideline of including a moderate amount of lean protein in the precompetition meal about 2 to 4 hours before is sufficient. In the immediate precompetition time frame (30 to 60 minutes before), little to no protein is recommended. It is also not typically necessary to consume protein during an event, with the exception of a possible benefit in response to small amounts of protein consumed during endurance activities lasting longer than 2.5 hours.[2] The main emphasis on protein consumption should occur immediately after the training or competition has finished. The athlete should focus on consuming approximately 15 to 30 g of protein immediately after in combination with the carbohydrate in a ~3:1 ratio of grams of carbohydrate to grams of protein.[2,3] This practice will help to start the glycogen repletion process, as well as initiate tissue repair and muscle protein synthesis.

Table 10-2

Guidelines for Before, During, and After Exercise Fueling and Hydration

TIMING	CARBOHYDRATE		PROTEIN	FAT	FLUID/ELECTROLYTES	
Before Easy to digest and will not upset stomach Familiar foods only	1 hour before	1 g/kg	Moderate protein included in the pre-event meal about 2 to 4 hours before Little to no protein 30 to 60 minutes before	Low fat in the pre-event meal about 24 hours before Little to no fat 30 to 60 minutes before	15 minutes before	8 to 16 ounces
	2 hours before	2 g/kg				
	3 hours before	3 g/kg			2 hours before	16 to 24 ounces
	4 hours before	4 g/kg				
DURING Exercise up to 2.5 hours: ~1 g/minute of glucose is the maximum amount absorbed or ~1.8 g/minute of both glucose and fructose is the maximum amount absorbed Exercise ≥2.5 hours: ~1.8 g/minute of both glucose and fructose is the maximum amount absorbed	Less than 30 minutes	None	Not necessary	Not necessary	Water	
	High intensity (30 to 75 minutes)	Small amount	Not necessary	Not necessary	Water (6 to 12 ounces) every 15 minutes (plus carbohydratres and electrolytes as needed when >1 hour).	
	Endurance and intermittent, high intensity (1 to 2 hours)	30 g/hour	Not necessary	Not necessary	Water (6 to 12 ounces) plus carbohydrates (and electrolytes as needed) every 15 minutes.	
	Endurance (2 to 3 hours)	60 g/hour	Not necessary	Not necessary	Water (6 to 12 ounces) plus carbohydrates (and electrolytes as needed) every 15 minutes.	
	Endurance (≥2.5 hours)	90 g/hour	Small amounts may be beneficial	Not necessary	Water (6 to 12 ounces) plus carbohydrates (and electrolytes as needed) every 15 minutes.	
After Liquid options best for those with poor appetite after exercise	Body weight in pounds/2=g of carbohydrates needed to replenish glycogen stores after glycogen-depleting activity; starting ~30 minutes after and then every hour x 4 if next activity session is in less than 8 hours		3:1 ratio of carbs-to-protein (~15 to 30 g/athlete)	Focus on healthy fat such as monosaturated and omega-3	Replace every pound lost with 24 fluid ounces. Replace lost electrolytes. Continue to hydrate until urine is pale.	

Fat Intake Before, During, and After Activity

Athletes typically focus the least on the timing of their fat consumption in relation to activity, but fat is a vital component of the diet and should not be ignored. The timing of fat intake matters and high fat before, during, or after exercise can inhibit both the utilization of glycogen stores and the glycogen repletion process afterward by slowing digestion and transit time through the digestive tract.[2,3] Prior to a competitive event or training session, athletes should include only small amounts of fat in their meals and little to no fat in the 30- to 60-minute window right beforehand. Fat consumption during activity is not necessary and typically not recommended, with the exception to this rule being some potential benefits for ultra-endurance events. However, the evidence

Sidebar 10-4

Pitfall #4: Inadequate fluid and electrolyte intake leading to frequent leg cramps. A male professional soccer player was consistently developing leg cramps shortly into the second half of games. The player was typically on the field for every minute of the first half and started the second half, but would have to leave the field due to the leg cramps. Upon investigation, it was revealed that the player did not properly hydrate before the games, did not find opportunities to hydrate during the first half, and did not maximize the half-time period to refuel and rehydrate. Once a structured hydration plan that included electrolytes was put in place, the leg cramps resolved.

is still limited and not yet fully supported.[7] In the immediate post-training or post-competition period (the first 30 to 60 minutes afterward), fat intake should be limited so as not to interfere with the glycogen repletion process.[2,3] As the time after ceasing activity increases, fat intake is encouraged and should focus on healthy fat such as monounsaturated and omega-3 that have an anti-inflammatory and regenerative effect to aid in performance gains and recovery.[2,3]

Fluid and Electrolyte Intake Before, During, and After Activity

Fluid intake varies widely between individuals, and recommendations should be considered simply a starting point.[2-4] Each athlete has their own sweat rate, and this rate should be evaluated on an individual basis. In order to more accurately anticipate fluid needs, athletes should undergo sweat testing, and pre-/post-activity weigh-ins should become part of any active individual's routine. This practice of weighing in before and after will provide the athlete with valuable information as to how much fluid they are typically losing through sweat. This amount can then be replaced, which helps to avoid progressive dehydration. General guidelines to use as a starting point are to consume approximately 16 to 24 ounces of hydrating fluid about 2 hours before.[2] An additional 8 to 16 ounces should be consumed within 15 minutes of the training session or competition.[2] During exercise, a good rule of thumb is to consume approximately 6 to 12 ounces of fluid every 15 minutes throughout the activity (Sidebar 10-4).[2] Plain water is usually sufficient as the hydrating beverage for activities lasting less than 1 hour, and either sports beverages or water plus a carbohydrate food source and electrolytes is preferred for longer activities.[2] Once the activity has ended, the athlete should immediately start to replace losses with a hydrating beverage such as water or a sports drink. The athlete can gauge exactly how

much fluid needs to be replaced by calculating the amount of body weight lost. Then, for every pound of body weight lost the athlete should consume 24 ounces of fluid.[2] The athlete should continue to hydrate until the urine is pale.[2]

Nutrition Strategies for the Active Adult (Nonathlete)

Proper fueling and hydration do not only apply to competitive athletes. With the population aging and individuals living a longer life, the number of adults who want to remain active is also increasing.[8] Nutrition is just as important for these active individuals as it is for competitive athletes. Without proper nutrition, active adults may experience decreased strength, energy, and may be more prone to injuries and illness. Further, inadequate nutrition can hamper one's ability to perform activities of daily living, job-related activities, and intentional exercise such as gardening, mowing the lawn, participating in an aerobics class, or walking to the store to run an errand. The National Academies of Sciences, Engineering, and Medicine developed the Dietary Reference Intakes, which include acceptable macronutrient intake levels.[4] Based on these recommendations, active adults should consume 45% to 65% of their total calories from carbohydrates such as brown rice, whole grain bread, pasta, potatoes, and fruit.[4] Carbohydrates will provide the energy necessary to complete everyday activities such as cooking, as well as allow for participating in intentional exercises such as walking around a nearby track. Protein should be consumed as 15% to 35% of total calories (or 0.8 to 1 g/kg of body weight) from sources such as lean meat, fish, low-fat dairy, legumes, nuts, and seeds.[4] Adequate protein will help to preserve lean body mass, repair body tissues, support the immune system, and prevent injuries.[4] The remaining calories should come from fats and oils and should equate to 20% to 35% of total calories, with <10% of total calories coming from saturated fats and <1% from *trans* fatty acids.[4] While some individuals may fear consuming fats at all given the attention placed on reducing cardiovascular disease risk, it is important to consume an appropriate level of fat. Fats provide important functions in the body such as serving as insulation to help regulate body temperature, providing a protective layer for our internal organs, supplying a concentrated energy reserve, aiding in the absorption of fat-soluble vitamins, and serving as a precursor for important hormones in the body. Active adults should also make sure to stay hydrated throughout the day and avoid dehydration. It is recommended that adult women consume at least 2.7 L and adult men consume at least 3.7 L of water or hydrating fluids per day.[4] A helpful visual aid to illustrate this recommended eating pattern for the active adult is MyPlate (Figure 10-2). MyPlate is the visual representation of the *Dietary Guidelines for Americans*[9] and provides a breakdown of what a plate should look like in order to maintain a balanced intake from all of the food

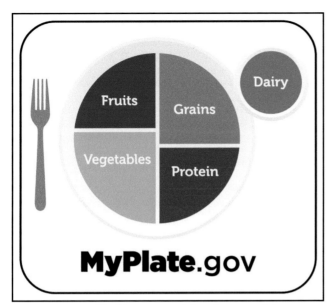

Figure 10-2. Overall healthy eating guidelines for active adults. (Reproduced with permission from the USDA.)

groups. MyPlate suggests that half of the plate should come from fruits and vegetables and the other half should be divided up between grains (with half of the grains from whole grain sources) and lean protein. In addition, hydrating fluids such as water or low-fat milk should accompany each meal. Fats and oils are intended to be used sparingly at each meal. An active individual needs to also plan proper fueling and hydration around specific activities (Sidebar 10-5). Similar to the competitive athlete, active adults will need to consume small amounts of quick-absorbing carbohydrates and hydrate prior to exercise. If the exercise lasts more than 60 minutes, the active individual is encouraged to consume a small amount of carbohydrates along with hydrating fluids. Refueling and rehydrating after the exercise is completed is also encouraged and can typically be accomplished by having a meal with rehydrating beverages such as water shortly after.

Conclusion

Athletic trainers are frequently asked questions by their clients on a wide array of sports-related topics, and one of the most common topic areas is nutrition and hydration. While sports dietitians are the recognized experts in the field of sports nutrition, athletic trainers should still have a solid foundation in basic nutrition concepts as it relates to athletic performance. The information presented in this chapter will help athletic trainers achieve the professional standards that they are expected to demonstrate for CAATE. It is the responsibility of the athletic trainer to ensure that the information they provide to clients is evidence based. Any information and recommendations should be individualized and must match the energy usage of the activity and training schedules.

Discussion Questions

1. How might the competition day nutrition and hydration plan differ between an athlete competing in the 100 m sprint versus an athlete competing in a half marathon?

2. How would you educate a soccer player who consumes a high-protein diet with very low carbohydrates because they believe that protein is the most important macronutrient for athletes?

3. If you have an athlete who is experiencing early fatigue and leg cramps during the second half of competitions, what are some of the key nutrition and hydration areas you should focus on to help eliminate those issues?

References

1. Commission on Accreditation of Athletic Training Education. *2020 Standards for Accreditation of Professional Athletic Training Programs.* CAATE; 2018.

2. Thomas DT, Erdman KA, Burke LM. Position of the Academy of Nutrition and Dietetics, Dietitians of Canada, and the American College of Sports Medicine: nutrition and athletic performance. *J Acad Nutr Diet.* 2016;116:501-528.

3. Kerksick C, Wilborn C, Roberts M, et al. ISSN exercise and sports nutrition review update: research and recommendations. *J Int Soc Sports Nutr.* 2018;15(38):1-57.

4. Institute of Medicine. *Dietary reference intakes.* National Academies Press. Accessed February 17, 2020. https://www.nal.usda.gov/fnic/dietary-reference-intakes

5. Stellingwerff T, Boit MK, Res PT. Nutritional strategies to optimize training and racing in middle-distance athletes. *J Sports Sci.* 2007;25:S17-28.

6. Stellingwerff T, Morton JP, Burke LM. A framework for periodized nutrition for athletics. *Int J Sport Nutr Exerc Metab.* 2019;29(2):141-151.

7. Tiller NB, Roberts JD, Beasley L, et al. International Society of Sports Nutrition position stand: nutritional considerations for single-stage ultra-marathon training and racing. *J Int Soc Sports Nutr.* 2019;16(1):50.

8. US Department of Health and Human Services, Administration on Aging. A profile of older Americans: 2018. US Department of Health and Human Services. https://acl.gov/sites/default/files/Aging%20and%20Disability%20in%20America/2018OlderAmericansProfile.pdf

9. US Department of Health and Human Services and US Department of Agriculture. *2015–2020 Dietary Guidelines for Americans.* 8th ed. 2015. Available at https://health.gov/our-work/food-nutrition/previous-dietary-guidelines/2015.

Chapter 11

Nutrition-Influenced Disorders

Tara LaRowe, PhD, RDN, CSSD, CD

Commission on Accreditation of Athletic Training Education *2020 Standards*

This chapter addresses the following *2020 Standards for Accreditation of Professional Athletic Training Programs*:

- Standard 55: Students must gain foundational knowledge in statistics, research design, epidemiology, pathophysiology, biomechanics and pathomechanics, exercise physiology, nutrition, human anatomy, pharmacology, public health, and health care delivery and payor systems.
- Standard 61: Practice in collaboration with other health care and wellness professionals.
- Standard 69: Develop a care plan for each patient. The care plan includes (but is not limited to) the following:
  - Assessment of the patient on an ongoing basis and adjustment of care accordingly
  - Collection, analysis, and use of patient-reported and clinician-rated outcome measures to improve patient care
  - Consideration of the patient's goals and level of function in treatment decisions
  - Referral when warranted
- Standard 79: Develop and implement strategies to mitigate the risk for long-term health conditions across the lifespan. These include (but are not limited to) the following conditions:
  - Cardiovascular disease
  - Diabetes
  - Obesity

Knoblauch M, ed. *Clinical Nutrition in Athletic Training* (pp 121-132).
© 2023 Taylor & Francis Group.

Introduction

Chronic disease is influenced by many factors, including genetics, environment, and lifestyle. Although having a strong family history may predispose individuals for being at higher risk for chronic disease, controllable factors (eg, weight, diet, and smoking) can significantly alter the path of disease development or progression. Suppose 2 individuals have the same genetic make-up and share the same environmental exposures. One of the individuals lives an active lifestyle and eats a well-balanced, nutritious diet, whereas the other individual lives a sedentary lifestyle and eats an energy-dense, nutrient-poor diet. Would they both have the same outcomes for disease? Most likely not. This chapter aims to discuss how diet can influence chronic disease, either through prevention or managing treatment of disease. While almost every chronic disease could be related somehow to diet, the focus for this chapter will be on those diseases that are most common, even among active populations: obesity, cardiovascular disease, hypertension, type 2 diabetes, metabolic syndrome, and osteoporosis. The chapter will conclude with a focus on nutrient-specific disorders. Like chronic disease, there are many nutrient-specific disorders that could warrant discussion, but anemia—particularly iron-deficient anemia—will be the highlighted disorder.

Genetics and Disease

Before focusing on diet's role in disease, it is important to first highlight the connection between genetics and disease. Each person's unique genetic make-up may explain why one person may develop heart disease and the other not, even though they both are physically active, nonsmoking, and eat a healthy diet. The field of genetics, as a result of the Human Genome Project, has expanded our understanding of genetic variation with human disease. It is important to understand the impact that genetics can have on health and disease, as science will continue to evolve with the aim to develop treatment and medications for conditions by using genetic testing.[1] The knowledge of specific genes linked to disease risk has led to opportunities in understanding how lifestyle factors such as diet interact with genes to mitigate risk for disease. For example, individuals with an A allele of the *FTO* gene (ie, the fat mass and obesity-associated gene) were found to have significantly less body fat after 2 years of consuming a high-protein diet, compared to individuals with the TT allele variant of *FTO* gene.[2,3] These same 2 variants of the *FTO* gene have also been shown to be influenced by dietary fat. Individuals with an A allele had significantly higher BMI and waist circumferences compared to TT homozygotes, but only when consumption of dietary saturated fat was high and polyunsaturated fat was low.[4] Genetic make-ups may set underlying conditions for disease, but also respond to dietary and nutritional interventions—showing the importance of lifestyle factors in the development of disease. The disorders that will be covered in this chapter are largely influenced by the interaction among genetics and diet, environment, and other lifestyle factors.

Obesity

The impact obesity has on chronic disease is extensive. According to the Centers for Disease Control and Prevention, nearly 93 million American adults (almost 40%) are obese.[5] Obesity can be thought simplistically as an energy balance problem, meaning increased body fat is the result of an imbalance of energy intake (ie, too many calories) and energy expenditure (ie, inactivity). However, obesity is much more complex and involves not only genetic predisposition but environmental factors such as access to healthy food, access and adequate places to play, and social norms around food and activity. Healthy lifestyle choices significantly play a role in obesity; however, healthy eating and activity can often be confined by the environment, which makes addressing obesity so difficult. Individuals with obesity compared to normal weight individuals have higher risk for cardiovascular disease and stroke, hypertension, type 2 diabetes, some cancers, and many other health consequences including poorer quality of life, mental illness, and low physical function.[6,7] Even more alarming is that the prevalence of obesity among children aged 2 to 19 years is 18.5%.[8] Children with obesity are more likely to become adults with obesity, leading to chronic disease. The causes of obesity are highly complex interactions between genetic and behavioral factors, including diet and physical activity. Preventive strategies for obesity have largely focused on behaviors related to dietary intake and activity patterns. Chapter 7 addresses nutrition's role in weight management extensively, as well as an overview of nutritional strategies for obesity prevention and treatment. In this chapter, the focus will be on chronic diseases that are strongly correlated with obesity—cardiovascular disease, hypertension, and diabetes.

Cardiovascular Disease

Heart disease is the leading cause of death among Americans and claims the lives of more than 600,000 individuals annually.[9] Advances in medical treatments have improved outcomes for many individuals affected by heart disease. More importantly, lifestyle factors, including diet, not only improve outcomes for those with disease but are the cornerstones for prevention.

Atherosclerosis cardiovascular disease (ASCVD) is a term that outlines the various types of heart disease including nonfatal myocardial infarction (heart attack), coronary heart disease death, and stroke. These diseases are caused by atherosclerosis. Atherosclerosis is a slow process, often developing over years, that deposits fat, cholesterol, and other substances into the walls of arteries. The build-up of plaque narrows the lumen of arteries, thereby restricting blood flow and potentially even causing ruptures as well as blockages that are induced by blood clots. Stroke, angina (chest pain), and myocardial infarction are all consequences of atherosclerosis.

Cholesterol and Atherosclerosis

Research attempting to establish the progression of ASCVD gained momentum in the 1960s. High blood cholesterol, or hypocholesterolemia, along with high blood pressure and smoking, were identified as primary risk factors for ASCVD. Additional research revealed that diets high in fat and cholesterol were associated with high blood cholesterol. This was the beginning of the "diet-heart hypothesis." However, total blood cholesterol is a composite of several lipoproteins; similarly, total dietary fat represents many different types of fatty acids in the diet. Therefore, the hypothesis that high dietary fat diet increases blood cholesterol is much more complex due to blood cholesterol fractions, or lipid profile. The major components of a lipid profile include total cholesterol, low-density lipoprotein (LDL), high-density

Table 11-1

Optimal Blood Cholesterol Levels

TOTAL CHOLESTEROL	<200 mg/dL
LDL CHOLESTEROL	<100 mg/dL
HDL CHOLESTEROL	≥60 mg/dL
TRIGLYCERIDES	<150 mg/dL

lipoprotein (HDL), and triglycerides. LDL, HDL, and triglyceride fraction found within blood cholesterol (ie, "total cholesterol") better predict risk for ASCVD. The National Cholesterol and Education Program of the National Heart, Lung, Blood Institute defines desirable lipid profile shown in Table 11-1.[10,11]

Risk Factors

Family history, or heredity, is a strong risk factor for development of ASCVD, but many of the risk factors are controllable through lifestyle choices. Some of the risk factors for developing ASCVD include:

- Age; 45+ for men and 55+ for women
- Family history of early heart disease (parent or sibling being diagnosed with heart disease before the age of 55 for men and 65 for women)
- High blood pressure
- High blood cholesterol
- Cigarette smoking
- Diabetes
- Overweight/obesity
- Physical inactivity

Dietary Management

What is known now about ASCVD, including risk factors, treatment, and management, has evolved over several decades. Current knowledge and evidence that is supported by the American College of Cardiology/American Heart Association (AHA/ACC) and implemented by the *Dietary Guidelines for Americans* are presented.

Diet and lifestyle remain the AHA's primary strategy for ASCVD prevention. In a joint 2013 publication, the ACC/AHA task force released guidelines on lifestyle management to reduce cardiovascular disease.[12] This publication emphasized and reviewed dietary recommendations with regard to lowering LDL cholesterol, whereas the updated 2019 publication focused on reducing ASCVD risk.[13] Both publications reflect current science and recommendations for clinical practice specific to lowering LDL cholesterol and reducing ASCVD risk. Dietary recommendations for reducing ASCVD risk include consuming a diet rich in vegetables, fruits, whole grains, and fish while minimizing saturated fat, processed meats, refined grains, and sodium.

Consume a Diet Emphasizing Vegetables, Fruits, Nuts, Whole Grains, and Fish

Diets higher in fruit and vegetable consumption are associated with decreasing one's risk for heart disease mortality by 30% to 40%.[14] However, it appears that overall diet patterns need to be considered regarding ASCVD risk. A diet pattern is defined as the combination of different foods and beverages in a diet and the frequency of which they are consumed (ie, habitual consumption). As such, the US Department of Health and Human Services and US Department of Agriculture's *Dietary Guidelines, 2020-2025* placed a large emphasis on plant-based and Mediterranean-style eating patterns.[14]

Plant-based and Mediterranean style diets, characterized by ample amounts of fruits, vegetables, nuts, legumes, lean vegetable or animal protein (ideally fish), and fiber from vegetables have been consistently associated with decreased risk for all-cause mortality.[15-17] The PREDIMED (Prevención con Dieta Mediterránea) trial that randomized participants who were already eating a traditional Mediterranean-style diet with extra supplementation of daily nut or olive oil consumption demonstrated 28% and 30% reductions, respectively, in combined cardiovascular endpoints of myocardial infarction, stroke, and cardiovascular mortality, compared to the control group.[15]

Replace Saturated Fat With Dietary Monounsaturated and Polyunsaturated Fats

Saturated fat has been associated with all-cause mortality.[18,19] Diets made up of less than 10% of total calories from saturated fat are shown to lower LDL cholesterol. Reducing the saturated fat content further to 7% of total calories results in even lower LDL cholesterol levels.[20] Currently, the AHA recommends saturated fat intake to be <7% of total daily calories.[14] Several randomized controlled trials showed significant reduction in LDL cholesterol when saturated fat was restricted to 7% of calories compared to a Western-type diet.[21-23] Furthermore, a meta-analysis of National Cholesterol Treatment Education Program Step 2 diet studies (<7% saturated fat)—along with weight loss (3 to 6 kg)—reported a reduction of LDL cholesterol by 16%.[24] However, it must be noted that when saturated fat intake is decreased, other components of the diet, such as carbohydrate or other fatty acids, will often increase to compensate for the reduction of saturated fat and to equalize total caloric intake. Replacing saturated fat with mono- and polyunsaturated fat (olive oils and other vegetables oils) reduces LDL cholesterol,[18,19] whereas

it has been shown that replacing saturated fat with refined carbohydrates (eg, simple sugars, white breads, pastas, rice) increases triglycerides and risk for stroke and mortality.[25]

Saturated fats can be thought as "solid fats" and come from animal products, including high-fat dairy cheeses, creams and butter, palm and coconut oils, and cocoa butter. Common sources of saturated fats in the American diet include regular cheese, pizza, grain-based desserts, mixed dishes with cheese and meats, hot dogs, sausages, and bacon.

Mono- and polyunsaturated fats are typically "liquid fats." Olive, canola, peanut, and safflower oil all have high proportions of monounsaturated fats, as well as nuts. Sunflower, corn, soybean, and cottonseed oil are sources rich in polyunsaturated fats. In addition to nuts and oils, fish also are rich sources of mono- and polyunsaturated fatty acids, specifically omega-3 fatty acids, that assist in reducing blood triglycerides as well as blood pressure and can slow the progression of atherosclerosis.[15]

Minimize the Intake of Processed Meats, Refined Carbohydrates, and Sweetened Beverages

High consumption of processed meats, refined carbohydrates, and sweetened beverages is linked to cardiovascular death.[26] In a prospective study of health professionals, plant protein was associated with reduced cardiovascular mortality, whereas processed red meat was associated with 34% increase in mortality.[27]

Carbohydrate quality contributes to risk for ASCVD. Carbohydrate quality refers to the food's nutritive value, or nutrient density. High-quality carbohydrates are typically whole and unrefined grains, fruits, or vegetables, whereas poor-quality carbohydrates are refined grains (eg, white bread, pasta, rice) and products made with added sugar and sweeteners. The *Dietary Guidelines, 2020-2025* recommends that half of grain intake comes from whole grain sources. Fiber from fruits, vegetables, and whole grains will help achieve the adequate intake (AI) of fiber (14 g per 1000 kcal), which is based on the amount shown to reduce ASCVD.[14] Added sugar in food products has increased substantially in the past 20 years. The additional sugar found in many diets contributes little nutrients to the diet with excess calories. The *Dietary Guidelines, 2020-2025* recommends limiting calories to less than 10% of total daily calories from added sugar. Although overall added sugar in the diet may increase risk for ASCVD and other diseases, most of the risk has specifically been linked to sugar-sweetened beverages.[25] Consumption of sugar-sweetened beverages leads to a number of health consequences, including weight gain and cardiovascular risk factors (eg, dyslipidemia).[28,29]

While quality of carbohydrate is related to ASCVD risk, the total amount of carbohydrate has also been associated with risk. As discussed previously, diets with excessive carbohydrate intake related to refined sources and sugar-sweetened beverages contribute to weight gain and lipid disorders.

Diets low in carbohydrate and high in animal fat and protein have been shown to increase cardiac and noncardiac mortality rates.[30,31] These types of diets have cycled in and out of public interest for several decades. Although they may have short-term benefits related to weight loss or control of blood glucose, these diets are not recommended for those with risk for ASCVD or whom already have existing disease.

Avoid Intake of *Trans* Fat

Trans fat, found in stick margarine and used pervasively in fast food and baked goods, has been shown to increase risk for ASCVD by increasing LDL cholesterol and lowering HDL cholesterol, while also being shown to increase mortality in several prospective studies.[19,32] Due to the adverse effects of *trans* fat, regulations to ban the use of *trans* fat in the food supply have been initiated; however, removing all trans fat, including partially hydrogenated oils, remains a public health priority.[33]

Reduce Amounts of Cholesterol and Sodium

The *Dietary Guidelines, 2020-2025* does not have a specific recommendation related to dietary cholesterol, whereas previous guidelines have set an amount to <300 mg/day.[14] The primary reason was in the understanding that dietary saturated fat and unsaturated fats influence blood cholesterol more so than dietary cholesterol and that foods in high dietary cholesterol are often high in saturated fat and sodium (eg, red processed meats like bacon and sausages and high-fat cheeses). With a reduction in the consumption of foods that are high in saturated fat and sodium, dietary cholesterol will naturally lower.

The recommendation to reduce sodium in the diet is linked to its connection with hypertension, which is a strong risk factor for ASCVD, and will be presented in more detail. The AHA and *Dietary Guidelines, 2020-2025* recommends no more than 2300 mg of sodium, or 1 teaspoon, in the diet per day.

Fat Facts and Myths

The controversy around diet and cardiovascular disease has extended over decades. It is no wonder that the public is confused about diet and health when opposing messages are reported constantly in the media. Three common food controversies related to cardiovascular disease are discussed here.

1. **Is coconut oil heart healthy?** Coconut oil behaves like a solid fat because of its saturated fat content (about 80% to 90%). In a recent meta-analysis, coconut oil compared to vegetables oils increased LDL cholesterol by 10.47 mg/dL, decreased HDL by 4.0 mg/dL, and did not significantly improve glycemic control, inflammation, or adiposity.[34] The bottom line is that coconut oil can add flavor to foods, but should not be used as the primary cooking fat. Individuals with no risk for cardiovascular disease could probably be more liberal with coconut oil, whereas individuals with existing ASCVD (or are at risk) should restrict use.

2. **Do eggs need to be limited because they are high in cholesterol?** Eggs are high in cholesterol (about 185 mg per egg). However, dietary cholesterol such as what would be consumed from eating eggs does not influence LDL cholesterol levels as much as saturated fat. Eggs, albeit high in cholesterol, have less saturated fat than unsaturated fats, provide high-quality protein, and are rich in vitamin D, riboflavin, vitamin B$_{12}$, iron, zinc, and 8 other essential nutrients. One egg per day within a nutritious diet is appropriate for most healthy individuals. However, special considerations among different populations may influence egg consumption due to the following: (1) vegetarians inherently eat less saturated fat and need good sources of protein, so egg consumption could be liberalized, (2) older individuals with normal cholesterol levels could also benefit from increased egg intake (2 eggs/day) to increase protein intake, which usually declines in older adults, and (3) egg intake should be restricted or limited among individuals with high cholesterol levels, dyslipidemia, or for those who have heart failure or diabetes mellitus.

3. **Does dairy increase risk for ASCVD?** Dairy foods might be the trickiest to navigate. The ACC/AHA 2019 guidelines did not include dairy in its report because of the unclear relationship between dairy consumption and ASCVD.[13] In one study of more than 130,000 individuals from 21 countries, dairy consumption—predominantly in milk and yogurt—was associated with 23% lower mortality rate from cardiovascular outcomes.[35] In a meta-analysis of 29 cohort studies (~1 million participants), there was no association between full or low-fat dairy and mortality or ASCVD outcomes.[36] However, when researchers specifically assessed fermented sources of dairy, such as some cheeses and yogurt, they found a 2% lower risk for cardiovascular disease.[36] Lastly, a randomized crossover study tested the effects of a Mediterranean diet supplemented with dairy. This study revealed that this eating pattern lowered blood pressure, increased HDL cholesterol, and lowered triglycerides.[37] The conclusion is that dairy foods remain neutral in relation to risk for ASCVD. Therefore, individual preferences and other considerations must be made on how to incorporate dairy into a healthy diet. For example, many patients with cardiac morbidities may also have other conditions such as osteoporosis. A cardiac patient with osteoporosis might be told by physicians and dietitians to consume milk and yogurt as a source of calcium to slow the progression of bone loss. In this scenario, it would be important to incorporate calcium-rich foods in the diet, but perhaps choose low-fat milk and yogurt to limit saturated fat intake.

Hypertension

Hypertension is defined as blood pressure consistently higher than 130 mm Hg systolic and 80 mm Hg diastolic. Hypertension affects nearly half of adults in the United States (108 million people) and of the deaths reported in 2017, half a million were due to hypertension as the primary or contributing cause.[38] Dubbed the "silent killer," having high blood pressure often occurs without any obvious symptoms or clinical complication, and many individuals live years without being diagnosed. Even when diagnosed, those with hypertension have poor control; only about 1 in 4 adults (24%) control their hypertension through medication, diet, or both.[39]

Untreated hypertension can lead to serious damage to the heart, brain, kidney, and eyes. Major complications from hypertension include congestive heart failure, myocardial infarction, stroke, end-stage renal disease, and retinopathy. The causes of hypertension are not fully known, but share similar risk factors that were discussed for ASCVD. Some modifiable risk factors include:

- Obesity (BMI of 30 kg/m²)
- High-sodium diet
- Lack of physical activity
- High alcohol intake

Hypertension differs between ethnicity and race. Black individuals develop high blood pressure earlier in life and with more severity than White individuals (ACC/AHA). Family history and age are also known risk factors. Blood pressure increases with age; therefore, risk increases with age.

Dietary Factors to Reduce Hypertension

Sodium is an essential nutrient responsible for maintaining fluid volume outside the cell and has a role in normal nerve and muscle function. Sodium's functions can be found in Chapters 3 and 5. Excessive sodium intake holds fluid in the body and increases the blood volume to be pumped throughout the body, creating a harder workload for the blood vessels, heart, and kidney. The increased pressure within vessel and tissues causes hypertension and damage over time. The *Dietary Guidelines, 2020-2025* recommends no more than 2300 mg per day of sodium in the diet.[14] Ninety percent of Americans meet or exceed the recommended intake for sodium (the average sodium intake for Americans is around 3400 mg/day), making sodium a prime target for prevention efforts. The ACC/AHA guidelines for dietary approaches to prevent and treat hypertension in adults recommends initial reductions in sodium to 2300 mg per day with a goal of no more than 1500 mg per day of sodium.[40]

The salt shaker often gets the blame for too much salt in the diet; however, 75% of sodium intake comes from processed foods rather than what is added from the salt shaker. Processed foods, along with increased meals and food consumed outside of the home (eg, restaurants), contribute to a food culture that is excessive in sodium, with this excess often not realized by the average consumer. Top sources of sodium in the US diet includes breads, pizza, sandwiches, cold cuts/cured meats, soups, burritos/tacos, savory snacks, chicken, cheese, eggs, and omelets.[14]

Dietary prevention and management of hypertension goes beyond targeting single nutrients such as sodium. As discussed previously with cardiovascular disease, the influence of healthy dietary patterns appears to have larger impact on health outcomes. The Dietary Approaches to Stop Hypertension (DASH) diet tested the effects of a diet pattern low in sodium on blood pressure and cardiovascular events.[41] The DASH trial along with 3 other trials funded by the National Heart Lung and Blood Institute, DASH-Sodium Trial, OmniHeart Trial, and OmniCarb Trial demonstrated that adhering to a DASH-style eating pattern was associated with lower blood pressure and LDL cholesterol.[41-44] The DASH dietary eating pattern is based on a diet rich in:

- Vegetables, fruits, whole grains
- Fat-free or low-fat dairy products, fish, poultry, beans, nuts, and vegetable oils

And limited in:

- Sodium (2300 mg)
- Foods high in saturated fat, including fatty meats, full-fat dairy, butter, coconut, and palm oils
- Sugar-sweetened beverages and sweets

Specific details on the DASH diet are shown in Table 11-2. Adhering to a DASH eating pattern ensures adequate fiber, protein, and food sources rich in magnesium, calcium, and potassium. These qualities combined with lower sodium and saturated fat intake result in desired health outcomes.

Diabetes

Diabetes results when blood glucose (ie, blood sugar) levels are too high. Cells in the body rely on glucose for energy, and when insulin is not properly produced (ie, type 1 diabetes) or utilized glucose (ie, type 2 diabetes) cannot enter the cell, thus causing interruptions in carbohydrate metabolism. Over time, high blood glucose leads to heart disease, stroke, kidney disease, and nerve damage, often affecting eyes and feet.

More than 30 million people in the United States have diabetes, defined as fasting blood glucose of >126 mg/dL, and nearly 25% with diabetes are unaware they have the disease.[45,46] The number of Americans with prediabetes, defined as fasting blood glucose between 100 to 126 mg/dL, is almost 3 times as those with diabetes (84.1 million).[45,46] If left untreated, those with prediabetes are highly likely to develop diabetes.

Table 11-2

Daily and Weekly DASH Eating Plan*

DASH DIET COMPONENT	DAILY SERVINGS	SERVING EXAMPLES
Sodium	2300 mg for standard DASH 1500 mg for lower sodium DASH	Foods that are part of the DASH diet are naturally low in sodium. Further reduce sodium by: • Seasoning food with herb/spices instead of salt • Choose low- or reduced-sodium options
Grains	6 to 8	1 slice whole grain bread, 1 ounce dry cereal, 1/2 cup cooked cereal, rice, or pasta • Choose whole grain options
Vegetables	4 to 5	1 cup leafy green vegetables, 1/2 cup cut-up raw or cooked vegetable such as carrots, tomatoes, broccoli, and sweet potatoes
Fruit	4 to 5	1 medium piece of fruit, 1/2 cup fresh, frozen or canned fruit, 4 ounces of 100% juice
Dairy-low fat or fat-free	2 to 3	1 cup skim or 1% milk, 1 cup low-fat yogurt, or 1 1/2 ounces part-skim cheese
Lean meat, poultry, and fish	6 1-ounce servings or less	1 egg or 1 ounce of cooked meat, poultry, or fish
Fats and oils	2 to 3	1 teaspoon margarine, 1 tablespoon mayonnaise, 2 tablespoons salad dressing
DASH DIET COMPONENT	**WEEKLY SERVINGS**	**SERVING EXAMPLES**
Nuts, seeds, and legumes	4 to 5	1/3 cup nuts, 2 tablespoons seeds or nut butter, 1/2 cup cooked beans or peas
Sweets	5 or fewer	1 tablespoon sugar, jelly or jam, 1/2 cup sorbet, 1 cup lemonade • Limit added sugars from beverages including soda, sweet teas, and juices

*Targets for a 2000 calorie/day diet.

Risk Factors

Type 2 diabetes differs from type 1 not only by pathophysiology but by risk factors. An established risk factor for type 1 is inherited risk from parents or siblings. Family history of diabetes is also a risk factor for type 2 diabetes, but other risk factors align closely with those similar to cardiovascular disease, hypertension, and other chronic conditions. These include:

- Age 45 or older (although, type 2 is becoming more common among young people)
- Overweight (BMI ≥25 kg/m²)
- Sedentary lifestyle
- Ethnicity: Black, Latino, Native American, Asian American, Pacific Islander
- Having prediabetes or gestational diabetes
- Hypertension
- Lipid disorder (HDL <35 mg/dL and triglycerides ≥250 mg/dL)
- History or existing vascular disease

Lifestyle and Diet for Prevention and Management of Diabetes

The management of type 1 diabetes relies on insulin therapy whereby individuals must learn how to balance the amount of insulin they need in proportion to their food intake. The management of type 2 diabetes, on the other hand, focuses more on preventive strategies as lifestyle modifications have significant implications on long-term complications.

The Diabetes Prevention Program (DPP), a type 2 diabetes prevention study, was a landmark trial comparing the effects of metformin, a drug to control high blood glucose, to an intensive lifestyle intervention among high-risk individuals.[47] Key features in the lifestyle intervention included (1) modest weight loss, (2) physical activity for 30 minutes, 5 times per week, and (3) improving heathy food choices with the assistance of counseling from registered dietitians.[48] In this large US multicenter, randomized controlled trial, diabetes incidence decreased by 58% among those in the intensive lifestyle intervention and 31% with metformin, compared to control group.[47] Ten-year follow-up since DPP randomization showed that diabetes incidence was 34% reduced for the lifestyle intervention group and 18% in the metformin group, compared to control.[49] Clearly, lifestyle changes are beneficial for the prevention and management of diabetes.

The DPP showed that changes in 3 modifiable risk factors—body weight, physical activity, and nutrition—work synergistically together to mitigate risk for diabetes. Weight management is often the primary goal for diabetes prevention. Even a small amount of weight loss (2 to 5 kg or 5% of initial body weight) can impact risk by lowering blood glucose levels and blood pressure and produce a more favorable blood lipid panel. Weight loss can be achieved through diet and activity. Physical activity is a component of diabetes management because of exercise effects on blood glucose. Exercising muscles enhance the transportation of glucose uptake into the cell. Dietary changes for people with diabetes include following a healthy diet within an appropriate calorie amount to produce or maintain weight loss. Nutritional needs for individuals with diabetes are similar with those without; however, individuals with type 2 diabetes are at higher risk for have existing cardiovascular disease, hypertension, and obesity. Recommendations for a healthy diet align closely with those suggested by the ACC/AHA guidelines for cardiovascular disease and the DASH diet for hypertension. The Mediterranean diet, DASH, and vegetarian/vegan diets have all been shown to assist with weight loss and improve blood glucose control among those with type 2 diabetes.[14] Fiber-rich sources of carbohydrates, including vegetables, fruits, and whole grains, release glucose more slowly into the blood thus producing a lower insulin response, especially when eating in a mixed meal (eg, along with protein and healthy fat) as opposed to refined carbohydrates. Additionally, sugar-sweetened beverages and artificially sweetened beverages have shown strong association with type 2 diabetes risk.[14]

Osteoporosis

Osteoporosis is a significant public health concern. An estimated 53 million people already have osteoporosis or are at risk for developing the disease.[50] Women disproportionately are affected by osteoporosis than men: 25% (1 in 4) of women aged 65 years or older compared to 5% (1 in 20) of men aged 65 years and older.[51] Osteoporosis, which means "porous bone," leads to frail bones due to a decrease in bone mass and bone quality. It is often associated with older individuals, as this is the life stage when physical complications from the disease occur including fractures in the hip, spine, and wrist. The timeline leading up to these events starts much earlier in life, and preventive strategies of diet and lifestyle changes can significantly lessen the burden of osteoporosis in old age. Until about age 30, bones are still in the formation and building phase, or referred to as peak bone mass. Thereafter bone breakdown occurs at a faster rate than formation. Maximizing peak bone mass during early life's critical period means bones will be further away from low density and fractures during the later years of life.

Risk Factors Associated With Osteoporosis

Bone loss is common in older age, but the magnitude of loss often depends on whether peak bone mass was achieved during childhood and adolescence. Risk factors for bone loss include the following:

- Female
- Advanced age
- Family history of disease
- Thin or small body frame
- Cigarette smoking
- Abnormal or loss of menstrual periods (amenorrhea)
- Early menopause
- Disordered eating that decreases adequate energy and nutrients, such as anorexia and bulimia nervosa
- Medications (corticosteroids and anticonvulsants) and medical conditions (thyroid disease and anticonvulsants) that may inhibit calcium absorption
- Excessive alcohol or caffeine intake
- Insufficient calcium and vitamin D intake

Influences of Diet and Lifestyle to Reduce Risk

Bone mineralization and maintenance require many nutrients including protein; vitamins D, K, and A; and the minerals calcium, phosphorus, fluoride, and magnesium. When it comes to bone health, calcium and vitamin D are 2 key nutrients that receive the most attention as they are important in building and maintaining bone strength and integrity.

Calcium and vitamin D work together to achieve maximum absorption, but only work optimally when both exist within the body in adequate amounts. Recommended calcium intakes depends on life stage groups: 1000 mg/day for children ages 4 to 8 years, adults ages 19 to 50 years, and adult men ages 51 to 70 years; 1200 mg/day for women ages 51 to 70 years and adults 70 years or older; and 1300 mg/day for children ages 9 to 18 years.[52] Vitamin D recommendations are 600 IU/day for ages 1 to 70 years and increases to 800 IU/day after age 70.[52] The *Dietary Guidelines, 2015-2020* have consistently recommended that sources of dairy be part of a healthy diet, partly due to dairy being a rich source of calcium and vitamin D.[14] Foods rich in calcium, apart from fluid milk, include yogurt, cheese, calcium-fortified beverage, soybeans, calcium-fortified tofu, kale, and broccoli. Vitamin D, which is converted in the body from sunlight exposure, is found naturally in few foods, but are in fatty fish (eg, salmon) and mushrooms (if grown under ultraviolet light) and smaller amounts in beef liver, cheese, and egg yolk. The best sources of vitamin D from the diet are in fortified dairy products including milk and yogurt.

Achieving peak bone mass occurs earlier in life, reflecting the increased calcium requirements during adolescence, yet current trends indicate that fluid milk intake, a rich source of calcium and vitamin D, is decreasing among young individuals. According to the National Risk Behavior Survey, youth in grades 9 to 12 who attend public schools exhibited daily milk consumption that decreased significantly in years 2011 to 2015, from 44.3% to 27.2%.[53] Continuing this trend of lower dairy intake will likely have major health consequences related to osteoporosis risk. Therefore, promotion of dietary intake rich in calcium and vitamin D is essential, especially among young individuals.

Weight-bearing activity is also encouraged to maintain strong bones. Exercising our bones is just as important as exercising our heart and muscles. Weight-bearing and strength-training activity activates the remodeling and strength processes of the bone, and if they are not exercised they will become weak and frail. Fitness experts recommend the following to promote bone health:

- Perform weight-bearing activities including walking, hiking, jogging, dancing, tennis, or team sports such as basketball or soccer.
- Add strength-training exercise, or resistance exercise, to one's fitness routine. This includes 20 to 30 minutes of training 2 to 3 times per week, using body-weight exercises, weight machines, or free weights to stress the bone and increase bone-building capacity.
- Other forms of exercises such as yoga or tai chi are not as effective for improving bone health, but do increase flexibility and balance and can contribute to overall health by preventing bone and joint injuries.

Anemia

Anemia is a condition when there is lower than normal red blood or hemoglobin to carry oxygen to cells and tissues. Several types of anemia are caused by vitamin or mineral deficiencies of iron, vitamin B_6, vitamin B_{12}, and folate. Iron-deficiency anemia is one of the most common deficiencies in the world, affecting 30% to 70% of populations in economically developing nations of Africa, Aisa, and

Latin America. It is also present in 30% to 40% of populations in industrialized countries of North America, Europe, and Australasia, including the United States.[54] Life stages that are at increased risk for deficiency include childhood, pre-pregnancy, pregnancy, and post-pregnancy, especially if breastfeeding. During pregnancy, iron is needed in greater amounts to support growth and development of a child and fetus in addition to that iron loss that occurs through menstruation and breastfeeding.

Iron is a component of hemoglobin and myoglobin, which transports oxygen in the blood and holds oxygen for muscle use, respectively. Iron also plays roles in many enzymatic reactions of energy metabolism and immune function. Iron is closely regulated within the body such that when iron is low absorption increases. Without adequate iron intake, deficiency may occur. Iron deficiency occurs in 3 stages:

1. **Iron stores depletion:** Blood ferritin is low due to depleted iron stores, but physiological impairments are not seen.
2. **Iron-deficiency erythropoiesis:** Serum ferritin remains low, and serum transferrin increases, while hemoglobin remains the same. Functional signs will occur, including fatigue.
3. **Iron-deficiency anemia:** Ferritin and hemoglobin levels are low, resulting in insufficient red blood cells that are small and pale in color. This is the most severe stage where many clinical symptoms present including cold intolerance, low energy levels, decreased performance among athletes, and pale skin.

Athletes and Iron-Deficiency Anemia

Oxygen use for working muscles and lungs is critical during aerobic and endurance training. This may be one reason why athletes are more likely to have iron-deficiency anemia than the nonathlete. Based on research conducted by Beard and Tobin, 3 groups of athletes appeared to be at greatest risk: women, vegetarians, and distance runners.[55] Some research has reported between 26% to 60% of female athletes are affected by iron-deficiency anemia.[56-58] Because of the large proportion of athletes at risk, iron is a nutrient of concern. Athletes are commonly assessed for adequate intake of iron, especially if they are of high risk and presenting with symptoms of fatigue and low energy.

Dietary Management of Iron-Deficiency Anemia

Iron requirements are largely based on life stages and gender. Children will require more iron during growth and maturation and women will start requiring more than their male counterparts once menstruation begins. For men and women ages 19 to 50 years, the requirement is 8 mg/day and

18 mg/day, respectively, while pregnant persons require 27 mg/day.[59]

Iron in food is found in 2 types: heme and nonheme iron. Heme iron is the iron in hemoglobin and myoglobin found in animal foods. Nonheme iron is present in both animal and plant foods, but is not part of hemoglobin or myoglobin. Beef, chicken, and fish contain approximately 40% heme iron and 60% nonheme iron. Plant foods including beans, fortified cereals, and green leafy vegetables are sources of only nonheme iron. Heme iron is much more bioavailable (ie, the body absorbs iron more efficiently) than nonheme iron. Therefore, vegetarians and vegans need more iron from foods than do those that eat foods with heme iron. Iron bioavailability, in both heme and nonheme foods, can be enhanced by vitamin C. Eating fruits and vegetables, which are rich sources of vitamin C, along with iron-containing foods can enhance iron absorption. An example would be to pair blueberries with fortified cereal or steamed broccoli with chicken breast. Iron's absorption, like other minerals, can be influenced by other food component interactions. For example, iron absorption can compete with calcium intake and can be inhibited by tannins in tea, phytic acid in grains, and excessive caffeine intake.

Supplementation may be needed if iron amounts cannot be achieved from diet alone. The upper limit of iron intake is 45 mg/day, and there is risk for toxicity if iron intake is not monitored properly. Therefore, iron supplementation should only occur after confirmation of iron-deficiency anemia, through hematologic analysis, and under the care of a physician and dietitian.

Conclusion

Nutrition and diet are the cornerstone to maintaining health and preventing disease. Imbalances of calories leads to obesity, resulting in large increases of chronic disease including cardiovascular disease, hypertension, and diabetes. These 3 diseases share many of the same risk factors and typically receive the same dietary recommendations for prevention and management. A shift in nutrient-based recommendations to diet pattern recommendations allows research to better understand the complexities and interactions from food and better application of diet recommendations. Adherence to a healthy diet pattern—one that is rich in plant-based foods, lean proteins, and healthy fats—ensures that nutrient requirements are being met, decreasing risk for nutrient-specific deficiencies such as vitamin D, calcium, and iron and preventing many chronic diseases.

Discussion Questions

1. Family history is a common among risk factor for many of the conditions discussed in this chapter. Investigate your risk for disease by asking family members and knowing your numbers (blood lipid panel and blood pressure). Further assess your risk for heart disease using the ACC/AHA Heart Risk Calculator: https://www.cvriskcalculator.com/

2. Record and analyze your diet using a mobile app or other nutrition software program. Compare it to the recommendations from the *Dietary Guidelines, 2020-2025*; ACC/AHA; and DASH diet guidelines. Think about the dietary changes you would have to make to adhere to diet recommendations discussed in this chapter.

3. Compare and contrast the Mediterranean and DASH diet eating patterns. How do they both serve to prevent risk for chronic conditions? Are there certain individuals who would adapt better to one eating pattern over the other? Why?

4. A 16-year-old distance runner reports that she lost 10 pounds over a year to be "lighter and faster." She has been amenorrheic for 3 months and says her energy is low and her running times have increased. Besides a concern for overall energy intake, what specific micronutrients would be of concern for this runner? Why?

References

1. US Department of Energy Office of Science. Office of Biological and Environmental Research. Human Genome Project Information Archive 1990-2003. Last modified March 26, 2019. Accessed April 24, 2020.

2. Merritt DC, Jamnik J, El-Sohemy A. FTO genotype, dietary protein intake, and body weight in a multiethnic population of young adults: a cross-sectional study. *Genes Nutr.* 2018;13(1):4.

3. Zhang X, Qi Q, Zhang C, et al. FTO genotype and 2-year change in body composition and fat distribution in response to weight-loss diets. *The POUNDS LOST Trial.* 2012;61(11):3005-3011.

4. Phillips CM, Kesse-Guyot E, McManus R, et al. High dietary saturated fat intake accentuates obesity risk associated with the fat mass and obesity–associated gene in adults. *J Nutr.* 2012;142(5):824-831.

5. Hales CM, Carroll MD, Fryar CD, Ogden CL. Prevalence of obesity and severe obesity among adults: United States, 2017-2018. NCHS Data Brief, no 360. National Center for Health Statistics; 2020.

6. US Department of Health and Human Services, National Heart, Lung, and Blood Institute. Managing overweight and obesity in adults: systematic evidence review from the obesity expert panel, 2013. Accessed April 24, 2020.

7. Bhaskaran K, Douglas I, Forbes H, dos-Santos-Silva I, Leon DA, Smeeth L. Body-mass index and risk of 22 specific cancers: a population-based cohort study of 5.24 million UK adults. *Lancet.* 2014;384(9945):755-65.

8. Hales CM, Carroll MD, Fryar CD, Ogden CL. Prevalence of obesity among adults and youth: United States, 2015–2016. NCHS data brief, no 288. National Center for Health Statistics; 2017.

9. Benjamin EJ, Muntner P, Alonso A, et al. Heart disease and stroke statistics—2019 update: a report from the American Heart Association. *Circulation.* 2019;139(10):e56-e528.

10. National Cholesterol Education Program. Third report of the national cholesterol education program (NCEP) expert panel on detection, evaluation, and treatment of high blood cholesterol in adults (adult treatment panel III) final report. NIH Pub. No. 02-5215. National Heart, Lung, and Blood Institute; 2002.

11. Grundy SM, Stone NJ, Bailey AL, et al. 2018 ACC/AHA/AACVPR/AAPA/ABC/ACPM/ADA/AGS/APhA/ASPC/NLA/PCNA guideline on the management of blood cholesterol: a report of the American College of Cardiology Foundation/American Heart Association task force on clinical practice guidelines. *Circulation.* 2019;139:e1082–e1143.

12. Goff DC, Lloyd-Jones DM, Bennett G, et al. 2013 ACC/AHA Guideline on the assessment of cardiovascular risk. *Circulation.* 2014;129(25_suppl_2):S49-S73.

13. Arnett DK, Blumenthal RS, Albert MA, et al. 2019 ACC/AHA guideline on the primary prevention of cardiovascular disease: executive summary: a report of the American College of Cardiology/American Heart Association task force on clinical practice guidelines. *Circulation.* 2019;140(11):e563-e595.

14. US Department of Agriculture and US Department of Health and Human Services. 2020-2025 *Dietary Guidelines for Americans.* 9th ed. December 2020. Available at DietaryGuidelines.gov. Accessed July 7, 2022.

15. Estruch R, Ros E, Salas-Salvadó J, et al. Primary prevention of cardiovascular disease with a Mediterranean diet supplemented with extra-virgin olive oil or nuts. *N Eng J Med.* 2018;378(25):e34.

16. Kim H, Caulfield LE, Rebholz CM. Healthy plant-based diets are associated with lower risk of all-cause mortality in US adults. *J Nutr.* 2018;148(4):624-631.

17. Reedy J, Krebs-Smith SM, Miller PE, et al. Higher diet quality is associated with decreased risk of all-cause, cardiovascular disease, and cancer mortality among older adults. *J Nutr.* 2014;144(6):881-889.

18. Phillips CM, Kesse-Guyot E, McManus R, et al. High dietary saturated fat intake accentuates obesity risk associated with the fat mass and obesity–associated gene in adults. *J Nutr.* 2012;142(5):824-831.

19. Wang DD, Li Y, Chiuve SE, et al. Association of specific dietary fats with total and cause-specific mortality. *JAMA Internal Medicine.* 2016;176(8):1134-1145.

20. Linda VH. A summary of the science supporting the new national cholesterol education program dietary recommendations: what dietitians should know. American Dietetic Association. *J Am Diet Assoc.* 2001;101(10):1148-1154.

21. Lichtenstein AH, Ausman LM, Jalbert SM, et al. Efficacy of a therapeutic lifestyle change/step 2 diet in moderately hypercholesterolemic middle-aged and elderly female and male subjects. *J Lipid Res.* 2002;43:264-273.

22. Jenkins DJA, Kendall CWC, Marchie A, et al. Effects of a dietary portfolio of cholesterol-lowering foods vs lovastatin on serum lipids and C-reactive protein. *JAMA.* 2003;290(4):502-510.

23. Obarzanek E, Kimm SYS, Barton BA, et al. Long-term safety and efficacy of a cholesterol-lowering diet in children with elevated low-density lipoprotein cholesterol: seven-year results of the Dietary Intervention Study in Children (DISC). *Pediatrics.* 2001;107(2):256.

24. Yu-Poth S, Zhao G, Etherton T, Naglak M, Jonnalagadda S, Kris-Etherton PM. Effects of the National Cholesterol Education Program's Step I and Step II dietary intervention programs on cardiovascular disease risk factors: a meta-analysis. *Am J Clin Nutr.* 1999;69(4):632-646.

25. Yang Q, Zhang Z, Gregg EW, Flanders WD, Merritt R, Hu FB. Added sugar intake and cardiovascular diseases mortality among US adults. *JAMA Internal Medicine.* 2014;174(4):516-524.

26. Micha R, Peñalvo JL, Cudhea F, Imamura F, Rehm CD, Mozaffarian D. Association between dietary factors and mortality from heart disease, stroke, and type 2 diabetes in the United States. *JAMA.* 2017;317(9):912-924.

27. Song M, Fung TT, Hu FB, et al. Association of animal and plant protein intake with all-cause and cause-specific mortality. *JAMA Internal Medicine.* 2016;176(10):1453-1463.

28. Malik VS, Popkin BM, Bray GA, Després J-P, Hu FB. Sugar-sweetened beverages, obesity, type 2 diabetes mellitus, and cardiovascular disease risk. *Circulation.* 2010;121(11):1356-1364.

29. Hu FB. Resolved: there is sufficient scientific evidence that decreasing sugar-sweetened beverage consumption will reduce the prevalence of obesity and obesity-related diseases. *Obes Rev.* 2013;14(8):606-619.

30. Seidelmann SB, Claggett B, Cheng S, et al. Dietary carbohydrate intake and mortality: a prospective cohort study and meta-analysis. *Lancet Public Health.* 2018;3(9):e419-e428.

31. Noto H, Goto A, Tsujimoto T, Noda M. Low-carbohydrate diets and all-cause mortality: a systematic review and meta-analysis of observational studies. *PloS One.* 2013;8(1).

32. Kiage JN, Merrill PD, Robinson CJ, et al. Intake of trans fat and all-cause mortality in the Reasons for Geographical and Racial Differences in Stroke (REGARDS) cohort. *Am J Clin Nutr.* 2013;97(5):1121-1128.

33. Mozaffarian D. Dietary and policy priorities for cardiovascular disease, diabetes, and obesity: a comprehensive review. *Circulation.* 2016;133(2):187-225.

34. Neelakantan N, Seah JYH, van Dam RM. The effect of coconut oil consumption on cardiovascular risk factors: a systematic review and meta-analysis of clinical trials. *Circulation.* 2020;141(10):803-814.

35. Dehghan M, Mente A, Rangarajan S, et al. Association of dairy intake with cardiovascular disease and mortality in 21 countries from five continents (PURE): a prospective cohort study. *Lancet.* 2018;392(10161):2288-2297.

36. Guo J, Astrup A, Lovegrove JA, Gijsbers L, Givens DI, Soedamah-Muthu SS. Milk and dairy consumption and risk of cardiovascular diseases and all-cause mortality: dose–response meta-analysis of prospective cohort studies. *Eur J Epidemiol.* 2017;32(4):269-287. doi:10.1007/s10654-017-0243-1

37. Wade AT, Davis CR, Dyer KA, Hodgson JM, Woodman RJ, Murphy KJ. A Mediterranean diet supplemented with dairy foods improves markers of cardiovascular risk: results from the MedDairy randomized controlled trial. *Am J Clin Nutr.* 2018;108(6):1166-1182.

38. Centers for Disease Control and Prevention, National Center for Health Statistics. Underlying cause of death, 1999–2017. CDC WONDER Online Database. Centers for Disease Control and Prevention; 2018. Accessed March 29, 2020.

39. Centers for Disease Control and Prevention (CDC). *Hypertension Cascade: Hypertension Prevalence, Treatment and Control Estimates Among US Adults Aged 18 Years and Older Applying the Criteria From the American College of Cardiology and American Heart Association's 2017 Hypertension Guideline—NHANES 2013–2016.* US Department of Health and Human Services; 2019.

40. Flack JM, Calhoun D, Schiffrin EL. *The New ACC/AHA Hypertension Guidelines for the Prevention, Detection, Evaluation, and Management of High Blood Pressure in Adults.* Oxford University Press US; 2018.

41. Sacks FM, Svetkey LP, Vollmer WM, et al. Effects on blood pressure of reduced dietary sodium and the Dietary Approaches to Stop Hypertension (DASH) diet. *N Eng J Med.* 2001;344(1):3-10.

42. Appel LJ, Brands MW, Daniels SR, Karanja N, Elmer PJ, Sacks FM. Dietary approaches to prevent and treat hypertension. *Hypertension.* 2006;47(2):296-308.

43. Appel LJ, Sacks FM, Carey VJ, et al. Effects of protein, mono-unsaturated fat, and carbohydrate intake on blood pressure and serum lipids: results of the OmniHeart randomized trial. *JAMA.* 2005;294(19):2455-2464.

44. Sacks FM, Carey VJ, Anderson CA, et al. Effects of high vs low glycemic index of dietary carbohydrate on cardiovascular disease risk factors and insulin sensitivity: the OmniCarb randomized clinical trial. *JAMA*. 2014;312(23):2531-2541.

45. Centers for Disease Control and Prevention. National Diabetes Statistics Report, 2020. Centers for Disease Control and Prevention, US Department of Health and Human Services; 2020.

46. American Diabetes Association. Classification and diagnosis of diabetes. *Diabetes Care*. 2016;39(Suppl 1):S13-S22.

47. The Diabetes Prevention Program Research Group. Achieving weight and activity goals among Diabetes Prevention Program lifestyle participants. *Obes Res*. 2004;12(9):1426-1434.

48. The Diabetes Prevention Program Research Group. The Diabetes Prevention Program (DPP): description of lifestyle intervention. *Diabetes Care*. 2002;25(12):2165-2171.

49. The Diabetes Prevention Program Research Group. 10-year follow-up of diabetes incidence and weight loss in the Diabetes Prevention Program Outcomes Study. *Lancet*. 2009;374(9702):1677-1686.

50. National Institutes of Health Osteoporosis and Related Bone Disease National Resource Center. Bone health for life: health information for you and your family. National Institutes of Health and U.S. Department of Health and Human Services. Accessed April 21, 2020.

51. Centers for Disease Control and Prevention. Office of Science (OS) Office of Genomics and Precision Public Health. Does Osteoporosis Run in Your Family? Published 2019. Accessed April 21, 2020.

52. Del Valle HB, Yaktine AL, Taylor CL, Ross AC. *Dietary Reference Intakes for Calcium and Vitamin D*. National Academies Press; 2011.

53. Miller G, Merlo C, Demissie Z, Sliwa S, Park S. Trends in beverage consumption among high school students-United States, 2007-2015. *MMWR Morb Mortal Wkly Rep*. 2017;66(4):112-116.

54. World Health Organization. Nutritional anaemias: tools for effective prevention and control. World Health Organization; 2017.

55. Beard J, Tobin B. Iron status and exercise. *Am J Clin Nutr*. 2000;72(2):594S-597S.

56. Balaban EP, Cox JV, Snell P, Vaughan RH, Frenkel EP. The frequency of anemia and iron deficiency in the runner. *Med Sci Sports Exerc*. 1989;21(6):643-648.

57. Pate RR, Miller BJ, Davis JM, Slentz CA, Klingshirn LA. Iron status of female runners. *Int J Sport Nutr Exerc Metabol*. 1993;3(2):222-231.

58. Nickerson HJ, Holubets M, Tripp A, Pierce WE. Decreased iron stores in high school female runners. *American Journal of Diseases of Children*. 1985;139(11):1115-1119.

59. Institute of Medicine, Food and Nutrition Board. *Dietary Reference Intakes for Vitamin A, Vitamin K, Arsenic, Boron, Chromium, Copper, Iodine, Iron, Manganese, Molybdenum, Nickel, Silicon, Vanadium, fnd Zinc: A Report of the Panel on Micronutrients*. National Academy Press; 2001.

Chapter 12

Disordered Eating Behaviors

Tabbetha D. Lopez, PhD, RD, LD
Tracey Ledoux, PhD, RD
Jon P. Gray, EdD

Commission on Accreditation of Athletic Training Education *2020 Standards*

This chapter addresses the following *2020 Standards for Accreditation of Professional Athletic Training Programs*:

- Standard 56: Advocate for the health needs of clients, patients, communities, and populations.

- Standard 57: Analyze the impact of health literacy and social determinants of health on patient care and outcomes to determine health care strategies that empower patients and improve outcomes.

- Standard 58: Incorporate patient education and self-care programs to engage patients and their families and friends to participate in their care and recovery.

- Standard 61: Practice in collaboration with other health care and wellness professionals. [Dietitians].

- Standard 70: Evaluate and manage patients with acute conditions, including triaging conditions that are life threatening or otherwise emergent. [Eating disorders or disordered eating behaviors.]

- Standard 71: Perform an examination to formulate a diagnosis and plan of care for patients with health conditions commonly seen in athletic training practice. [The development of disordered eating behaviors or eating disorders.]

- Standard 77: Identify, refer, and give support to patients with behavioral health conditions. Work with other health care professionals to monitor these patients' treatment, compliance, progress, and readiness to participate. [Disordered eating behaviors or eating disorders.]

- Standard 79: Develop and implement strategies to mitigate the risk for long-term health conditions across the lifespan. [Developed from disordered eating behaviors or eating disorders.]

- Standard 94: Develop and implement specific policies and procedures for the purposes of identifying patients with behavioral health problems and referring patients in crisis to qualified providers.

Knoblauch M, ed. *Clinical Nutrition in Athletic Training* (pp 133-139).
© 2023 Taylor & Francis Group.

Learning Objectives

After reviewing this chapter, readers will be able to:
- Identify individuals with disordered eating behaviors.
- Interpret and apply nutrition concepts to evaluate individuals with disordered eating behaviors.
- Provide recommendations to improve the nutritional health of individuals with disordered eating behaviors.

Introduction

This chapter will define disordered eating behaviors, discuss the factors that lead to disordered eating behaviors, describe the consequences of disordered eating behaviors, and provide recommendations for individuals identified with disordered eating behaviors.

Disordered Eating Behaviors

Disordered eating behaviors refer to a myriad of abnormal eating behaviors that often mirror symptoms of diagnosed eating disorders. The difference between disordered eating behaviors and a diagnosed eating disorder (ie, anorexia nervosa, bulimia nervosa) is the frequency of behaviors and the level of the severity of the behaviors. The development of disordered eating behaviors is multifactorial including genetic, personal factors, family and peer influences, sociocultural pressures, and body dissatisfaction.

Disordered eating behaviors often include:
- Preoccupation associated with food, weight, and body image
- Frequent dieting
- Chronic weight fluctuations
- Compulsive eating habits
- Obsessive calorie counting
- Anxiety associated with specific foods or eating with others
- Skipping meals regularly/fasting/chronic restrained eating
- Self-worth based on body shape and weight
- Rigid rituals or rules around food and exercise
- Feelings of guilt and/or shame associated with food
- Misuse of laxatives or diuretics
- Loss of control around food
- Binge eating
- Self-induced vomiting
- Making up for eating "bad" foods by excessive exercising, fasting, or purging

Disordered eating behaviors exist on a continuum ranging from unhealthy behaviors (ie, frequent dieting) to extreme behaviors (ie, self-induced vomiting). These behaviors are deleterious to the individual's mental and physical health. These behaviors can lead to obesity, bone loss, gastrointestinal disturbances, electrolyte and fluid imbalances, low heart rate, depression, anxiety, social isolation, and diagnosed eating disorders.[1] These individuals are also more susceptible to the addiction of caffeine, tobacco, drugs, and alcohol.[2] It is important for clinicians to be able to identify the characteristics of disordered eating behaviors in order to intervene before those behaviors increase in severity and frequency.

Consistent cultural and societal messages from fashion, cosmetic, fitness, insurance, pharmaceutical, and weight loss industries promoting the ideal body size has increased the prevalence of disordered eating behaviors.[3,4] Social networking sites have increased our exposure to society's beauty ideals, body comparisons, and self-objectification—increasing the internalization of these ideals.[4] Research has found that young adults with frequent use of social networking sites are at increased risk for developing weight dissatisfaction, self-worth based on appearance, drive for thinness, thin-ideal internalization, self-objectification, body surveillance, and diet behaviors.[4]

Disordered eating behaviors frequently begin during adolescence. The National Center on Addiction and Substance Abuse (CASA) reports that 62% of teenage girls are trying to lose weight, 59% are actively dieting, and 68% exercise with a specific goal of weight loss or weight maintenance.[5] In teenage boys 29% report trying to lose weight, 28% are actively dieting, and 51% exercise with the goal of losing weight or to avoid gaining weight.[5] Adolescents are more likely to engage in disordered eating behaviors (ie, dieting and binge eating) to control weight and body shape and are unlikely to engage in healthy behaviors (ie, regular exercise and fruit/vegetable intake), especially during critical periods such as puberty and identity formation.[6] This is important for clinicians to be aware; young adults who attempt unhealthy weight-control behaviors are at a higher risk for becoming involved with tobacco and alcohol use, suicide attempts, and unprotected sexual activity.[2,7]

Disordered eating behaviors are significantly more prevalent in adolescents who are overweight or obese.[1] Unhealthy weight control behaviors such as frequent dieting, compulsive eating habits, and restriction are present in 76% of girls with obesity and 55% of boys with obesity, and extreme weight control behaviors such as fasting, bingeing, and purging have been found in 18% of girls with obesity and 6% of boys with obesity.[7,8] These behaviors are more likely to continue into adulthood, increasing the risks for health and psychological problems such as heart disease, type 2 diabetes, metabolic syndrome, specific types of cancer, diagnosed eating disorders, depression, and anxiety.[1,8-10]

The most significant predictor of disordered eating behaviors is a negative body image such as a preoccupation of weight, body shape, size, self-worth based on appearance, weight dissatisfaction, drive for thinness, thin-ideal internalization, self-objectification, and body surveillance.[1,4,8]

Body Image

Body image is defined as a mental picture of one's body, including conscious and unconscious perceptions, attitudes, and feelings. It can be an evolving perception based on recent changes in weight, shape, eating behaviors, or mood and is often linked to the influence of one's shape and weight on self-worth.[1,8] The media has portrayed women as ultra-thin and men as muscular. The media portrays unrealistic beauty ideals of glamorous and Photoshopped women, encouraging other women to internalize and engage in appearance comparisons.[4] The consistent and repeated exposure to these images leads to the acceptance of these body images as normative, also known as "internalization." Much of the research on internalizing body ideals has focused on women; however, more research has focused on the importance of men's muscular ideals. Internalizing of body ideals can lead to body dissatisfaction.

Body Dissatisfaction

Body dissatisfaction is defined as a negative body image, a negative assessment of one's shape and/or weight. Individuals with high body dissatisfaction have frequent dieting behaviors, other disordered eating behaviors, low self-esteem, and depressive symptoms.[11] Body dissatisfaction is the most significant contributor to disordered eating behaviors and diagnosed eating disorders.[12] Negative body perceptions are formed as early as childhood with exposure to unrealistic ideals for men and women. For example, women are frequently pressured to achieve a thin ideal body shape, while men are often pressured to achieve a muscular phenotype; consequently, all genders can suffer from body dissatisfaction due to these unrealistic body ideals. Mass media is the most significant contributor to adolescent body dissatisfaction.[4] There is some evidence the internalization of thin-ideal can be different for different racial/ethnic groups; the adherence to socially prescribed body ideals may increase body dissatisfaction. It is also important to note that Asian and Hispanic adolescents often experience more body dissatisfaction than White adolescents."[11,13,14]

Adolescents are especially susceptible to body image pressures from their parents and peers. Research has shown that adolescents whose mothers both frequently diet and have body dissatisfaction are more likely to be dissatisfied with their weight and to become constant dieters.[3] There is also evidence that adolescents who perceive it is important to their father to be thin were more likely to become constant dieters.[3] Body dissatisfaction can also come from peer pressures, such as teasing, criticism, comparisons, judging, social conflict, and social exclusion.[18] Adolescents who experience weight-based teasing are more likely to have a higher BMI, binge eat, and have disordered eating behaviors in young adulthood as compared to other adolescents.[15] Research suggests that weight-based teasing in adolescence predicts obesity and disordered eating behaviors into adulthood.[14]

Gender has been shown to influence body dissatisfaction in adolescents. In adolescent girls, as BMI increases so does their level of body dissatisfaction. This relationship between BMI and body dissatisfaction tends to increase an adolescent girl's risk of engagement in disordered eating behaviors as well as their risk for developing a diagnosed eating disorder.[16] A study found that almost 50% of adolescent girls who were overweight or obese were dissatisfied with their bodies, and 9.5% of those individuals met criteria for frequent binge eating.[16] Interestingly, the prevalence of body dissatisfaction among adolescent boys has increased significantly in the last decade. In male adolescents, body dissatisfaction is largely related to "muscularity."[15,16] Therefore, men often engage in unhealthy behaviors such as muscle-building supplements (eg, androstenedione) or hormone-related therapy (eg, growth hormone, anabolic steroids) to achieve ideal muscularity.[17] A study found that 18% of young men were extremely concerned about their weight and shape and 7.6% of them were actively using unhealthy means to achieve their ideal muscularity.[17] Excessive use of creatine supplements, growth hormone derivatives, and anabolic steroids to achieve desired muscle gains and fat losses can lead to the development of eating disorders.[17,18]

Weight Discrimination

Weight discrimination is unequal or unfair treatment, and weight bias is negative weight-related attitudes toward individuals with excess weight. Discrimination or bias can come from parents, peers, educators, medical professionals, or the media.[19] Weight discrimination often leads to a lack of quality health care, education, and support.[20] Individuals experiencing weight discrimination or weight bias are more likely to binge eat and are less motivated to lose weight.[16] To help reduce the risk of weight discrimination and bias, clinicians should treat obesity as a disease, accept body size diversity, and promote health as opposed to weight loss.

The internalization of body ideals, teasing, and weight discrimination shapes the negative thoughts and feelings individuals have of their bodies. These perceptions of the ideal body lead to a desire to achieve this body. Unfortunately, adolescents are not equipped with the knowledge of health and fitness to achieve their perception of an "ideal body" healthily. Therefore, they begin unhealthy disordered eating behaviors, some of which come from mirroring adults around them as well as from social media or peers. Disordered eating behaviors can increase in frequency and severity when adolescents have feelings of inadequacy, and unobtainable body ideal goals can lead to diagnosed eating disorders.

Eating Disorders

Eating disorders are diagnosed by characteristics specified in the *Diagnostic and Statistical Manual of Mental Disorders, Fifth Edition* (DSM-5).[21] In general, eating disorders are characterized by severe and frequent levels of disordered eating behaviors, excessive exercise, and/or unhealthy preoccupation with one's weight or shape. It is estimated that 20 million women and 10 million men in America have suffered from an eating disorder.[20] Risk factors for developing eating disorders include history of dieting, perfectionism, body dissatisfaction, behavioral inflexibility, weight stigma, appearance ideal internalization, and teasing. Each disorder is characterized by specific factors that arise from within an individual's brain chemistry, personality, family, peer group, or social environment. There are severe health consequences of eating disorders such as muscle wasting, heart failure, cardiovascular complications, gastroparesis, constipation, pancreatitis, bone loss, and kidney failure. Eating disorders take on many different forms; anorexia nervosa, bulimia nervosa, and binge eating disorder are the most common. It is important to remember each individual experiences eating disorders uniquely.

Anorexia Nervosa

Anorexia nervosa is defined by weight loss, difficulties maintaining appropriate weight, restrictive eating patterns, fear of weight gain, and severe body image distortion. Individuals with anorexia nervosa often have a fear of gaining weight, which is manifested through an excessive restriction of food as well as excessive participation in physical exercise or laxative use. Individuals with anorexia nervosa often extremely restrict caloric intake and have rigid food rules; this can range from refusal to eat carbohydrates to restricting to 1 cup of raw vegetables a day.[20] These behaviors may also present as restricting calories, including excessive exercise or laxative use to compensate for the calories consumed. Other behaviors could include self-induced vomiting, excessive exercise, or the misuse of laxatives, diuretics, and/or enemas.

Diagnostic Criteria According to the DSM-5[21]

1. Restriction of energy intake relative to requirements leading to a significantly low body weight in the context of age, sex, developmental trajectory, and physical health.
2. Intense fear of gaining weight or becoming fat, even though underweight.
3. Disturbance in the way in which one's body weight or shape is experienced, undue influence of body weight or shape on self-evaluation, or denial of the seriousness of the current low body weight.

Warning Signs

Warning signs and symptoms include severe and frequent disordered eating and body dissatisfaction as well as intense fear of gaining weight, feeling out of control, mood swings, suicidal thoughts, impaired school performance, and secretive behavior around food. Physical symptoms include gastrointestinal complaints, menstrual irregularities, dental problems, dry skin and hair, the growth of fine hair on the body (lanugo), yellow skin, and poor wound healing.

Health Consequences

In anorexia nervosa, the intense cycles of malnutrition deny the body access to essential nutrients to function normally. Some of the more severe consequences include muscle wasting, heart failure, gastroparesis, neurological problems, and death. Muscle tissue throughout the body is broken down for energy including the heart, skeletal, and gastrointestinal systems. The cardiovascular system slows down as it has less energy to pump blood, increasing the risk for heart failure. Gastroparesis, constipation, and bacterial infections are due to gastrointestinal muscle loss and long-term inadequate nutritional intake. The extreme calorie deficiency leads to neurological problems including problems concentrating, fainting, dizziness, and numbness in appendages. Electrolyte imbalances can cause seizures, muscle cramps, heart failure, and kidney failure. Overall, individuals suffering from anorexia nervosa have a 6-fold increase in mortality compared to those without the disorder.[20]

Bulimia Nervosa

Bulimia nervosa is a characterized by recurrent binge eating behavior. Binge eating is defined as intake of excessive amounts of food in a short period with a loss of control over their actions. Binge eating with loss of control episodes are followed by feelings of guilt and shame for the behavior, which leads to patterns similar to anorexia nervosa such as self-induced vomiting, fasting, overexercising, or the misuse of laxatives, enemas, or diuretics.[22] Unlike anorexia nervosa, an individual with bulimia nervosa is typically just above or below average weight. This often makes the diagnosis of bulimia somewhat challenging.

Diagnostic Criteria According to the DSM-5[21]

1. Recurrent episodes of binge eating. An episode of binge eating is characterized by both of the following:
   - Eating, in a discrete period of time (eg, within any 2-hour period), an amount of food that is definitely larger than most people would eat during a similar period of time and under similar circumstances.
   - A sense of lack of control overeating during the episode (eg, a feeling that one cannot stop eating or control what or how much one is eating).
2. Recurrent inappropriate compensatory behavior in order to prevent weight gain, such as self-induced vomiting; misuse of laxatives, diuretics, or other medications; fasting; or excessive exercise.
3. The binge eating and inappropriate compensatory behaviors both occur, on average, at least once a week for 3 months.
4. Self-evaluation is unduly influenced by body shape and weight.
5. The disturbance does not occur exclusively during episodes of anorexia nervosa.

Warning Signs

Warning signs of bulimia nervosa include difficulties eating with others, disappearing after meals often to go to the restroom, fad diets, excessive use of mouthwash/mints/gum, changes in personality, emotional outbursts, depression, self-harm, substance abuse, suicide attempts, guilt, self-disgust, self-loathing, frequent trips to the bathroom, erratic behavior, or mood swings. Physical symptoms include weight fluctuations, stomach cramps, menstrual irregularities, yellowing teeth, calluses on fingers due to self-induced vomiting, dry skin and hair, the growth of fine hair on the body (lanugo), and poor wound healing.

Health Consequences

Recurrent binge and purging cycles impact chemical and electrolyte balances in the body. These imbalances lead to heart failure, rupture of the stomach or esophagus, pancreatitis, seizures, muscle cramps, and death. Heart failure in bulimia is often cause by electrolyte imbalances of potassium, sodium, and chloride during purging cycles. Frequent purging can also lead to rupturing of the stomach, ulcers, acid reflux, and rupturing of the esophagus. The electrolyte imbalances also lead to seizures and muscle cramps. Due to lack of follow-up, the death rates of bulimia are not as well known as anorexia; however, the rates are approximately that 4% of individuals with a diagnosis of bulimia die from it. Bulimia is known to have the highest suicide rates of any eating disorder.

Binge Eating Disorder

Binge eating disorder is characterized by recurrent episodes of excessive food intake, often in a 2-hour period, resulting in physical discomfort. The individual often feels a sense of loss of control over their actions and experiences shame for the actions or distress or guilt after the actions, and it occurs at least 1 time per week.[23] Individuals with this disorder tend to be normal weight or higher than average weight. However, health risks are similar to those of with clinical obesity. This is the newest eating disorder added to the DSM in 2013.

Diagnostic Criteria According to the DSM-5[21]

1. Recurrent episodes of binge eating. An episode of binge eating is characterized by both of the following:
   - Eating, in a discrete period of time (eg, within any 2-hour period), an amount of food that is definitely larger than most people would eat during a similar period of time and under similar circumstances.
   - A sense of lack of control overeating during the episode (eg, a feeling that one cannot stop eating or control what or how much one is eating).
2. The binge eating episodes are associated with 3 (or more) of the following:
   - Eating much more rapidly than normal.
   - Eating until feeling uncomfortably full.
   - Eating large amounts of food when not feeling physically hungry.
   - Eating alone because of feeling embarrassed by how much one is eating.
   - Feeling disgusted with oneself, depressed, or very guilty afterward.
3. Marked distress regarding binge eating is present.
4. The binge eating occurs, on average, at least once a week for 3 months.
5. The binge eating is not associated with the recurrent use of inappropriate compensatory behaviors (eg, purging) as in bulimia nervosa, and does not occur exclusively during the course of bulimia nervosa or anorexia nervosa.

Warning Signs

Warning signs of binge eating disorder are the disappearance of large amounts of food in short periods of time, fear of eating in public, hiding food, eating in secret, eating only specific foods, fad diets, sporadic dieting, and withdrawing from friends or activities. Physical symptoms include fluctuations in weight, stomach cramps, gastrointestinal complaints, and difficulties concentrating.

Table 12-1

NEDA Recommendations for Preventing Body Dissatisfaction in Adolescents and Young Adults[28]

Be positive	Set a positive example, avoid talking about dieting, weight loss, or good versus bad foods.
Encourage acceptance	Teach respect, love, and acceptance of their and other unique bodies.
Build self-esteem	Encourage character building, self-assurance, and decision-making.
Open communication	Encourage open, honest communication and acknowledge their feelings and opinions.
Critical thinking	Discuss brainstorming and challenging media messages. Teach them how to think, not what to think.
Personal values	Encourage self-worth, wisdom, loyalty, fairness, curiosity, self-awareness, and relationships.
Deal with emotions	Assist with dealing with emotions without food, using alternative methods such as journaling or physical activity.

Table 12-2

NATA Recommendations for Preventing, Detecting, and Managing Disordered Eating in Athletes[24]

Departmental recommendations	Identify a health care team within your facility to provide detection and treatment, develop a compressive management plan, and establish screening procedures and policies.
Identification	Proper training is required for the identification of disordered eating behaviors and DSM-5 disorders. Trainers need to be mindful of changes in dietary intake or weight control behaviors.
Complications	Athletes can suffer serious medical consequences due to disordered eating behaviors such as cardiovascular complications, bradycardia, hypotension, hypothermia, reproductive issues, and electrolyte imbalances.

Health Consequences

The health consequences of binge eating disorder are commonly associated with those of clinical obesity. Consequences including weight gain, high blood pressure, high cholesterol, heart disease, type 2 diabetes mellitus, and emotional and mental distress.

Disordered Eating and Eating Disorders in Athletes

Disordered eating behaviors and diagnosed eating disorders are common in athletes due to the pressures to achieve a high level of success. Sports emphasizing size, weight, and appearances, such as body building, gymnastics, figure skating, wrestling, rowing, and horse racing, especially put athletes at risk. It is estimated that nearly 62% of female athletes and 33% of male athletes suffer from disordered eating behaviors.[24] Due to the intense physiological demands of high intensity and volume sport, the effects of these behaviors can be detrimental. A study of female high school athletes found that 42% had disordered eating behaviors, and they were

8 times more likely to incur an injury than athletes who did not report disordered eating behaviors.[19] College athletes are at an increased risk for developing eating disorders; one study found 35% of women and 10% of men had anorexia nervosa, while 58% of women and 38% of men had bulimia nervosa.[20,25] Another study of Division II female athletes reported that 25% showed disordered eating behaviors, 26% menstrual dysfunction, 10% low bone density, and 3% had all 3 symptoms.[20,26] Unfortunately, 91% of athletic trainers working with female athletes report working with athletes with eating disorders or the symptoms, while only 27% felt confident identifying an athlete with an eating disorder.[27]

Prevention

As clinicians, athletic trainers should be able to provide prevention, early detection, and management of disordered eating behaviors. The National Eating Disorder Association (NEDA) provides tools and resources to learn and provide support to individuals and clinicians (Table 12-1). The National Athletic Trainers' Association provides recommendations for preventing, detecting, and managing disordered eating in athletes (Table 12-2).

Discussion Questions

1. A female long distance runner is 101 pounds, 66 inches tall, and has a BMI of 16. She trains twice a day, plus workouts at the campus fitness center. You notice she is self-isolating, she has no friends or social connections, and she is also not doing well academically. You are concerned about her—how do you approach these sensitive topics?

2. A successful friend is 45 years old, weighs 200 pounds, and is 55 inches tall. She has decided to make a dramatic lifestyle change and has asked for your help. You help her with a training plan and discuss healthy eating with her. She agrees and says she will follow the plan. After 3 weeks of weekly training, you notice the client's weight is not decreasing. She states she is eating small healthy meals most of the time. However, during recalls there are very large gaps and you notice she reports feeling ill around those gaps. How do you approach this topic and help your friend?

References

1. Goldschmidt AB, Aspen VP, Sinton MM, Tanofsky-Kraff M, Wilfley DE. Disordered eating attitudes and behaviors in overweight youth. *Obesity.* 2008;16(2):257-264.

2. Cattarin JA, Thompson JK. A three-year longitudinal study of body image, eating disturbance, and general psychological functioning in adolescent females. *J Eat Disord.* 1994;2(2):114-125.

3. Field AE, Camargo CA, Jr., Taylor CB, Berkey CS, Roberts SB, Colditz GA. Peer, parent, and media influences on the development of weight concerns and frequent dieting among preadolescent and adolescent girls and boys. *Pediatrics.* 2001;107(1):54-60.

4. Holland G, Tiggemann M. A systematic review of the impact of the use of social networking sites on body image and disordered eating outcomes. *Body Image.* 2016;17:100-110.

5. Califano JA, Bollinger LC, Bush C, Chenault KI, Curtis JL, Dimon J. *Food for Thought: Substance Abuse and Eating Disorders.* The National Center on Addiction and Substance Abuse at Columbia University; 2003.

6. Neumark-Sztainer D, Paxton SJ, Hannan PJ, Haines J, Story M. Does body satisfaction matter? Five-year longitudinal associations between body satisfaction and health behaviors in adolescent females and males. *J Adolesc Health.* 2006;39(2):244-251.

7. Neumark-Sztainer D, Story M, Hannan PJ, Perry CL, Irving LM. Weight-related concerns and behaviors among overweight and nonoverweight adolescents: implications for preventing weight-related disorders. *Arch Pediatr Adolesc Med.* 2002;156(2):171-178.

8. Hayes JF, Fitzsimmons-Craft EE, Karam AM, Jakubiak J, Brown ML, Wilfley DE. Disordered eating attitudes and behaviors in youth with overweight and obesity: implications for treatment. *Curr Obes Rep.* 2018;7(3):235-246.

9. Singh AS, Mulder C, Twisk JW, van Mechelen W, Chinapaw MJ. Tracking of childhood overweight into adulthood: a systematic review of the literature. *Obes Rev.* 2008;9(5):474-488.

10. Llewellyn A, Simmonds M, Owen CG, Woolacott N. Childhood obesity as a predictor of morbidity in adulthood: a systematic review and meta-analysis. *Obes Rev.* 2016;17(1):56-67.

11. Bucchianeri MM, Fernandes N, Loth K, Hannan PJ, Eisenberg ME, Neumark-Sztainer D. Body dissatisfaction: do associations with disordered eating and psychological well-being differ across race/ethnicity in adolescent girls and boys? *Cultur Divers Ethnic Minor Psychol.* 2016;22(1):137-146.

12. Stice E, Whitenton K. Risk factors for body dissatisfaction in adolescent girls: a longitudinal investigation. *Dev Psychol.* 2002;38(5):669-678.

13. Quick V, Eisenberg ME, Bucchianeri MM, Neumark-Sztainer D. Prospective predictors of body dissatisfaction in young adults: 10-year longitudinal findings. *Emerg Adulthood.* 2013;1(4):271-282.

14. Paterna A, Alcaraz-Ibáñez M, Fuller-Tyszkiewicz M, Sicilia Á. Internalization of body shape ideals and body dissatisfaction: a systematic review and meta-analysis. *Int J Eat Dis.* 2021;54(9):1575-1600. doi:10.1002/eat.23568

15. Puhl RM, Wall MM, Chen C, Bryn Austin S, Eisenberg ME, Neumark-Sztainer D. Experiences of weight teasing in adolescence and weight-related outcomes in adulthood: a 15-year longitudinal study. *Prev Med.* 2017;100:173-179.

16. Sonneville KR, Calzo JP, Horton NJ, Haines J, Austin SB, Field AE. Body satisfaction, weight gain and binge eating among overweight adolescent girls. *Int J Obes.* 2012;36(7):944-949.

17. Field AE, Sonneville KR, Crosby RD, et al. Prospective associations of concerns about physique and the development of obesity, binge drinking, and drug use among adolescent boys and young adult men. *JAMA Pediatr.* 2014;168(1):34-39.

18. Lavender JM, Brown TA, Murray SB. Men, muscles, and eating disorders: an overview of traditional and muscularity-oriented disordered eating. *Curr Psychiatry Rep.* 2017;19(6):32.

19. Ramos Salas X, Alberga AS, Cameron E, et al. Addressing weight bias and discrimination: moving beyond raising awareness to creating change. *Obes Rev.* 2017;18(11):1323-1335.

20. Keski-Rahkonen A, Hoek HW, Susser ES, et al. Epidemiology and course of anorexia nervosa in the community. *Am J Psychiatry.* 2007;8(64):1259-1265.

21. American Psychiatric Association. *Diagnostic and Statistical Manual of Mental Disorders.* 5th ed. Author; 2013.

22. Favaro A, Caregaro L, Tenconi E, Bosello R, Santonastaso P. Time trends in age at onset of anorexia nervosa and bulimia nervosa. *J Clin Psychiatry.* 2009;12(70):1715-1721.

23. Hudson JI, Hiripi E, Pope HG Jr, Kessler RC. The prevalence and correlates of eating disorders in the National Comorbidity Survey Replication. *Biol Psychiatry.* 2007;61(3):348-358.

24. Bonci CM, Bonci LJ, Granger LR, et al. National Athletic Trainers' Association position statement: preventing, detecting, and managing disordered eating in athletes. *J Athl Train.* 2008;43(1):80-108.

25. Johnson C, Powers PS, Dick R. Athletes and eating disorders: the National Collegiate Athletic Association study. *Int J Eat Disord.* 1999;26(2):179-188.

26. Jankowski C. Associations between disordered eating, menstrual dysfunction, and musculoskeletal injury among high school athletes. *Yearbook of Sports Medicine.* 2012:394-395.

27. Greenleaf C, Petrie TA, Carter J, Reel JJ. Female collegiate athletes: prevalence of eating disorders and disordered eating behaviors. *J Am Coll Health.* 2009;57(5):489-496.

28. National Eating Disorders Association. Developing & modeling positive body image. https://www.nationaleatingdisorders.org/learn/general-information/developing-positive-body-img

Chapter 13

Nutritional Considerations for Travel

Mandy Tyler, MEd, RD, CSSD, LD, LAT
E. Joanna Soles, DHSc, ATC, LAT

Commission on Accreditation of Athletic Training Education *2020 Standards*

This chapter addresses the following *2020 Standards for Accreditation of Professional Athletic Training Programs*:

- Standard 55: Students must gain foundational knowledge in statistics, research design, epidemiology, pathophysiology, biomechanics and pathomechanics, exercise physiology, nutrition, human anatomy, pharmacology, public health, and health care delivery and payor systems.
- Standard 59: Communicate effectively and appropriately with clients/patients, family members, coaches, administrators, other health care professionals, consumers, payors, policy makers, and others.
- Standard 83: Educate and make recommendations to clients/patients on fluids and nutrients to ingest prior to activity, during activity, and during recovery for a variety of activities and environmental conditions.

Learning Objectives

After reviewing this chapter, readers will be able to:

- Examine the potential roles and responsibilities of the athletic trainer in meal planning and nutritional considerations while traveling.
- Discuss menu planning strategies and best nutritional options for before and after events, and identify how these strategies can be adapted to a variety of restaurant types.
- Outline common nutritional concerns and considerations associated with travel, including airline nutrition, hotels, altitude, heat concerns, food safety, and travel to foreign countries.

Knoblauch M, ed. *Clinical Nutrition in Athletic Training* (pp 141-150).
© 2023 Taylor & Francis Group.

Role of the Athletic Trainer

When it comes to nutrition, whether traveling or not, the athletic trainer's role may vary significantly from one job to the next, and even from one sport to the next (Sidebar 13-1). Professional sports and some universities may have the support of a sports dietitian, so athletic trainers may have a very limited role, while high school athletic trainers may be tasked with all aspects of meal planning. Research has shown that athletic trainers generally have significantly more nutrition knowledge than coaches and athletes,[1] so athletic trainers should be ready to be involved to best serve their athletes.

Plan Ahead

Regardless of how the team is traveling, planning ahead is essential to ensuring good nutrition options are available. A general daily schedule should be constructed to include regular meals and snacks; it is important that mealtimes are similar to the team's usual daily routine. If the team has an early flight or a late-night bus trip, ensure plans are made for how meals will be provided. In addition, ensure the foods provided are similar to what the athletes are accustomed to eating. A road trip for a tournament may not be the best time to try the local cuisine if it is outside the team's normal diet.

When going on a long bus ride that encompasses a normal mealtime, athletic trainers should evaluate the route to see what towns will be encountered during that mealtime.

Without prior planning, teams often default to a fast food option that may have limited healthy selections. While this may be a convenient option to turn to occasionally on the return trip, when the athletes will have several days to recover before competing again, burgers and fries are not ideal before a game or event. It is also a good idea to travel with an ice-chest on bus trips where athletes can store snacks and extra beverages. For a minimal price, athletic trainers can easily add the makings for peanut butter and jelly sandwiches and stock up on healthy snacks such as string cheese, fruit, and Greek yogurt.

Trips requiring long flights can present unique circumstances for athletes. In general, athletes are not wired to sit stationary for long periods of time. Flights may lead to boredom, which can lead to grazing, or mindless snacking throughout the flight. On the other end of the spectrum, relying on in-flight catering is unlikely to meet an athlete's high energy demand. Packing healthy snacks (ie, trail mix, dried fruit, granola bars) can help ensure an athlete arrives at the destination with optimal fuel. Athletic trainers should make sure to remind athletes that snacks should be packed in their carry-on bag and comply with airline travel restrictions (discussed later in this chapter).

Menu Planning

A fundamental aspect of menu planning is being proactive and making meal arrangements ahead of time, instead of being reactive and trying to plan meals while on the trip. As an athletic trainer, there are several factors to consider when planning meals for a trip; these include budget, mode of transportation, available restaurant options, any special dietary needs or restrictions, and the general food preferences, likes, and dislikes of the team for which the meal is being planned.

If planning for a bus trip, it is likely the team will stop at a gas station or convenience store at some point. Following are recommendations that athletic trainers can share with athletes specific to items that can help fuel their sports performance that are found at most gas stations.[2] Providing the team with a list of ideas can help the athletes resist the temptation to grab candy, chips, and soda during the stop (Table 13-1).

Similar to providing athletes with a list of suggested items for snacks at gas stations, it is a good idea to provide them with guidance on the best meal selections at various fast food restaurants. Below are general recommendations that can be shared with athletes to equip them with the knowledge needed to make healthier choices when eating fast food.

- Select whole grain sources of carbohydrates when possible—ask for burgers and sandwiches to be made on a wheat bun and choose baked chips or pretzels when possible.

Table 13-1

Gas Station Recommendations

CARBOHYDRATES	PROTEINS	HYDRATION
• Pretzels, pita chips, Chex Mix (General Mills), dry cereal • Granola bars, sports bars • Snack crackers such as animal crackers, Goldfish (Pepperidge Farms), Cheez-Its (Kellogg Company), graham crackers, Ritz (Mondelēz International) • Baked chips • Fig Newtons (Nabisco), SkinnyPop Popcorn (Amplify Snack Foods), trail mix, dried fruit	• Mixed nuts • Peanut butter • Hummus • Beef jerky • Tuna fish packet	• Bottled water • Sparkling water • Sports drinks • 100% fruit juice • Chocolate milk

*Note—These suggestions can also apply to recommended options out of vending machines.

• Choose healthy side items: Fruit and yogurt parfaits, baked chips, apple slices, baby carrots, and side salads are all great choices that many restaurants offer.

• Limit fried foods, including French fries, onion rings, tater tots, chicken nuggets, and fried fish sandwiches. Instead choose options that are baked, grilled, or steamed.

• Avoid sodas, sweet tea, lemonade, and other sugar-sweetened beverages that provide calories but little nutritional value. The athlete's best option is to choose water with the meal; however, many restaurants now offer 100% fruit juice as well as sports drinks.

• Watch portion sizes and do not value-size the meal. It is better to have a healthy snack later in the day than to fill up on nutrients that are not supporting the athlete's sports nutrition goals.

Pre-Event Options

A general rule of thumb with pregame meal planning is that the closer the meal is to the time of the competition, the lighter the meal should be. If the schedule allows, aim to schedule the team's pregame meal 3 to 4 hours prior to competition. This will allow players adequate time to digest their food, use the restroom, and allow the athletes time to rest before the event. The pregame meal should contain a good source of carbohydrates, a moderate amount of lean protein, and be relatively low in fat and fiber content. Below are ideas for pre-event meals:

• Breakfast: French toast, turkey sausage, fresh sliced fruit, 100% orange juice

• Italian food: Pasta with marinara sauce and grilled chicken, Italian bread, salad with light dressing

• Casual dining: Grilled chicken breast or salmon filet, rice pilaf, mixed vegetables, fresh sliced fruit cup

• Deli sandwiches: 6-inch sub sandwich with turkey, ham, or roast beef; pretzels; apple slices; sports drink

• Fast food: Grilled chicken wrap, Greek yogurt and fruit parfait, sports drink

In the event that the team has a reduced amount of time between the pregame meal and competition, it is necessary to plan a smaller meal or snack, focused around easily digested carbohydrates (Figure 13-1). This meal/snack could be as simple as:

• Fruit smoothie
• Granola bars
• Bagel
• Banana
• Peanut butter and jelly sandwich

The key to successful menu planning lies in knowing what the athletes like and will eat. Having foods that are familiar and accepted by the athletes is important not only to ensure they are well fueled but also to keep their game-day fueling plan as consistent as possible.

Recovery Nutrition

When working on the meal schedule, do not forget about the importance of planning for a healthy meal following the activity. This meal is especially relevant when the athletes are planning to compete again on the same day or the following day. The goal of the recovery meal is to replace the carbohydrate stores used during the activity, to provide protein to assist with muscle repair and rebuilding, and to provide fluid to help the athlete restore hydration levels.[3]

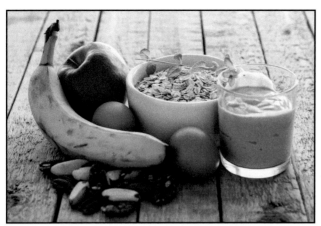

Figure 13-1. Example of healthy pre-event options. (BLACKDAY/Shutterstock.com.)

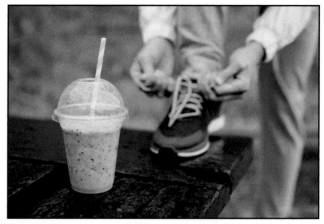

Figure 13-2. Post-exercise nutrition option—Select items with a quick source of carbohydrates and a good source of protein. (Dirima/Shutterstock.com.)

Example meals:

- Pasta with marinara sauce and grilled chicken, breadsticks, and salad
- Build your own burrito bowl: Chicken or steak fajita meat, rice, black beans, corn, lettuce, tomato, salsa, guacamole
- Teriyaki chicken and vegetables, steamed rice, wonton soup
- Grilled salmon or chicken breast, sweet potato, steamed vegetables, dinner roll
- Turkey sub sandwich, pretzels, fruit and yogurt parfait, sports drink

Ideally, the postexercise meal should be consumed within the first 2 hours after an event. If the meal is delayed, encourage athletes to supplement with a snack containing a quick source of carbohydrates, to optimize glycogen synthesis, and 20 to 25 g of protein for muscle repair (Figure 13-2).[4] Some quick and easy options include:

- Chocolate milk and granola bars
- Greek yogurt and fruit parfait
- Bagel with peanut butter and jelly
- Protein bar and sports drink
- Fruit smoothie made with Greek yogurt
- Crackers and cheese with low-fat milk

Meal Delivery Options

With the advancements in technology, meal planning has been made more convenient in recent years. The use of apps such as UberEats, GrubHub, and DoorDash provide athletic trainers with a new method for arranging meal delivery to a specific location at a specific time. Learning to utilize technology resources not only saves time and adds convenience, it also expands meal options to restaurants that previously may not have been possible to logistically coordinate for the team.

In addition to becoming familiar with meal delivery apps, it is recommended to research area grocery stores before the trip in order to purchase fresh fruits and vegetables, as well as cold items such as milk, 100% fruit juice, deli meat, cheese, and Greek yogurt. Many grocery stores also offer food delivery services, which adds convenience and allows for fresh foods to be delivered directly to the team's hotel or event venue.

Hotel Dining

Advanced communication with the hotel is essential. Even if the team only plans on utilizing the free continental breakfast, the hotel management needs to be made aware of the quantity of food the athletes may consume at the meal. Many hotels will cater meals for large groups, which may be a good option for a convenient dinner. The athletic trainer should also find out if there are refrigerators in the players' rooms for the storage of perishable snacks. If not, many hotels often have a limited number of mini refrigerators they can provide to rooms when requested in advance. Encouraging athletes to have healthy snacks in their rooms can prevent late-night trips to hotel vending machines.

Continental Breakfast (Best Pregame Options)

When traveling frequently with teams, it quickly becomes evident that hotels can vary greatly in terms of both the types and quality of food included in the free continental breakfast (Figure 13-3).

If you are counting on the continental breakfast to serve as the pre-event meal, it is recommended to notify the hotel management ahead of time to ensure there will be quality options available. Teaching athletes the best pregame options from the continental breakfast layout is important. The following is a list of recommended options as well as items to limit.

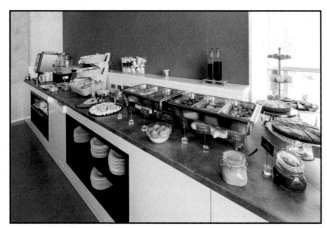

Figure 13-3. Example of hotel continental breakfast—Center the meal around carbohydrates and lean proteins. (Edvard Nalbantjan/Shutterstock.com.)

Best Options

- Carbohydrates: Encourage athletes to center their meal around carbohydrates to help top off glycogen stores in the body.
  - Oatmeal: Try mixing in peanut butter or nuts for added protein and dried fruit for added carbohydrates.
  - Bagels and toast: Try topping with peanut butter rather than cream cheese.
  - Pancakes, waffles, French toast: Encourage athletes to limit the amount of butter and syrup added to the top.
  - Breakfast cereal (limit the sugary varieties): Suggest athletes try topping their yogurt with dry breakfast cereal for an added crunch and consider taking a box of cereal for a snack later.
  - Fruit: Enjoy fruit with breakfast and grab a piece for the road.
- Proteins: Encourage athletes to choose lean protein options with their breakfast; a general goal is to include 20 to 25 g of protein with the meal.
  - Eggs: An egg contains approximately 6 g of protein. Many hotel buffets offer hard-boiled or scrambled eggs that provide a good way to help athletes meet their protein needs.
  - Turkey sausage, turkey bacon: If available, turkey sausage and turkey bacon both provide protein with less fat than the regular variety.
  - Nut butters (peanut, almond), mixed nuts: Nuts are a nutritious option at breakfast, as they contain protein and unsaturated fatty acids. Consider using nut butters as a spread in place of cream cheese, butter, or margarine and mixing nuts into oatmeal and cereal for added protein.
  - 1% or fat-free milk: Each cup of milk provides 8 g of protein along with calcium and vitamin D.

  - Greek yogurt: Greek yogurt contains approximately 20 g of protein per cup; it is also a good source of calcium. A fruit and yogurt parfait is a great breakfast option for athletes.
  - Cottage cheese: Cottage cheese is an excellent source of protein, containing approximately 23 g per cup. Try topping cottage cheese with fresh berries for additional nutritional benefits.

Options to Limit

- Carbohydrates: Encourage athletes to limit carbohydrate-based foods that contain excess amounts of added sugar and/or fat.
  - Donuts, pastries, biscuits
  - Sugary breakfast cereals
- Proteins: Limit protein sources that are greasy or high in saturated fat and may lead to gastrointestinal distress during the activity.
  - Bacon, sausage, cheesy/greasy eggs
- Fats: Limit saturated fats with breakfast; high-fat meals may slow down the digestive process and result in gastrointestinal distress during the activity.
  - Gravy (ie, biscuits and gravy)
  - Cream cheese
  - Butter, margarine

Travel Concerns Impacting Nutrition and Health

Airline Travel

Promoting optimal nutrition for athletes and teams traveling via the airlines can present unique challenges the athletic trainer needs to consider in advance (Figure 13-4). First, when preparing for a trip that requires air travel, it is useful to be aware of airline travel restrictions. The current airline restrictions require that any liquid, gel, or paste an athlete plans to take on board in their carry-on bag must be smaller than 3.4 ounces in size. In addition, all the 3.4-ounce size containers an individual carries onto the flight must be placed inside one quart-sized, resealable bag to go through security (ie, https://www.tsa.gov/travel/security-screening/liquids-rule).

Practically speaking, these regulations mean athletes will not be allowed to carry on bottles of water, juice, or sports drinks. The 3.4-ounce size limit also applies to dips, spreads, peanut butter, honey, jam/jelly, hummus, and yogurt, as these items are classified by the airlines as liquids, gels, creams, or pastes. Educating athletes on what is/is not allowed to be carried through security is an important aspect of preparing for the flight. Remind athletes that larger-sized containers of

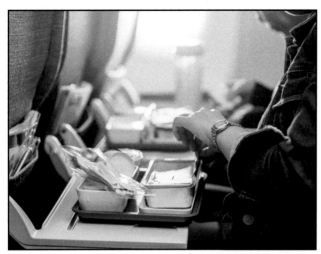

Figure 13-4. Prepackaged airline meal—Plan ahead by packing healthy snack options to eat during the flight. (shutter_o/Shutterstock.com.)

items, such as peanut butter, can be placed in their checked baggage to have upon arrival. When in doubt, it is always best to check the Transportation Security Administration (TSA) website for guidance on whether a food or beverage is allowed in carry-on luggage (ie, https://www.tsa.gov/travel/security-screening/whatcanibring/food). Encourage athletes to carry an empty water bottle on flights that can be refilled once they are through security. The small cups provided on flights are inadequate for ensuring proper hydration.

A second aspect of planning for airline travel is considering what meal/snack options will be available at the airports. Flight delays and long layovers can result in athletes spending a long period of time in airport terminals. Athletic trainers should work with athletes to come up with a list of healthy snack options they can carry with them when traveling.

Ideas include:
- Dry cereal or trail mix (packed in individual resealable bags)
- Beef jerky
- Granola bars, sports bars
- Dried fruit, raisins
- Snack-size containers of peanut butter or hummus (1-ounce cup)
- Crackers, pretzels, pita chips

Educating athletes on the best meal options from airport restaurants is equally important. Fast food, cinnamon rolls, ice cream, and other sweet treats are common in airport terminals. Guiding athletes on how to make the healthiest choices from the options available is key to avoiding poor nutrition. Prior to traveling, it may be helpful to research what restaurants are available at the airports that the team will be traveling through and provide suggestions to the team about the best meal options. In addition to equipping athletes with knowledge on travel restrictions and airport food selections, it is good to provide them with general nutrition

tips for the actual flight. For long flights, encourage athletes to get up and walk regularly throughout the flight and also to stay hydrated. The dryness of pressurized cabin air can lead to fluid loss and contribute to dehydration[5]—thus, athletes should be reminded to consume fluids throughout the flight. The Aerospace Medical Association recommends consuming 8 ounces of water each hour to prevent dehydration, especially if the flight is more than a few hours long.[6]

Altitude

When traveling to a location that is a different altitude than what the athlete/team is used to performing in, it is important to be aware of the physiological impact exercising at a higher altitude can have on the body. Within the first few hours of altitude exposure, the body begins to experience a reduction in plasma volume and therefore must make adaptations to compensate for a reduced flow of oxygen to the muscles. To do this, the body increases the production of red blood cells, which results in an increase in hemoglobin concentration, the oxygen-carrying component of red blood cells.[7,8]

Nutrition is of great importance when the body is making adaptations to being at a higher altitude. The primary nutrient of concern is iron, which is necessary for the production of red blood cells. Therefore, athletes should be educated on proper iron-rich foods to include in their diet before and during altitude exposure.[8]

The following are key points to share regarding iron intake:
- Iron in the diet can come from both animal (heme iron) and plant (nonheme iron) sources. Our bodies absorb heme iron better than nonheme iron.
- Animal sources of iron include lean red meat, chicken, turkey, pork, and seafood.
- Plant sources of iron include beans, dark green leafy vegetables (spinach), whole wheat bread, fortified breakfast cereals, and enriched rice and pasta.
- Consuming plant sources of iron with vitamin C aids in the absorption of iron. For example, add strawberries to a spinach salad to aid with iron absorption from spinach.
- Consuming plant sources of iron along with animal sources of iron also helps to enhance the absorption of iron. For example, adding beans to chili or eating chicken with rice (Figure 13-5).

In addition to iron, ensuring adequate hydration is important when athletes are participating in activities at a higher altitude. Athletes are at an increased risk of dehydration when exercising at altitudes due to lower ambient humidity levels, increased fluid losses as a result of increased ventilation, and the diuresis that occurs with initial altitude exposure.[7] Working with athletes to ensure adequate fluid intake to offset these losses is important for the prevention of dehydration.

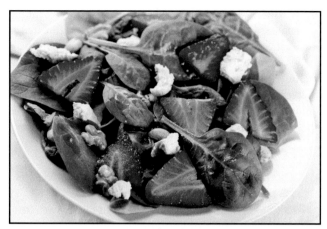

Figure 13-5. Strawberry spinach salad—Combining foods rich in vitamin C aids in the absorption of iron from plant sources. (Nitr/Shutterstock.com.)

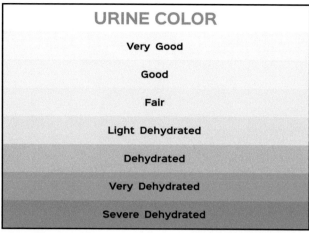

Figure 13-6. Example of urine color chart for monitoring hydration. (gritsalak karalak/Shutterstock.com.)

As a result of hypoxic conditions, sleep disturbances, and irregular training conditions, athletes exercising at high altitudes tend to be at a greater risk of illness and infection. Teams should be encouraged to consume a wide variety of fruits, vegetables, and anti-inflammatory foods throughout the travel season to promote overall health. Additionally, athletes exposed to high altitudes should consume a well-balanced diet with adequate total caloric intake to support training adaptations and increased energy needs.[8,9]

Hot/Humid Environments

When traveling to environments that are hot and/or humid, the primary nutritional concern is hydration. This concern is especially relevant when the athlete is not accustomed to exercising in hot and/or humid environments and will not have time to properly acclimatize to the environment before competition. Maintaining adequate hydration is essential for healthy cardiovascular and cognitive function. Athletes with fluid deficiencies as little as 1% to 2% may start showing compromised decision making and an elevated heart rate.[10] With the additional concern of heat-related illnesses, euhydration (or the state of optimal body water) should be emphasized to teams in the days prior to travel. To ensure proper hydration on a daily basis, athletes should be educated on monitoring their level of thirst, urine color, and frequency of urination (Figure 13-6).

During exercise, the goal is to maintain hydration and not lose more than 2% body weight.[7,8,10] While athletes should be mindful not to overhydrate, cool beverages should be consumed regularly during prolonged outdoor activities. Electrolytes (eg, sports drinks) may need to be included for individuals who are exercising for a prolonged period of time, who have higher-than-average sweat rates, or who have high sweat sodium concentrations.[7,8] Sweat rates of athletes can be highly variable, thus athletic trainers and sports dietitians should work with athletes to develop individualized hydration plans for their sports.

After exercise, hydration levels should be restored within 4 hours for optimal recovery.[10] While sports drinks are not always necessary to achieve euhydration, beverages that appeal to one's taste generally result in an increase in intake.[11] Weight assessment can be useful to ensure that hydration has been fully restored before the next competition or workout. Athletes should be encouraged to consume more fluid than the amount lost during the activity. A general goal is to consume 125% to 150% of the amount of fluid lost,[8] or 2.5 to 3 cups of fluid for each pound of body weight lost during the exercise session.

Food Safety

Food safety is of great importance to help ensure the overall health and well-being of athletes. The Centers for Disease Control and Prevention estimates that 1 in 6 Americans will get sick with a food-borne illness each year.[12] The symptoms of food-borne illness can range from mild stomach cramps to severe diarrhea, vomiting, and fever lasting in length from a few hours to several weeks.[13] Taking steps to prevent the consumption of contaminated food that can lead to food-borne illness is a necessity, especially when planning meals for traveling teams. The following are a few simple steps athletic trainers can take to help reduce the risk of food-borne illnesses amongst the athletes and teams they work with.

Handwashing

Ensure that athletes have the opportunity to wash their hands before eating. The athletic trainer may need to teach athletes how to properly wash their hands. Quick handwashing tips to share include:

- Use warm running water for handwashing.
- Scrub hands with antibacterial soap for 20 seconds, making sure to clean under the nails when washing.

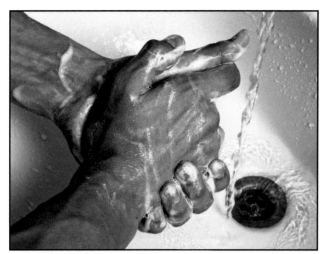

Figure 13-7. Proper hand washing to promote food safety. (ProStockStudio/Shutterstock.com.)

○ Tip: If the athlete sings "Happy Birthday" all the way through 2 times, this will take approximately 20 seconds.

- Dry using a clean towel or allow hands to air dry.[14]

If going on a bus trip to an event at an outdoor facility where there will not be handwashing opportunities, pack an alcohol-based hand sanitizer (containing at least 60% alcohol) for athletes to use prior to eating. Hand sanitizer will not remove dirt and debris that are on the hands, but it will help with killing germs and bacteria. Athletes should allow hand sanitizer to air dry on their hands and not wipe their hands with a towel, which may reduce the effectiveness of the sanitizer. One of the simplest and most critical steps for food safety is proper handwashing (Figure 13-7).[14]

Food Handling

Anyone responsible for meal preparation or serving needs to wash their hands before handling food. Single-use gloves and/or serving utensils should be used, rather than allowing individuals to directly handle food others will consume. In addition to handwashing, look for ways to limit the handling of food by team members.

For example:

- Buy individual serving size bags of pretzels rather than a large bag that everyone puts their hands in.
- When setting out grapes and other fruits, break into smaller segments for easy grabbing.
- Have tongs available for serving sandwiches, fresh cut fruit, and vegetables.
- Remember to ensure the necessary serving utensils are available when menu planning.

An added concern with food handling is the potential for cross-contamination of food allergens, which is of extreme importance if anyone traveling with the team has a food allergy. Following food-safety practices to prevent potential cross-contamination, such as having separate utensils

and dishware for preparing and serving allergen-containing food, must be practiced at all times. Also, ensure caterers used for meals on the trip are made aware of any food allergies so necessary precautions in food preparation/service can be made; ask caterers to clearly label all foods containing allergens. Remind those athletes with food allergies about the importance of traveling with an Epi-Pen (Mylan Inc, a Viatris Company) and having it readily available at all times.[5]

Food Temperature Control

Another aspect of food safety is making sure food is held at the appropriate temperatures.

- Hot food needs to be held hot: Should be held at a temperature of 140 °F or greater.
- Cold food needs to be held cold: Should be held at a temperature of 40 °F or lower.
- Any food held outside of the appropriate temperature control zone for more than 2 hours should be thrown away. If the outside temperature is >90 °F, food should not be kept out of temperature control longer than 1 hour (Figure 13-8).[15]

Watch for practices that may seem common among teams that could easily lead to food-borne illness due to being held at improper temperatures. For example:

- Athletes taking leftover pizza or sub sandwiches from a bus trip to the hotel room to eat later.
- Sliced melon held in the heat at a track meet or other outdoor event.
- Packing yogurt, cheese sticks, or milk for post-game snacks and not storing the items in an iced cooler.
- Keeping leftover breakfast tacos or deli sandwiches out and available all day for athletes to eat as snacks between events.

Traveling

Traveling to foreign countries may present a unique challenge to athletes. Foods that athletes are familiar with consuming may be difficult to locate, and local produce may differ from what the athlete is accustomed to consuming. Language barriers may make grocery shopping a challenge, as product packaging may look different, pricing may be difficult to determine, and athletes may be hesitant to ask questions and/or try new foods. In preparation for the trip, if it appears food options will be limited at your travel destination, consider shipping a box of nonperishable snacks to the hotel or event venue in advance to have available when you arrive.

It is important to note that not all countries have standards for food safety that are as comprehensive as those established in the United States, thus food safety must be taken into consideration when traveling abroad. To assist with this, the Centers for Disease Control and Prevention has established a Traveler's Health Website (ie, https://wwwnc.

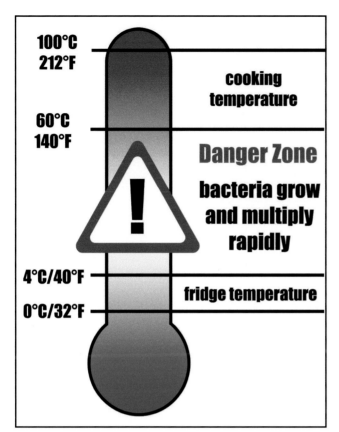

Figure 13-8. Food safety temperature danger zone chart. (desdemona72/Shutterstock.com.)

cdc.gov/travel/). This website allows individuals to review any health and safety concerns in the travel destination and includes recommendations for eating and drinking safely. Prior to traveling, athletes should be provided with guidance on whether the water is safe to drink. If the water is not safe to consume, athletes should be advised to drink bottled water from sealed containers only, avoid ice in drinks, avoid foods (produce) that have been washed in the water, and use bottled water for brushing teeth. Athletes should also be provided with a list of recommended area restaurants to eat and should be cautioned on possible food safety concerns with purchasing food from street vendors and open-air markets. Foods noted to be of high risk for food-borne illnesses include fresh produce (raw vegetables, salad, fruit that is not peeled before eating), unpasteurized milk/dairy products, raw eggs, and undercooked meat, seafood, and shellfish.[12] Athletes should also be cautioned against purchasing any supplements, herbal products, or medications abroad, especially if reading and/or speaking the native language is a barrier. Careful planning before the trip can help ensure athletes are nutritionally equipped to compete and enjoy the trip without the added concern of what food will be available to eat.

Conclusion

Travel can be a challenge for athletes and athletic teams. Changes to meal timing, food selections, and regular eating practices can cause problems from poor performance to severe food poisoning. Many of these challenges can be overcome with careful preparation and planning. It is important for athletic trainers to be prepared to assist with meal planning for the teams and athletes that they are working with and to be ready to provide athletes with guidance on best nutritional choices at convenience stores, fast food restaurants, airports, and hotel buffets. In addition, athletic trainers need to be aware of the unique nutrition concerns associated with airline travel, competing at altitude or in excessive heat, and traveling to foreign countries. With preparation and knowledge, athletic trainers will be able to assist the team and ensure athletes have good nutritional choices available throughout the trip to support their performance.

Discussion Questions

1. Describe 3 unique nutritional concerns an athletic trainer may encounter when planning meals for a traveling team.
2. Discuss precautions an athletic trainer can take to help minimize food safety concerns for their athletes when traveling.

References

1. Torres-McGehee TM, Pritchett KL, Zippel D, Minton DM, Cellamare A, Sibilia M. Sports nutrition knowledge among collegiate athletes, coaches, athletic trainers, and strength and conditioning specialists. *J Athl Train.* 2012;47(2):205-211.
2. Clark N. Traveling athletes & gas station nutrition. Nancy Clark RD Blog. Published November 19, 2015. Accessed April 29, 2020.
3. NCAA. Fueling for recovery factsheet. NCAA.org. Published 2013. Accessed February 29, 2020.
4. Pritchett KL, Pritchett RC, Bishop P. Nutritional strategies for post-exercise recovery: a review. *S Afr J Sports Med.* 2011;23(1), 20-25. doi:10.17159/2078-516X/2011/v23i1a370
5. Halson SL, Burke LM, Pearce J. Nutrition for travel: from jet lag to catering. *Int J Sport Nutr Exerc Metab.* 2019;29(2):228-235. doi:10.1123/ijsnem.2018-0278
6. Aerospace Medical Association. *Health Tips for Airline Travel.* https://www.asma.org/asma/media/asma/Travel-Publications/HEALTH-TIPS-FOR-AIRLINE-TRAVEL-Trifold-2013.pdf. Accessed February 29, 2020.
7. Saunders PU, Garvican-Lewis LA, Chapman RF, Périard JD. Special environments: altitude and heat. *Int J Sport Nutr Exerc Metab.* 2018;29(2):210-219. doi:10.1123/ijsnem.2018-0256
8. Thomas DT, Erdman DA, Burke LM, MacKilloop M. Position of the Academy of Nutrition and Dietetics, Dietitians of Canada, and the American College of Sports Medicine: nutrition and athletic performance. *J Acad Nutr Diet.* 2016;116(3):501-527.

9. Koivisto AE, Olsen T, Paur I, et al. Effects of antioxidant-rich foods on altitude-induced oxidative stress and inflammation in elite endurance athletes: a randomized control trial. *PLoS One.* 2019;14(6):e0217895. doi:10.1371/journal.pone.0217895

10. McDermott BP, Anderson SA, Anderson LE, et al. National Athletic Trainers' Association position statement: fluid replacement for the physically active. *J Athl Train.* 2017;52(9):887-895. doi:10.4085/1062-6050-52.9.02

11. O'Neal EK, Poulos SP, Bishop PA. Hydration profile and influence of beverage contents on fluid intake by women during outdoor recreational walking. *Eur J Appl Physiol.* 2012;112(12):3971-3982. doi:10.1007/s00421-012-2372-2

12. Centers for Disease Control and Prevention. Food safety: was it something I ate? https://www.cdc.gov/foodsafety/index.html. Updated February 19, 2020.

13. Centers for Disease Control and Prevention. Food poisoning symptoms. https://www.cdc.gov/foodsafety/symptoms.html. Updated February 18, 2020.

14. Centers for Disease Control and Prevention. Handwashing and hand sanitizer use factsheet. https://www.cdc.gov/handwashing/pdf/HandSanitizer-p.pdf. Accessed July 3, 2022.

15. USDA.gov. "Danger Zone". https://www.fsis.usda.gov/food-safety/safe-food-handling-and-preparation/food-safety-basics/danger-zone-40f-140f. Updated June 28, 2017. Accessed July 3, 2022.

Chapter 14

Deciphering Food Labels

Mark Knoblauch, PhD, LAT, ATC, CSCS

Commission on Accreditation of Athletic Training Education *2020 Standards*

This chapter addresses the following *2020 Standards for Accreditation of Professional Athletic Training Programs*:

- Standard 55: Students must gain foundational knowledge in statistics, research design, epidemiology, pathophysiology, biomechanics and pathomechanics, exercise physiology, nutrition, human anatomy, pharmacology, public health, and health care delivery and payor systems.

Learning Objectives

After reviewing this chapter, readers will be able to:

- Understand basic regulations associated with food packaging.
- Understand the types of food label claims found on food packages.
- Identify and understand the different components of the nutrition facts label and ingredient list.

Knoblauch M, ed. *Clinical Nutrition in Athletic Training* (pp 151-165). © 2023 Taylor & Francis Group.

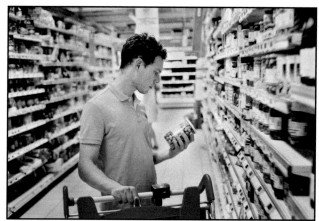

Figure 14-1. Competition between food manufacturers means consumers must often sort through an array of advertising tactics to determine which product is best for them. (Song_about_summer/Shutterstock.com.)

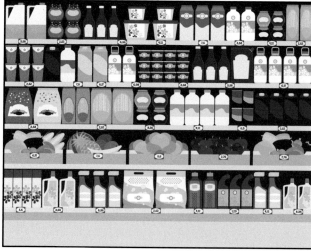

Figure 14-2. To separate their product from the competition, manufacturers often rely on bright colors, pictures, and attractive marketing with the intent of drawing the consumer's attention. (Sheila Fitzgerald/Shutterstock.com.)

Introduction

When it comes to food choices, consumers are often besieged by a variety of factors that can influence their decision as to what food to buy or consume. Certain scents, a particular memory, media advertisements, and even packaging labels can all play a role in the decision-making process involved in food consumption. Packaging labels might be considered a food manufacturer's final opportunity to convince a consumer to buy their particular product. This last chance effort can contribute to the attention-grabbing food labels that are often splashed with flashy colors and maybe even a smiling face, all with the intent of convincing the consumer that a particular manufacturer's product is better than the competition (Figure 14-1). While food marketing tactics are designed to play a key role in influencing a consumer's purchasing decisions, they often do not outline the less "sexy" aspects of a food item that can be found on those same labels, such as the food's nutritional content or quantity. That information is instead often relegated to the back of the package amidst jargon such as the manufacturer's contact information and the barcode. To an individual trying to stay healthy, however, the information contained on that back panel serves as an all-in-one source of facts that outlines important health-related data about the food. Unfortunately, the amount of information contained on the package label, as well as how it is presented, can be quite overwhelming amidst the vast array of food claims and nutritional information that is typically found on a label. To the average consumer, such as those wanting to start a diet or at least become healthier, the amount of information may be difficult at times to wade through.

Despite the array of information listed on a food package, only a few key items are essential for the customer when it comes to interpreting the food's nutritional information. This chapter discusses these important items, with the intent of highlighting relevant food label information so that athletic trainers can better help active individuals understand or be able to interpret for themselves some of the listed food claims, nutrition content, and ingredients of the food itself. Athletic trainers can play an important intermediary role for consumers who may be confused or even intimidated by the vast amount of information found on a food label. However, once the consumer is taught how to decipher the nutritional information, they can take advantage of this wealth of information that can, in turn, help them make better choices about the foods they buy as well as help them design a high-quality diet. Therefore, this chapter is designed to help athletic trainers better understand several key components of a food label—particularly those related to nutritional aspects of food—so that they can, in turn, educate their athletes, clients, and patients on how to use the information on the food label to help improve their diet.

Package Label

Anyone who has ever negotiated a grocery store aisle can attest to the seemingly overwhelming array of available food choices. Even within the same specific food category (eg, nonsweetened corn flakes), a consumer may have 3 to 5 or more options to choose from, which include choices that range from name brand to store brand to generic. To aid consumers in making their purchasing decision, manufacturers often design their packaging with eye-catching colors and graphics along with claims such as "fat-free" or "no added sugar," all of which are largely used to catch the consumer's attention (Figure 14-2). Some consumers may take it a step further and look specifically at the nutritional content of foods, perhaps finding that one brand is "fortified with vitamin A" or "contains 100% of the recommended intake of fiber." While it may seem as though the information shown on food labels appears somewhat random or perhaps even excessive, many of the items found on a food package are in fact quite highly regulated, leaving food manufacturers to be held to a particular set of standards that must be met in order for that food to enter the market. In some cases, these requirements are meant to protect the consumer by ensuring that certain claims (eg, "low in cholesterol") are applied consistently across foods as well as across manufacturers. In other cases, package labeling regulations ensure that specific information such as a food item's nutritional content or ingredients are made available. Given the amount of information contained on a food label, it is important that consumers are able to locate and decipher the pertinent information needed to understand the nutritional content of their food.

Parts of a Food Label

To truly understand the make-up of a package label, the most reliable source of information is that provided by the US Food and Drug Administration (FDA) that establishes the regulations required in order for a food item to be allowed on the market.[1] Unfortunately, the comprehensiveness and detail provided by the FDA's website can make it difficult to find any specific item of interest. Quite frankly, the information provided by the website is more geared toward food manufacturers, as they are the ones who must meet the FDA's extensive food labeling guidelines. Because of the labeling variations that could occur without specific and detailed regulations, the comprehensiveness of the FDA's regulations helps ensure that specific labeling requirements are met consistently across manufacturers who plan to sell their food in the United States. In addition, the detail required by the FDA serves to help protect consumers from false or misrepresented claims that, were less-stringent guidelines required, could be manipulated by the manufacturers and result in labeling practices that would potentially have detrimental consequences for consumers.

For the average consumer or health professional interested in understanding the basics of food labels, it is not necessary to read through the extensive food labeling guidelines provided by the FDA. Rather, a general understanding of a few of the more consumer-based regulations can provide enough information to help understand the complexities involved with food labeling regulations, particularly in helping consumers better understand the nutrition and/or health-related features of food packaging labels. Next, some of the regulations of the food packaging label that are most relevant to the athletes, patients, and clients that athletic trainers commonly interact with will be discussed, along with a general overview of what goes into designing a food package label.

Labeling Requirements

What we might see as a simple box or package on the store shelf has likely been through a series of design and redesign phases, as there is actually quite a bit of science involved with food package labeling. Terms such as *primary*

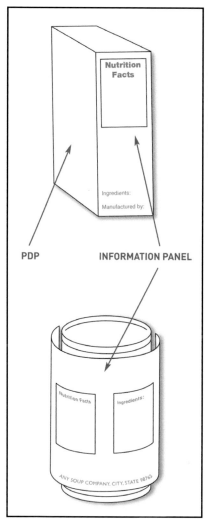

Figure 14-3. The PDP is that portion of the package label that is most likely to be seen by the consumer, while the information panel is that panel immediately to the right of the PDP on most packages. (Data source: Food and Drug Administration. *Food Labeling Guide.* 2013:6.)

display panel, information panel, and *alternative panel* are used to describe areas of the food container that are partitioned off for certain labeling sections.[1] Once the package type has been determined by the manufacturer, be it a box, jar, or other type, the appropriate labeling aspects must then be placed accordingly.

According to the FDA, 5 required components must be included on food labels, with very few exceptions.[1] These items include a statement of identity (ie, name of the food), the item's net weight, the address of the manufacturer, the nutrition facts label, and the ingredients. Each of these items must be placed in certain locations on the package to help maintain consistency across the wide variety of available food products and also aid the consumer in recognizing the appropriate labeling information. For example, the statement of identity and net quantity of food must appear on the primary display panel (PDP)—that front portion of the package most likely to be seen by the customer while on the shelf—as well as on the alternative display panel (ADP), which is an available panel that is deemed suitable for displaying required food information. Separately, the information panel is designated as the panel immediately to the right of the PDP (Figure 14-3).[1] In round containers such as a jar,

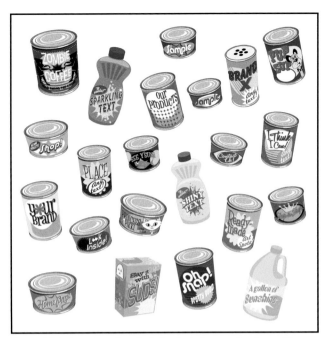

Figure 14-4. Aspects such as font size, text placement, color, and image use are all important aspects of a food package, yet are still somewhat regulated specific to what is allowed on a food label. (Sheila Fitzgerald/Shutterstock.com.)

the information panel would be the area of the label to the right of the main label display. And no matter the color palette, font size, or celebrity endorsement that a manufacturer decides on for a label, the FDA mandates that none of these allowances can impede the presence of any required label items. Specific to the aforementioned exceptions, single-ingredient items such as coffee or perhaps dehydrated plant material that is used as a condiment (eg, spices) do not typically need to have an ingredient list or a nutrition facts label due to the insignificant amount of nutrients in those food items.

When it comes to outlining how required items are going to be displayed on a food package, guidelines are provided by the FDA; however, there is some degree of freedom allowed to the food manufacturers specific to the overall presentation of that information. For example, font size on the information panel should not be less than 1/16 of an inch high, with the exception of very small labels.[1] In other words, the FDA does not necessarily mandate the exact size of words in certain areas of the package label, but it may set certain minimum standards (Figure 14-4). Other examples of labeling requirements include that the nutrition facts label maintain specific font requirements, or that lettering found on the package label must contrast with the background color so as to allow for easy reading by a consumer. There are also requirements specific to the location of certain label items, such as how images or phrases that are not required by the FDA to be on a package cannot be placed between particular required label items such as the nutrition facts label and the package ingredients.

As mentioned earlier, there is a wealth of details involved in the design of a food label. However, the design and requirements of a label are probably not as important for athletic trainers to be aware of as is an understanding of certain other label components, such as the nutrition facts label or the list of ingredients. Rather, the requirements specific to label design are more important for food manufacturers to ensure that their package design is allowed to be marketed. Any individual interested in the science of food label requirements and/or design are encouraged to read through the FDA's regulations specific to food packaging and labeling, as the FDA itself outlines the rules for the industry. For the purpose of this book, however, the remainder of the chapter will be spent focusing on a few key aspects of the food label that have a direct impact on consumers and their food choices. In particular, details regarding food label claims, the nutrition facts label, and the ingredients list will be outlined.

Food Label Claims

Given the degree of competition within the food industry, manufacturers are quick to highlight any advantage that may help "sway" a consumer away from the competition. Whereas most consumers are not familiar with the intricacies of food preparation regulations and may also not be aware of the specific health benefits of particular ingredients, manufacturers are often quick to point these aspects out on their packaging through the use of food claims. Examples of these claims might include "low in sodium," "heart healthy," or "helps keep you alert and awake!" and can often be found prominently highlighted on the PDP of a food package. Given the array of claims that can be made about a particular food item, it is important to understand the regulations that manufacturers are held to, particularly those standards that must be met in order to make such claims. In understanding these claims, patients, clients, and active individuals in general can be better informed as to the nutritional content of their food and be able to separate the hype from the pertinent information (Figure 14-5).

Types of Food Claims

To help delineate the range of food claims that can be used on a product, the FDA separates food claims into 1 of 3 categories: nutrient content claims, structure/function claims (SFCs), and health claims. The classification of a particular food claim is dependent upon what the manufacturer is attempting to highlight. For example, "fortified with vitamin D" would fall under nutrient content claims, while "heart healthy" is a type of health claim. And much like package labeling guidelines, food claims are also highly regulated as to the wording that a manufacturer can use. To help outline some of the intricacies involved in food label claims, a closer look at the requirements will be outlined next.

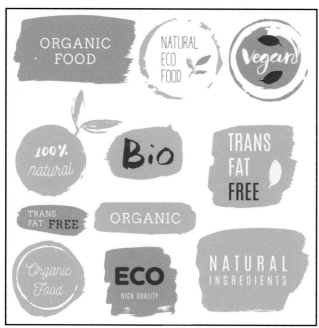

Figure 14-5. While there are a wide array of food claims made, those placed on food labels are regulated by the FDA and therefore must meet specific guidelines. (Ermine/Shutterstock.com.)

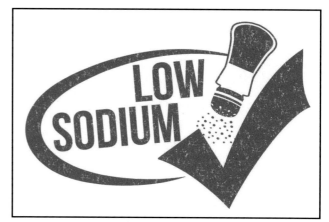

Figure 14-6. Nutrition content claims may seem simple in design, but often involve nutrition science, marketing ingenuity, and maintaining compliance with food regulations. (ducu59us/Shutterstock.com.)

Nutrient Content Claims

Arguably, nutrient content claims (NCC) are perhaps the most common type of food claim found on packaging given the wide range of available nutrients combined with the potential health benefits or risks associated with each. Nutrient content claims are typically utilized by a manufacturer to highlight a particularly beneficial aspect—or indicate a lack or low amount—of a particular ingredient or nutrient in the food product. Using sodium as an example, there is a well-known association between sodium consumption and risk for several fluid-based medical conditions (eg, hypertension). Therefore, any food product with an already low per-serving sodium content might benefit by including food claims such as "low sodium" or "less than 5 mg of sodium per serving," as long as the actual sodium content meets the FDA's labeling requirements for the chosen NCC. In other words, in cases where a product's ingredient content meets the threshold of qualifying for a certain health claim for that ingredient, it would not be unexpected for a manufacturer to take advantage of that aspect and include a related food claim on the package. Dry pasta, for example, often contains no sodium and is low in cholesterol. Capitalizing on this fact, a manufacturer could make associated claims such as "sodium-free" or "low in cholesterol" on the package's PDP in order to gain a consumer's business—provided that the nutrition content meets the FDA's requirements. Such highlighting of nutrient claims may be even more likely if a competing food product has a recipe with a higher content of a problematic ingredient (eg, sodium, cholesterol) or a lower content of a beneficial ingredient (eg, vitamin A), as any keen marketing department could see the benefit of promoting

their food product's health benefits over that of the competitor (Figure 14-6).

Nutrient content claims are strictly regulated by the FDA. So much so that only claims that are specifically approved by the FDA can be used on a product. While the regulations might seem restrictive at times, there is a viable purpose for maintaining strict regulation over NCCs, as consumers could easily become confused or potentially become misled if manufacturers were left to devise their own package claims. For example, without specific NCC regulation, one package might then be able to claim "lots of protein" without indicating just how much the word "lots" would indicate. By regulating the words used in food claims, consistency is maintained across food labels. This, in turn, helps limit any confusion on the part of the customer. Consequently a manufacturer cannot create their own claim such as *"still* low-fat after all these years," and instead must adhere to one of the approved—though somewhat unexciting—food claims such as "low in fat." A few NCC examples are shown in Table 14-1.

Along with the wording of an NCC, the appearance of the claim is regulated to some degree, and NCCs must be able to be verified by a consumer using the food label. For example, a printed food claim cannot be more than twice the size of the food's statement of identity,[1] and there must also be associated nutrition labeling for any NCC made.[1] In other words, a consumer must be able to verify the nutrition claim of "low in fat" by being able to view the actual fat content on the nutrition facts label.

Different NCCs can be further grouped according to the detail of the claim that is made.[1] For example, an "absolute" nutrition claim is one that states the particular content of a nutrient per serving (eg, "500 mg of calcium"). "Relative" NCCs, on the other hand, are those claims that compare a nutrient in a particular food item with an amount in a separate "reference" food item. For example, a food package claim such as "contains less than half the sodium of traditional potato chips" would qualify as a relative NCC. However, the type of reference claim made is dependent upon the comparison

Table 14-1

Nutrient Content Claim Requirements

CLAIM	REQUIREMENT
Calorie-free	Less than 5 calories per RACC and per labeled serving
Cholesterol-free	Contains less than 2 mg of cholesterol per RACC and per labeled serving
Excellent source of	Contains 20% or more of the daily value per RACC
Low sodium	140 mg or less of sodium per RACC
Sodium-free	Less than 5 mg of sodium per RACC and per labeled serving
Sugar-free	Less than 0.5 g of sugars per RACC and per labeled serving

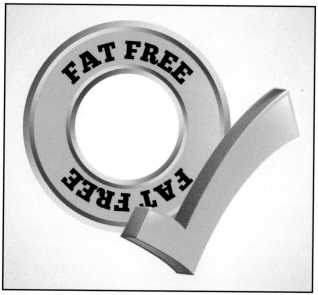

Figure 14-7. Despite the specific regulations required for nutrition content claims, food manufacturers must ensure that their packages project simple and easily understood information for the consumer. (Vectorfair.com/Shutterstock.com.)

food. For example, relative NCCs, such as those that include the terms "fewer" or "less," are allowable even when the comparison foods are not in the same category, such as when making a claim for a snack wafer against a cookie. However, when using the NCC "light," the comparison foods must be within the same category (eg, microwaveable popcorn against microwaveable popcorn). "Implied" NCCs are those that effectively "imply" that a particular nutrient's presence or absence can have beneficial health benefits. For example, a food product high in fiber may have an implied NCC of "a great source of fiber." Similarly, a food item that makes a comparison of nutrients (eg, "as much fiber as 6 slices of bread") would be considered an "equivalence" type of implied NCC (Figure 14-7).

It should be pointed out that, with few exceptions, NCCs are not permitted on foods intended for infants and children less than 2 years old. Those exceptions include listing the percent of vitamins and minerals in relation to percent daily value, certain NCCs on infant formula, using the terms "unsweetened" and "unsalted" as taste claims, and using "sugar-free" and "no added sugar" on dietary supplements.

Health Claims

A health claim is any package claim that highlights a relationship between a particular ingredient and a disease or health-related condition. An example of a health claim might be "This product contains 100% of the RDA for vitamin D. Adequate intake of vitamin D has been shown to reduce the risk of osteoporosis." In addition, an *implied* health claim can be made when the claim suggests that an ingredient or amount of ingredient in the food is related to a disease or health-related condition.

Health claims may appear at times to be similar to SFCs. However, the difference between the 2 types of claims is that health claims must be specific to a reduction in disease risk, whereas SFCs are limited to only describing the function of that nutrient within the body. More specifically, health claims require mention of both a particular substance (ie, ingredient or nutrient) and a disease. Even though health claims must outline a reduction in disease risk, they cannot infer diagnosis, treatment, or cure of any disease. Furthermore, health claims must be able to reference scientific evidence for the listed claim, with any claim meeting the *authorized* classification being required to show significant scientific agreement (SSA) among experts that there is strong evidence to support the claim.[2] To aid in the approval process, specific health claim categories have been developed by the FDA that outline a link between certain nutrients and health conditions, such as "sodium and hypertension" or "fruits and vegetables and cancer" (Sidebar 14-1).

When there is not significant agreement that a relationship exists between a disease and an ingredient, a qualified health claim (QHC) may be used instead. QHCs arose in the early 2000s due to legal challenges specific to the SSA standard required for health claims.[3] Many QHCs have arisen from manufacturer petitions for health claims that were later, after FDA review, found to have insufficient evidence to meet the SSA standard and in turn warranted a QHC.[4] The FDA review of a health claim is quite substantial in nature, and the outcome of that review ultimately determines the wording used for the QHC.[5]

When utilizing a QHC, manufacturers are indicating that some evidence of a relationship exists between a product/nutrient and a disease state, but not at a level that might be considered significant.[5] To highlight the fact that the claim may not be well accepted, a disclaimer must accompany any

QHC. For illustrative purposes only, an example of a QHC might be written as "evidence suggests, but does not prove, that eating 6 ounces of fish daily in conjunction with exercise and consuming a diet low in saturated fat and cholesterol may contribute to a reduction in one's risk of stroke."

Structure/Function Claims

Whereas NCCs are specific to individual ingredients/nutrients, SFCs reference how a particular nutrient or ingredient impacts the body. An example of a SFC might be used in a product that has a high level of vitamin A, such as "vitamin A promotes healthy vision." Whereas an SFC is pointing out a physiological use for a particular nutrient that is found in a food item, the FDA requires that the claim be factual in nature and is not misleading; however, SFCs do not need to undergo prereview and are not authorized by the FDA.[1] Unlike health-related claims, SFCs do not make reference to any disease and are only focused on how the nutrient is utilized by the body.

Dietary Guidance Claims

Dietary guidance claims are somewhat similar to health claims. However, whereas health claims must make note of both a substance and a disease, dietary guidance claims (DGC) do not have to mention both aspects but may mention one or the other. A DGC typically references a category of food (eg, nuts) rather than a specific nutrient that may be found in that food category (eg, omega-3 polyunsaturated fat). Any DGC used on food packaging must be truthful in nature, yet unlike other food claims does not have to go through FDA review prior to marketing the food product.[1] An example of a DGC might be "consuming a variety of nuts in moderation can have positive health benefits."

Consumers and Food Claims

Despite the relatively strict regulation of terminology available for food claims, there is still a possibility that athletes, patients, or clients misinterpret what a food claim is actually stating. For example, individuals on a low-carbohydrate diet may be drawn to a label's claim of "no sugar added" and assume that the food product is sugar-free. Unfortunately, their assumption would not be correct, as the claim is not stating that the product is sugar-free. Rather, the claim is highlighting the fact that no sugar was added to the food product during processing. The food may still contain a significant amount of sugar or other carbohydrate, but that sugar is inherent to the ingredients themselves rather than being added by the manufacturer. Similarly, "sodium-free" does not mean that there is zero sodium in the product, but rather that there is less than 5 mg of sodium per serving—not quite "zero" sodium, but at the same time a miniscule amount. Several nutrient claims regulated by the FDA have the potential to invite confusion or misinterpretation in a similar way that highlights the importance of ensuring that patients, clients, and active individuals are able to interpret a food claim properly.

Disclosure Statement

Disclosure statements are listed on a food label when the amount of a particular ingredient may contribute to increasing one's risk of disease. Specifically, any per serving (or per Reference Amount Customarily Consumed [RACC]) level that exceeds 4 g of saturated fat, 13 g of total fat, 60 mg of cholesterol, or 480 mg of sodium requires a disclosure statement that effectively directs the consumer to examine the specific content of that nutrient, usually outlined on the nutrition facts label. An example of a disclosure statement may be listed as "see nutrition information specific to saturated fat content." This is not to say that a disclosure statement is highlighting a particularly harmful level of a nutrient, but rather it directs the consumer to pay particular attention to a certain amount of an included nutrient.

Nutrition Facts Label

Food label claims are generally used as marketing tactics by manufacturers with the intent of highlighting certain aspects of a food product, such as "high in calcium" or "contains a significant amount of vitamin D, which has been shown to promote healthy bones." While label claims have a specific purpose behind their use, their presence is generally dependent upon whether the food manufacturer feels that the claim will help sell an item. The nutritional content of food, however, is not afforded the same arbitrary level of inclusion as food claims. Therefore, certain nutrient information consisting of both macro- and micronutrient make-up can be found on the food's nutrition facts label that must be clearly visible on one of the food package's display panels. The nutrition facts label lists the major nutrient groups (eg, carbohydrates) as well as a few of the more common micronutrients (eg, sodium) with the intent of providing the information in order to help consumers make more informed choices about their food.

Much like the requirements outlined for food claim terminology, the regulations associated with the nutrition facts

Sidebar 14-2

While most food is regulated by the FDA, certain products are under the authority of other regulating agencies. Meat and poultry products, for example, fall under the realm of the United States Department of Agriculture, while alcoholic beverages are regulated by the Alcohol and Tobacco Tax and Trade Bureau of the Department of the Treasury. Consequently, food labeling practices mandated by the FDA are not affected by the NLEA.

label are also quite extensive. The purpose in having such extensive regulations is to both protect the consumer by providing all nutrient information, as well as ensure consistency between food products. If a manufacturer was allowed to simply create its own nutrition facts label and include those items that it chooses, there would undoubtedly be vast fluctuations as to which nutrients were included, particularly among less-favorable aspects of certain foods (eg, such as those with a high sodium content). Such variation would be particularly problematic for consumers looking to monitor all aspects of their nutrition.

History of the Nutrition Facts Label

Up until the 1960s, nutritional content was not required on any food product except those outlined as "special dietary use" foods.[6] With most meals made at home, a general impression was formed that there was little need for requiring nutritional information.[7] However, with advancements in technology, processed foods became more accessible. The increased availability of processed foods served to drive an increased need for consumers to understand just what was in the processed foods. This, in turn, spurred the government into action, at first "recommending" that nutrient information be included on packages and only "requiring" label-based nutrient information when nutrients were added to the food or when specific nutrition claims were made.[6]

Legislation from 1973 first outlined what information should be on the early version of the nutrition facts label, in those particular cases where a label was required to be included on a food item. Total calories; total grams of protein, fats, and carbohydrates; and percent RDA of certain nutrients were all required to be listed by serving size. In addition, should the manufacturer choose to include them, sodium content as well as saturated and polyunsaturated fatty acid content were allowed to be listed on the label.[6]

In 1990, food labeling went through somewhat of an overhaul with the intent of allowing consumers to take advantage of the advancements that had been made in nutrition.

Under the belief that changes in eating habits—spurred in part by the use of nutrition labeling—could improve the health of Americans, the recommendation was made that uniform food labeling be required for almost all packaged foods. Eventually, the Nutrition Labeling and Education Act (NLEA) of 1990 was passed that affected all foods regulated by the FDA (Sidebar 14-2). The NLEA was a major progressive step in food nutrition labeling and set the standard for the majority of labeling requirements that are still in place today. For example, the NLEA outlined which nutrients must be listed in the nutrition label and specified that the required nutrients be presented relative to an individual's daily diet. The NLEA also mandated the development of specific definitions that could be used to outline the particular level of nutrients in a food item and also established that the FDA provides oversight for food health claims.

Recent Revisions to the Nutrition Facts Label

As information such as dietary influences on disease risk (eg, obesity) changes over time, consumers should have the opportunity to be made aware of such information in order to make healthy decisions about the foods that they consume. For many food items, the nutrition facts label provides consumers relevant information specific to serving size, calories, and nutritional content. Certainly, aspects such as disease risk as well as our understanding of nutrients undergoes change over time in response to new research findings, and any new information should be made available to consumers. Consequently, the nutrition facts label has itself continued to go through many changes over the years. Most recently, in 2016, the label was changed again with the intent of drawing attention to new information linking diet with obesity and heart disease.[8] In these latest changes, the listed serving size was updated and printed in larger font, an "added sugars" line was added to the panel, daily values were updated, and nutrient requirements were updated to include vitamin D and potassium as well as removing the heading of "calories from fat." Despite these numerous updates, the label itself was allowed to maintain its standard appearance overall (eg, black on a white background) as well as keeping its traditional layout (Figure 14-8, Sidebar 14-3).

Understanding the Components of the Nutrition Facts Label

At first glance, a patient or client who is unfamiliar with the content of a food package may find the nutrition facts label a somewhat intimidating mix of numbers and technical jargon. Depending on their understanding of nutrition, that is certainly understandable in the event that they do not understand what a calorie is, or if an understanding of saturated versus *trans* fat seems a foreign concept. To the average

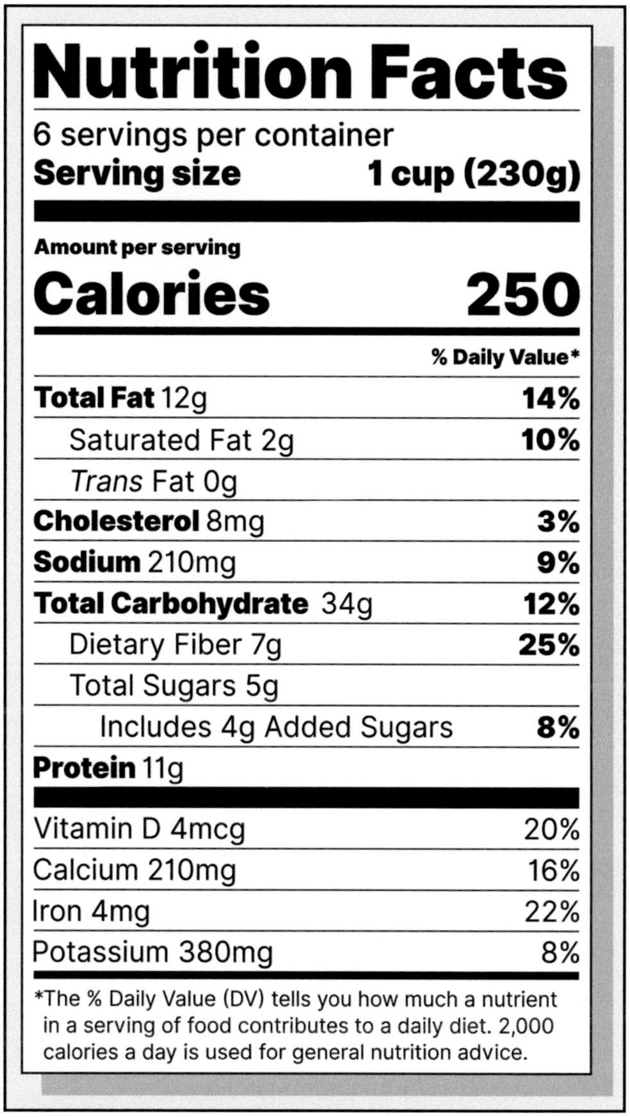

Nutrition Facts
6 servings per container
Serving size 1 cup (230g)
Amount per serving
Calories 250
% Daily Value*
Total Fat 12g 14%
Saturated Fat 2g 10%
Trans Fat 0g
Cholesterol 8mg 3%
Sodium 210mg 9%
Total Carbohydrate 34g 12%
Dietary Fiber 7g 25%
Total Sugars 5g
Includes 4g Added Sugars 8%
Protein 11g
Vitamin D 4mcg 20%
Calcium 210mg 16%
Iron 4mg 22%
Potassium 380mg 8%
*The % Daily Value (DV) tells you how much a nutrient in a serving of food contributes to a daily diet. 2,000 calories a day is used for general nutrition advice.

Figure 14-8. The newest version of the FDA's nutrition facts label, required on all food packages printed after January of 2021, is designed to highlight important information that will in turn help allow consumers to make more informed choices about their food. (marasdaisy/Shutterstock.com.)

> **Sidebar 14-3**
>
> Designing and printing a food package comes with significant cost to the manufacturer. When the FDA updates food labeling requirements such as a new design for the nutrition facts panel, manufacturers must comply with the new design—at significant cost. Due to design and printing costs, among other expenses, it has been estimated that the most recent changes to the nutrition facts panel and updates to the RACC will cost the food industry $2.3 billion, though the recommended benefits are expected to exceed these costs.[17]

consumer who might be considered as having a general understanding of nutrition, the nutrition facts label holds quite a bit of valuable information, and when used properly, the label provides a wealth of data that can be valuable for planning and better understanding one's diet. The athletic trainer can have a huge impact in this area as they can serve as a valuable resource for helping consumers decipher the extensive amount of information that can be found on the nutrition label.

Serving Size

At the top of the nutrition facts label is perhaps the most contextual bit of information presented to consumers—the *serving size* and the *servings per container.* Almost every informational component listed on the nutrition facts label is relevant only to the listed serving size (Figure 14-9). Therefore, it is important for consumers to be able to interpret all nutritional information on the label within the context of the serving size itself. For example, one serving of a processed food item may be listed on the package label as only consisting of 6 ounces of the item. However, the package itself may contain 30 total ounces of food, or the equivalent of 5 servings. When looking over the sodium content on the nutrition facts label, it may list 380 mg of sodium per serving, which in itself is not particularly problematic for most healthy individuals. But if the entire contents of the package are eaten in one sitting, the consumer would have taken in 1900 mg of sodium—nearly their whole day's recommended allowance!

Contributing to the problem of how much is consumed is that serving size can vary widely across products (Figure 14-10). For example, one 12-ounce soft drink can is considered one serving. Yet, one 20-ounce bottle of soft drink can also be labeled as one serving. Unfortunately, ounces or any other measure are not the determinant of a serving size across all products. While a 20-ounce soft drink might be considered as one serving, a smaller 14.5-ounce can of vegetables (eg, corn, green beans) is typically equivalent to 3.5 servings (at ½-cup per serving). Depending on a consumer's eating patterns, ½ cup of green beans may seem unrealistic as a serving size in the same way that 20 ounces of soft drink may be more than some consumers drink. But, that in itself does not change the listed serving size for a particular food item. What is more important is when a package such as a small bag of chips is not equivalent to one serving. In such cases, a "big eater" that eats much more than one serving size must perform a slight bit of math to ensure that they are accurately accounting for the proper amount of nutrients and calories in a particular food item.

So why is it that items such as soft drinks can be found in a variety of sizes, all of which are equal to a single serving? It has to do with the FDA's requirements for an item to be designated as "single serving." According to the FDA's food regulations, a single-serving container is generally considered as

Nutrition Facts

3 servings per container
Serving size   **1 cup (180g)**

	Per serving		Per container	
Calories	**245**		**735**	
		% DV*		% DV*
Total Fat	12g	**14%**	36g	**43%**
Saturated Fat	2g	**10%**	6g	**30%**
Trans Fat	0g		0g	
Cholesterol	8mg	**3%**	24mg	**8%**
Sodium	210mg	**9%**	630mg	**27%**
Total Carb.	34g	**12%**	102g	**36%**
Dietary Fiber	7g	**25%**	21g	**75%**
Total Sugars	5g		15g	
Incl. Added Sugars	4g	**8%**	12g	**24%**
Protein	11g		33g	
Vitamin D	4mcg	20%	12mcg	60%
Calcium	210mg	16%	630mg	48%
Iron	3mg	15%	9mg	45%
Potassium	380mg	8%	1140mg	24%

* The % Daily Value (DV) tells you how much a nutrient in a serving of food contributes to a daily diet. 2,000 calories a day is used for general nutrition advice.

Figure 14-9. It is important for the consumer to understand that the information listed on the Nutrition Facts panel is specific to the serving size listed on the package. Some food labels include nutrition information specific to the entire quantity of food in the package rather than just a single serving. (maradaisy/Shutterstock.com.)

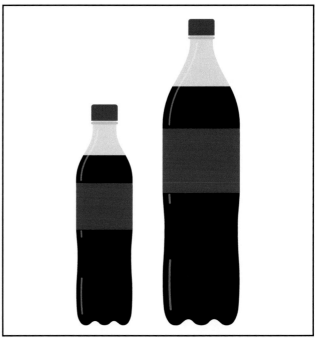

Figure 14-10. Varying serving sizes can complicate one's interpretation of what a food or drink item's nutritional content. Therefore, it is important for consumers to understand the Nutrition Facts label to ensure that they are accounting for all calories and nutrients consumed. (Africa Studio/Shutterstock.com.)

Sidebar 14-4

It is important to point out that serving sizes listed on a food label are not *recommended* intake levels; rather, they represent the amount of food that people are known to consume "per eating occasion," which today might be termed "in one sitting" such as a snack or at a meal. The amounts listed in these serving sizes are actually derived from consumer surveys that were conducted in the 1970s and 1980s. Those surveys established RACCs that manufacturers still use today to indicate a particular food item's serving size.

an individually packaged item that contains less than 200% of the RACC. A regular-sized cookie packaged individually, for example, would be considered as single sized if the cookie weighed 55 g, as the RACC (Sidebar 14-4) for cookies is 30 g and a 55 g cookie would not exceed 200% of the RACC. So even if a container holds more than the RACC—or even over twice the RACC—manufacturers are allowed discretion in labeling a product as "single serve" if it can reasonably be consumed in a single eating session.[1] This explains why a product such as a 20-ounce soft drink can be labeled as "one serving" even though the RACC for beverages is just 240 mL, or 8 fluid ounces, as it is assumed that the soft drink is typically consumed in a single eating session.

It should be noted that any food packages that meet the requirements for "single serve" will not likely contain all information typically required on the standard nutrition facts label. For example, the "servings per container" can be omitted from the nutrition facts label for single-serve food items. Also, metric weight is not required on the panel. Therefore, "1 package" is an acceptable serving size for a snack bag of chips, rather than listing any specific weight requirement such as "8 g" (Sidebar 14-5).

Calculating nutrient or calorie intake associated with the serving size is not particularly problematic as long as the athlete, patient, or client logs the items immediately, such as when preparing their meal. The bigger problem occurs when an individual tries to record the calories, carbohydrates, or other nutrients from memory. Research has shown that caloric intake estimation can vary quite significantly. Generally, recalling caloric intake from memory results in an under-reporting of calories.[9,10] However, one study found that both overweight and normal weight individuals exhibited a high range of over- or underestimation of caloric intake,[11] yet individuals who were overweight who were not trying to lose weight overestimated caloric intake by 37%. Therefore,

Sidebar 14-5

For foods that are not typically consumed in one sitting that contain at least 2 times the RACC yet less than or equal to 3 times the reference amount, such as a bag of chips at the convenience store, the food label for these items must include nutrition information *per serving* as well as *per package*. In other words, consumers must be provided nutrition information that is specific to their consuming either the recommended serving or the entire package of food. For larger packages where it would not be expected for the consumer to eat the entire package of food (eg, a large bag of chips), this dual-format label is not required.

Sidebar 14-6

Although RACC's were established through consumer surveys, a few can at times seem unrealistic. Take, for example, the serving size for cooking spray. The listed serving size on a cooking spray label is often listed as equivalent to a 1/4- to 1/3-second spray—much shorter than most consumers use in coating the bottom of their cooking pans!

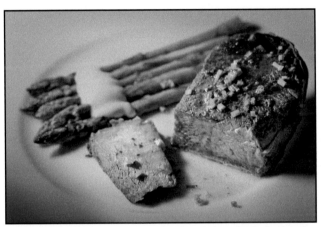

Figure 14-11. Portion size can vary significantly by individual as it is the amount customarily eaten in one sitting. This amount differs from serving size, which is standard for all foods. (supercat/Shutterstock.com.)

sitting they chose to eat 2 servings of mashed potatoes at 1 cup per serving, then their portion size would be equivalent to 2 cups. Understanding portion sizes and correctly estimating portion sizes are critical for accurately recording caloric and nutrient intake.

Calorie Content

The next primary component of the food label is the calorie content. Calories indicate the amount of energy that a food provides, and the calorie content section of the nutrition facts label can help consumers monitor their overall energy intake, which can, in turn, aid in weight management. Alongside the calories value is the "calories from fat," which provides a breakdown of fat's contribution to the overall calorie content. The calorie amount printed on the panel is not always exact but is relatively close to exact, as a serving with 50 or fewer calories is listed in increments of 5 while servings that contain more than 50 calories will be listed in increments of 10.

As stated earlier, the values listed on the nutrition facts label are relevant only within the context of the serving size. Therefore, the calorie amount listed on the label is specific to each serving and is not necessarily representative of the entire package—unless of course the package contents are equivalent to one serving. Any individual interested in recording daily caloric intake would need to multiply the total number of servings consumed in a sitting by the "calories per serving" value (Figure 14-12, Sidebar 14-7).

Individual Nutrients

Located under the calorie section of the nutrition facts label is information regarding a series of nutrients that includes both macro- and micronutrients. The government requires that certain nutrients be listed in a specific order, but does not necessarily require *all* nutrients found in a food to be listed. After the serving size and calorie headings, nutrients found on the nutrition facts label are listed in order by classification: macronutrients and sodium and mandatory public health nutrients such as vitamin D, calcium, and iron. More specifically, the required nutrients that must be outlined on the panel include *total* fat, saturated fat, *trans* fat, cholesterol, sodium (the only vitamin or mineral listed in the top portion of the panel), *total* carbohydrates, dietary

without the use of food labels to indicate the precise caloric amount (along with the reference amount of food), consumers can end up with quite a degree of fluctuation in estimating actual calories consumed. Over time, such incorrect estimations may contribute to why a patient or client is not losing or gaining weight, as their consumed calorie amounts are incorrect. To correct this potential error, patients and clients should be recommended to use the nutrition facts label as a guide and also pay close attention to serving sizes (Sidebar 14-6).

As discussed earlier, serving size is a predetermined amount of food that is based upon what surveys revealed as the amount of food typically eaten. This is in contrast, however, to *portion size*, which is the amount of food that an individual actually eats for a meal or snack (Figure 14-11). This may be confusing for some patients or clients as they may misinterpret a serving size for a portion size. Technically, if they elected to eat the exact amount of a serving size, their portion size would be the same amount. However, if in one

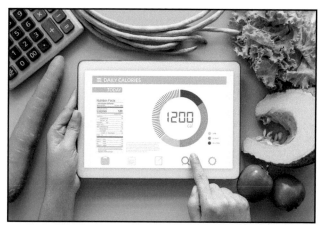

Figure 14-12. While apps have made it easier to monitor nutrition intake, it is essential that consumers are fluent on how to accurately interpret nutrition facts components such as serving size so that proper quantities can be entered into the app. (asiandelight/Shutterstock.com.)

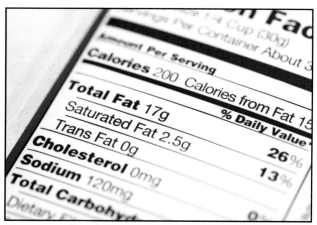

Figure 14-13. The individual nutrients and % daily value data can be found amongst the lower half of the nutrition facts label. This information is structured so that macronutrients and some micronutrients are listed first, followed by certain vitamins and minerals in the lowest section. (asiandelight/Shutterstock.com.)

fiber, sugars, and *protein*, followed by a secondary panel that lists the required vitamin D as well as minerals. Any voluntarily included vitamins or minerals (eg, folate) would then be listed as well.[12]

To help ensure consistency, each nutrient outlined on the nutrition facts label has its own unit of measure that must be followed. For example, the total quantity of fat must be listed up to the nearest 0.5 g increment (eg, 10.5 g), while fiber quantity is listed to the nearest gram. Vitamins and minerals, however, are listed in specific milligram or microgram quantities (eg, vitamin A = mcg, calcium = mg).

Based on the available space on a package, manufacturers are permitted in some cases to abbreviate nutrients. For example, when a package has 40 or less square inches, abbreviations may be used in the nutrition facts label *and* a horizontal nutrition facts label may be used rather than the more common vertically oriented label.[12] Such an orientation is commonly seen on smaller packages, such as condiment jars or candy bars (Figure 14-13).

Percent Daily Value

To the right of most nutrients on the nutrition facts label will be a number under the heading of "% daily value." These numbers are tied to the daily value recommendations for certain nutrients and can be used as a guide to indicate what percent of the recommended intake is supplied per serving of the labeled food. However, it is important to note that, as is shown at the bottom of the nutrition facts label, these percentages are in the context of a 2000-calorie diet (see Figure 14-13). Therefore, individuals who are not intending to consume 2000 calories would need to adjust the % daily value number to reflect their own diet. For example, an individual striving for a 3000-calorie diet per day would find that the listed % daily value numbers are lower than what they would need to maintain their 3000-calorie diet. Still, by illustrating a 2000-calorie diet directly on the label, consumers are provided with a general framework for how much each serving of food supplies for their diet. By providing the % daily value, consumers can see a quick-reference guide that outlines the contribution of a particular nutrient. If, for example, a serving provides 23% of the % daily value for total fat, consumers can more easily recognize that value as a high percentage as opposed to calculating out just how the listed *total fat* grams contribute to the consumer's daily caloric intake.

It is vital for consumers to be aware that the % daily value, like almost all nutrient amounts on the nutrition facts label, is tied in with the serving size. Therefore, while a particular nutrient content may not seem high as listed on the nutrition facts label, if more than one serving—or the entire package—is consumed, it could have a significant effect on the consumer's dietary intake. Using the previous example, if the *total fat* % daily value was 23% for the specified serving size, but the individual ate 3 servings, the total contribution for that one meal would be 69% of their recommended total fat intake. And, if the consumer miscalculates how much

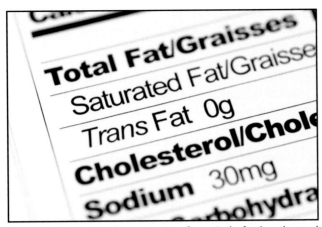

Figure 14-14. Knowing the serving size of a particular food product and how much of that food was consumed is essential for ensuring accurate estimation of key nutrients. (JohnKwan/Shutterstock.com.)

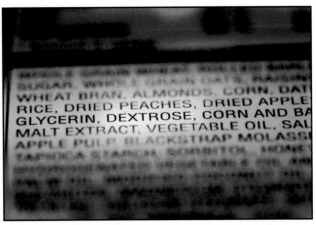

Figure 14-15. The ingredient list requires all ingredients used in a packaged food product to be listed in descending order by weight. Therefore, ingredients with the highest quantity in the food product will be listed first, while those with the least will be listed near the end of the ingredient list. (Benoit Daoust/Shutterstock.com.)

they actually consume, such as might occur by underestimating their intake, it could ultimately result in consistently exceeding their recommended fat intake. This highlights the importance of consumers ensuring that they factor in a food item's serving size when using the nutrition facts label to help guide their diet (Figure 14-14).

Certain nutrients such as *trans fat, sugars,* and *protein* do not have an associated % daily value on the nutrition facts label. This came about through multiple factors.[13] Specific to *trans* fat, a daily value could not be established by the FDA. Furthermore, *trans* fats have been banned by the FDA since 2018 for all foods sold in grocery stores and restaurants.[14] Protein does not contain a % daily value on the nutrition facts label, as protein intake is not considered a public health concern for individuals over the age of 4 years. Similarly, there is no % daily value for "sugars" (not to be confused with *total carbohydrate),* as no recommendation has been set specific to how much sugar to consume per day.

Ingredient List

Food items can be made up of what seems to be a limitless supply of ingredients. Manufacturers take advantage of ingredients to create marketable foods that will hopefully create a flavor that consumers will want to buy. However, in this time of increased health awareness, certain food ingredients may cause consumers to consider the impact of those ingredients. Sodium is a relevant example. Manufacturers will often include sodium in the ingredient list as it is both a flavor enhancer as well as a quite inexpensive preservative. Consumers, however, have been made well aware of sodium's influence on negative health events such as heart disease and hypertension, and may limit themselves to foods that do not have high sodium levels. The FDA itself outlines more than 3000 individual ingredients, food additives, and flavoring substances in a database known as *Substances Added to Food.*[15] Because of FDA regulations, consumers are now

made aware of all ingredients found in their processed foods thanks to the required inclusion of the ingredients list on food packages (Figure 14-15).

While the nutrition facts label is targeted largely at nutrient information, the ingredients label is designed to outline exactly of what the food item is comprised. For relatively simple foods like certain brands of butter, the ingredient list may be quite short—with only 3 or 4 ingredients. Processed foods, however, can have an extensive ingredient list that takes up a significant portion of the package label. The information contained within the ingredient list is vital for individuals seeking to avoid or limit certain ingredients in their diets, as well as for those consumers who are allergic to a specific food item. Of particular interest are those ingredients that are not common allergens, as other more common allergens (eg, gluten, peanuts) may be prominently displayed elsewhere on the food label.

Typically, a food's ingredient list will be found below the nutrition facts label when room allows. The FDA defines the ingredient list as " ... the listing of each ingredient in descending order of predominance." Therefore, items found on the ingredient list are ordered from highest content to lowest by weight; in other words, ingredients weighing the most are listed first and those weighing the least are listed last. While this does make it somewhat simple to determine the quantity of ingredients, such an ordering system does not always tell the consumer the whole story. The ingredient list only details the ingredients used to make the food product—it does not, however, summarize the total quantity of nutrients. Therefore, certain nutrients such as sodium may appear further down an ingredient list, which makes it appear as though the item is included in the food in relatively small amounts. However, there may in fact be 2, 3, 5, or more ingredients that contain sodium. Because of the total weight of sodium in the food item, sodium itself may qualify to be higher up on the ingredient list based on *total quantity,* but because

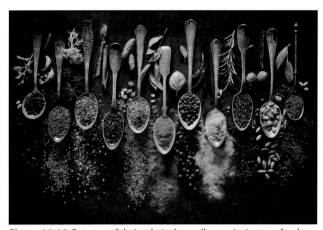

Figure 14-16. Because of their relatively small quantity in most food products, an array of herbs and spices as well as food additives like preservatives are typically the last few items found on an ingredient list. (Alexander Raths/Shutterstock.com.)

sodium was a part of several separate ingredients it may appear to be a relatively small portion of the food. Realistically, the actual sodium content listed on the nutrition facts label should be the primary reference for total sodium content, but a consumer wanting to separate out their salt intake from say, sodium bicarbonate, would find the relevant information listed on the ingredients label. Similarly, "sugar" may be included in a food listed as sugar itself or as high-fructose corn syrup or cane sugar, among other sources.

There are times when a food's nutrient content may not appear to match what is in the ingredients. This typically occurs when certain ingredients supply nutrients in very small amounts, such as for *trans* fat or sodium. In the case of *trans* fat specifically, the nutrition facts label may list the content of *trans* fat as "0," yet list partially hydrogenated vegetable oil in the ingredients list—a known contributor of *trans* fats. This apparent mismatch can occur when the manufacturer takes advantage of an FDA regulation that allows *trans* fat to be listed as "0" on the nutrition facts label if the actual *trans* fat content is 0.5 g or less.[1] Therefore, a listing of "0" on the nutrition facts label indicates that while there may indeed be *trans* fat in the product, the total amount is very low.

So what happens when an ingredient list contains items that are themselves made up of several ingredients? In such cases, the individual ingredients should be listed in parentheses next to the primary food item. For example, a food product that contains noodles cannot simply state "noodles" on the label. Rather, the manufacturer must list the separate ingredients used to make those noodles. Therefore, the ingredients list specific to those noodles may appear as follows: "enriched pasta (wheat flour, ferrous sulfate, niacin, thiamin mononitrate, riboflavin, folic acid)."

Flavoring agents, color enhancers, and preservatives are typically listed among the final few items of an ingredient list, and the set of regulations that outline their use are quite extensive—as are the qualifications for each.[16] For example, to qualify as an *artificial flavor* or *artificial flavoring,* the FDA

defines it as "... any substance, the function of which is to impart flavor, which is not derived from a spice, fruit or fruit juice, vegetable or vegetable juice, edible yeast, herb, bark, bud, root, leaf or similar plant material, meat, fish, poultry, eggs, dairy products, or fermentation products thereof." Color and flavoring agents have several regulations that they must be held to, such as a particular font size to indicate "artificially flavored." Preservatives that are considered as any chemical except salt, sugars, vinegars, spices, or oils extracted from spices that when added to food prevents or retards deterioration of that food. When used, preservatives must be listed using their common name and must include a description of that preservative's function such as "to help protect flavor" or "to retard spoilage" (Figure 14-16).

Conclusion

Although there is a wealth of marketing and sales tactics involved in the design of a food label, consumers have been afforded access to an abundance of nutritional information on food labels that can be invaluable when planning a healthy diet. Despite having some degree of freedom to design their packaging, manufacturers must still adhere to a variety of specific labeling standards that, in turn, helps maintain uniformity across food products and helps to ensure that consumers are presented information about a food product in a consistent yet understandable way. Font size requirements, food claim phrasing, and the ordering of a food's nutrients must all adhere to the FDA's guidelines in order for a food to be marketed. The nutrition facts label, as well as the ingredients list, provides vital information for consumers; however, the complexity of some of the information found in these sections of a food label may be daunting for some individuals. Athletic trainers can play a key role in relaying to consumers both the value and the importance of these areas of the food label, as these label components can be invaluable for athletes, patients, and clients in successfully planning a healthy diet.

Discussion Questions

1. How might an individual's health or fitness goals influence which part(s) of the nutrition facts label they pay the most attention to?

2. When making portion size adjustments based on the listed serving size of a food item, what impact might small errors (such as rounding up to "100 calories" from "85" to make the calculations easier to perform) have on an individual's health or diet plan over time?

3. What information do you feel should be listed on a nutrition facts label that is not currently listed? Why?

References

1. US Food and Drug Administration. *A Food Labeling Guide: Guidance for Industry.* 2013.

2. US Food and Drug Administration. *Authorized Health Claims That Meet the Significant Scientific Agreement (SSA) Standard.* US Department of Health and Human Services; 2018.

3. Hooker NH, Teratanavat R. Dissecting qualified health claims: evidence from experimental studies. *Crit Rev Food Sci Nutr.* 2008;48(2):160-176.

4. US Food and Drug Administration. *Qualified Health Claims: Letters of Enforcement Discretion.* 2017. https://www.fda.gov/food/food-labeling-nutrition/qualified-health-claims-letters-enforcement-discretion

5. US Food and Drug Administration. *Questions and Answers on Health Claims in Food Labeling.* 2017.

6. Boon CS, Lichtenstein AH, Wartella EA. *Front-of-Package Nutrition Rating Systems and Symbols: Phase I Report.* National Academies Press; 2010.

7. Kessler DA. The federal regulation of food labeling. *N Eng J Med.* 1989;321(11):717-725.

8. US Food and Drug Administration. *Changes to the Nutrition Facts Label.* US Food and Drug Administration; 2016. https://www.fda.gov/Food/GuidanceRegulation/GuidanceDocumentsRegulatoryInformation/LabelingNutrition/ucm385663.htm

9. Carels RA, Harper J, Konrad K. Qualitative perceptions and caloric estimations of healthy and unhealthy foods by behavioral weight loss participants. *Appetite.* 2006;46(2):199-206.

10. Krall EA, Dwyer JT. Validity of a food frequency questionnaire and a food diary in a short-term recall situation. *J Am Diet Assoc.* 1987;87(10):1374-1377.

11. Brown RE, Canning KL, Fung M, et al. Calorie estimation in adults differing in body weight class and weight loss status. *Med Sci Sports Exerc.* 2016;48(3):521.

12. US Food and Drug Administration. *Industry Resources on the Changes to the Nutrition Facts Label.* US Food and Drug Administration; 2020. https://www.fda.gov/food/food-labeling-nutrition/industry-resources-changes-nutrition-facts-label

13. US Food and Drug Administration. *How to Understand and Use the Nutrition Facts Label.* 2020.

14. US Food and Drug Administration. *Final Determination Regarding Partially Hydrogenated Oils (Removing Trans Fat).* 2018.

15. US Food and Drug Administration. *Substances Added to Food (formerly EAFUS).* 2018.

16. US Food and Drug Administration. *Title 21—Food and Drugs. Chapter I—Food and Drug Administration, Department of Health and Human Services. Subchapter B—Food for Human Consumption, Part 101 Food Labeling.* 2019.

17. Fortin ND. *Food Regulation: Law, Science, Policy, and Practice.* Wiley; 2007.

Chapter 15

Nutrition Counseling for Athletic Trainers

Penny Wilson, PhD, RDN

Commission on Accreditation of Athletic Training Education *2020 Standards*

This chapter addresses the following *2020 Standards for Accreditation of Professional Athletic Training Programs*:

- Standard 55: Students must gain foundational knowledge in statistics, research design, epidemiology, pathophysiology, biomechanics and pathomechanics, exercise physiology, nutrition, human anatomy, pharmacology, public health, and health care delivery and payor systems.
- Standard 59: Communicate effectively and appropriately with clients/patients, family members, coaches, administrators, other health care professionals, consumers, payors, policy makers, and others.
- Standard 83: Educate and make recommendations to clients/patients on fluids and nutrients to ingest prior to activity, during activity, and during recovery for a variety of activities and environmental conditions.

Learning Objectives

After reviewing this chapter, readers will be able to:

- Understand why nutrition counseling can be an important part of an athletic trainer's role.
- Prepare for nutrition counseling sessions.
- Identify where the client is in the Stages of Change Model.
- Gain tools to conduct a nutrition counseling session and follow-up sessions.

Knoblauch M, ed. *Clinical Nutrition in Athletic Training* (pp 167-178). © 2023 Taylor & Francis Group.

Introduction

Intercollegiate student athletes "perceived athletic trainers to have strong nutrition knowledge."[1] This perception is likely to be held by others with whom athletic trainers work. Athletic trainers should be able to provide nutrition counseling as an added service to their clients, as long as the athletic trainer is comfortable with providing this type of counseling and that nutrition counseling is allowed by state licensure laws. This chapter will help athletic trainers understand the basics of nutrition counseling, the models of offering counseling, and how to structure and conduct nutrition counseling sessions. If at any time the athletic trainer is not comfortable providing nutrition counseling, the client should be referred to a registered dietitian.

What Is Nutrition Counseling?

Nutrition counseling is defined as "advising and assisting individuals and groups on appropriate nutrition intake by integrating information from the nutrition assessment with information on food and other sources of nutrients and meal preparation consistent with cultural background and socioeconomic status."[2]

An athletic trainer can work with a client to assess the client's current nutrition status and eating patterns, and help make improvements to one or both. This may also include a review and assessment of any dietary supplements the client is using.

Why Is Nutrition Counseling Important?

Finding nutrition information these days is easy. A quick internet search can provide most anyone a degree of nutrition information; however, the information found may or may not be accurate. Athletic trainers can be one trusted source for evidence-based nutrition information. In fact, athletic trainers have been cited by collegiate athletes as their primary source of nutrition information.[1] Being a trusted source for nutrition information does not mean that an athletic trainer needs to know "everything" related to nutrition. Rather, athletic trainers can provide guidance specific to the information they are comfortable with, yet still recommend that a client see a registered dietitian for more in-depth information or information with which they are uncomfortable. If any time an athletic trainer is uncomfortable with the nutrition questions being asked or the overall nutrition status of the client, that client can be referred to a registered dietitian.

Can Athletic Trainers Provide Nutrition Counseling?

If the athletic trainer has concerns about conducting nutrition counseling, state licensure laws and the defined Scope of Practice can be checked. Some states have strict licensure laws that govern who can provide nutrition counseling. The Commission on Dietetic Registration has a list of nutrition counseling licensure requirements that can be used check basic licensure requirements. The athletic trainer should understand their state's licensure laws prior to conducting nutrition counseling sessions.

Preparing for the Session

Conducting an effective nutrition counseling session requires time to prepare for both the athletic trainer and the client. Once the athletic trainer and client agree to meet, any or all of the following forms could be provided to the client:

- Nutrition and health history
- Food and drink log
- Medication and dietary supplement listing (may be included on the nutrition history form)

Ideally, the client should return the completed forms well before the session, thereby allowing ample time for the athletic trainer to thoroughly review the forms prior to the meeting. Researching a client's medications and supplements takes time, and in order to conduct an effective session this time should be factored into the preparation time.

Nutrition and Health History Form

A nutrition history form captures information about the client's physical status and health history. The form usually includes the following information, and should be customized based on the athletic trainer's experience and goals:

- Birthdate
- Injuries and surgeries (including dates of each)
- Health history, including any illnesses or diseases
- Food allergies or intolerances and the reaction experienced when eaten
- Favorite foods
- Least favorite foods

The nutrition history form gives the athletic trainer basic information about the client as well as any medical and food issues to be aware of, and provides a starting place for the counseling session.

Time	What	How Much	Hunger Scale		Symptoms/ Mood/Thoughts/How You Feel
			Before Meal*	After Meal*	

Figure 15-1. A sample food and drink log.

Food and Drink Log

Having 3 to 5 days of food log information can help the athletic trainer understand what the client is eating and drinking and when. A food and drink log (Figure 15-1) typically includes 1 to 3 days of weekday eating and 1 to 2 days of weekend eating. Having weekdays and weekend days included in the log provides a more complete picture of the client's eating patterns as most people eat and drink differently on weekdays and weekends.

Including beverages on the log helps the athletic trainer understand the client's total intake of calories and water. The client should be encouraged to include everything that is consumed on the days for which they are logging.

A food and drink log should contain the following information:

- Date and time of eating or drinking
- What was consumed
- Amount
- Notes (This area can be used for any notes that the client wants to make about what the client ate or how they felt. It can be also used to record how hungry the client was when starting eating and how full or satisfied they were when they stopped eating. A discussion of hunger and fullness can be found later in this chapter.)

If prior to a nutrition session the athletic trainer suspects that the client may have an eating disorder, the benefits of having a food log should be weighed against the potential negative effects of asking the client to keep a food log. Please refer to Chapter 12 for more information on eating disorders.

Medication and Dietary Supplement Form

A full listing of any medications, dietary supplements, or other drugs (Figure 15-2) that the client is using is important for the athletic trainer to have so that a full picture of the client's health can be understood. The medication and dietary supplement listing could be included in the nutrition history form or a separate form. The medication and dietary supplement listing form should include the following information:

- Name of the medication
- Dosage
- Frequency
- Reason for use
- When started
- Any improvements or side effects experienced

This form typically needs ample time for review prior to the meeting. Specifically, research on medication and dietary supplements should be done prior to the meeting if at all possible so that the athletic trainer can enter the session fully informed of the client's needs. If the client is subject to doping control (eg, drug testing), all medications and dietary supplements (including all ingredients of those products) should be checked against the banned supplement list for the organization under which they compete.

Research has estimated that 88% of intercollegiate student athletes use at least one dietary supplement.[1] Asking a client about their supplement use helps the athletic trainer understand if the client is taking dietary supplements

Figure 15-2. A sample medication and supplement log.

Medication or Supplement Name	Dosage	Frequency	Why taking	Date started	Any benefits? Any side effects?

because they are concerned about their macronutrient and micronutrient intake or if they are taking supplements to enhance sport performance. For more information about dietary supplements, see Chapter 6.

Alcohol and Drug Use

The athletic trainer may want to collect information about alcohol and illicit drug use during the session. Drinking alcohol and using illicit drugs can impact the client's eating and drinking. The client may or may not disclose this information depending on the level of trust achieved with the athletic trainer.

Physical recording of information about alcohol and illicit drug use needs to be carefully considered. If written records of the counseling session are subject to disclosure to others, the athletic trainer should decide whether or not to record this information because it may be released outside of the counseling session with the client.

Client Goals for the Session

The client should be asked either on the nutrition history form or at the beginning of the session what their goals are for the individual session as well as for the longer term, if appropriate. Asking the client to provide goals, either in the initial meeting or on the nutrition history form, helps the client think through what they want to achieve. Having 1 and no more than 3 goals helps the client focus on what is most important to them, without having a large number of goals that may be overwhelming. If the client does have a large number of goals, the athletic trainer can work with the client to prioritize the goals and determine which one they

would like to focus on first. As the goals are achieved, the list can be reviewed to determine what goals should be targeted next. The client's goals should be kept in mind by the athletic trainer when preparing for and conducting the session.

Understanding the Body's Hunger and Fullness Signals

American culture is obsessed with diets and dieting. This obsession has led to a disconnect from the body's hunger and fullness signals. Helping the client understand hunger and fullness signals can help them learn to eat when their body needs food and stop when full.

While the ability to quantify hunger and fullness may be included on a client's food log, the athletic trainer may want to spend time in the session understanding whether the client is responding to their body's hunger and fullness cues or not. For example, the food log may show that the client is eating when they are not hungry. The athletic trainer can then talk with the client about what made them choose to eat at that time. The athletic trainer may discover that the client is eating due to boredom. The athletic trainer and client can work together toward a goal of having the client eat when hungry and stopping when full.

Understanding Hunger

Helping a client understand and respond to biological hunger—the body's signal that food is needed—can help the client eat when their body needs food rather than when they *think* they should eat.

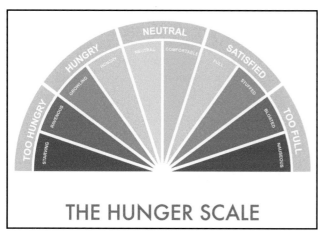

THE HUNGER SCALE

Figure 15-3. Basic hunger and fullness scale that can be used with clients to help them identify their hunger and fullness levels. (Evgenia.B/Shutterstock.com.)

As Evelyn Tribole, MS, RD and Elyse Resch, MS, RD, FADA state in their book *Intuitive Eating: A Revolutionary Program that Works:*

> Food and energy are so essential to the survival of the human species that if we don't eat enough, we set off a biological fuse that turns on our eating drive, both physically *and* psychologically. The hunger drive is truly a mind–body connection. Eating is so important that the nerve cells of appetite are located in the hypothalamus region of the brain. A variety of biological signals triggers eating. What many people believe to be an issue of willpower is instead a *biological drive.* The power and intensity of the biological eating drive should not be underestimated.[3]

When the biological drive that hunger creates is ignored or silenced, overeating—even bingeing—can result. Helping clients listen to and honor their body's hunger signals, and eating when hungry, can assist in their achievement of many of their goals.

Hunger can be classified either using a scale of 0 to 10 with 0 being "starving and beyond," 5 being "neutral," and 10 being "uncomfortably full, even painfully full" (Figure 15-3). A second scale to classify hunger can ask the client if the hunger is comfortable, uncomfortable, or neutral.

Explaining the difference between biological hunger and other types of hunger—such as cravings or eating for emotional reasons—helps the client start to identify biological hunger. Having a client indicate their hunger on the food log, using either one of these scales, can be helpful in understanding if the client is eating when they are biologically hungry.

When a client learns to honor their hunger, episodes of overeating/bingeing may cease because they, and their body, learn that hunger signals will be listened to. The process of learning to hear one's hunger signals can take time. Any progress toward hearing hunger signals and eating when actually hungry should be celebrated with the client.

Understanding Fullness

Just as a lack of hearing the body's hunger signals exists for many clients, they may also lack the ability to feel and understand their body's fullness signals. Many people have been brought up to be members of the clean-plate club, which leads to an inherent need by a client to eat all of the food on their plate regardless of whether they feel full or not. Just as learning to hear and respond to the body's hunger signals can be a challenge, so can stopping eating when comfortably full.

In order for a client to understand that they can stop eating when they are full, they first need to understand that they can eat when their body signals that it needs food—this is known as "biological hunger." Responding to the body's hunger and fullness signals go hand-in-hand. If the client is not confident that they can eat when their body is hungry, then stopping when they are full can also be a challenge to learn. For example, if someone does not know when they will get their next meal, they may overeat to be sure they have enough food to last for a while.

The 0 to 10 scale mentioned previously can also be used for fullness. Additionally, fullness can be classified as comfortable, uncomfortable, or neutral. Having the client record their fullness levels on their food log can help the athletic trainer understand the fullness level to which the client is eating. Usually, eating to a level of fullness that allows a client to go without eating another meal for 3 to 4 hours is considered normal. This will vary depending on the client's age, growth status, and amount and intensity of workouts that are being done. Just as with hunger signals, it can take time for a client to learn to determine the level of fullness that is appropriate for them.

Counseling Tools

When conducting a nutrition counseling session, the primary consideration to keep in mind is what are the client's goals for the session and for the long term. The athletic trainer will want to understand the client's level of motivation for making the changes being discussed. A variety of counseling tools exists to help determine factors, such as patient motivation. The athletic trainer should choose the tools they are comfortable with as well as those tools that will provide the best outcomes.

The Stages of Change Model, also known as the Transtheoretical Model, discussed later in this chapter, helps the athletic trainer identify the client's readiness to change their behavior. Once the athletic trainer understands what stage of change the client is in, they can then choose a counseling approach. An overview of 4 counseling approaches is discussed in the Stages of Change Model—instructive, guided, cognitive behavior therapy (CBT), and motivational interviewing (MI). The discussion of each approach also includes pros and cons of each, so that the athletic trainer will

Sidebar 15-1

Stages of Change. Sam had been working with his athletic trainer for a few months to put on lean mass, stay injury-free, and improve his eating. During the winter break, his mother was diagnosed with breast cancer and began treatment. After his mom's diagnosis, Sam talked with his athletic trainer and explained that he couldn't really concentrate on his workouts and eating right now. He was spending a lot of time helping take care of his little sister, cooking for the family, and helping around the house while his mom was receiving treatment. He said he didn't know how long her treatment was going to last.

Sam was in the action step—making changes and planning on continuing to make changes until his mother's diagnosis. Then, due to the change in his family and his need to do more to help, he moved into the precontemplation phase.

Betty, another student athlete, went to see her athletic trainer to talk about her eating because her coach told her she needed to. At the start of the session she says, "I don't know why I'm here. My eating is fine. Coach made me come."

Betty is in the precontemplation phase because she doesn't see any problems and is not willing to make any changes at this point.

While the Stages of Change Model is not perfect, it can help when talking with a client to understand how ready they are to make a change.

have a basic understanding of some of the skills needed to conduct a counseling session and is able to choose the most appropriate approach for the client, goals, and session length.

The athletic trainer should strive to take a nonjudgmental approach and use appropriate terminology with the client.

Taking a Nonjudgmental Approach

Choosing foods and beverages has become fraught with guilt and judgment. Clients need a safe place, and person, to talk about their choices. The athletic trainer can be this person by taking a nonjudgmental approach during counseling sessions with the client.

A nonjudgmental approach is achieved when a counselor (eg, athletic trainer, dietitian) does not judge or criticize their client for their choices. During nutrition counseling sessions, athletic trainers should listen actively and be curious about why the client made the decisions they made. Judgments about whether a client is "good" or "bad," or that

the choices they have made are "good" or "bad," should be avoided in the counseling session and in any contact with the client. If they feel they are being judged, they likely will not be honest during the session and may choose not to attend additional counseling sessions.

The Stages of Change Model

The Stages of Change Model can be helpful in identifying how ready a client is to making changes. The Stages of Change in this model are:

- **Precontemplation:** The client does not plan to take action or make changes within the next 6 months.
- **Contemplation:** The client is beginning to think about making changes within the next 6 months.
- **Preparation:** The client is ready to take action within the next 30 days and may start taking small steps to change.
- **Action:** The client has made changes and will continue making changes.
- **Maintenance:** The client has maintained their new behavior for a while and intends to maintain the changes they have made.
- **Termination:** The client has no desire to return to their previous state.[4]

A client may move through the steps sequentially, but usually they will move back and forth between them. For example, a client may be in the action phase at one point, but then an event happens and they move into the precontemplation phase (Sidebar 15-1).

Counseling Approaches

Helping clients change their eating behavior can be challenging. Understanding how and why a client chooses to eat or drink certain foods and beverages and then helping them change how they make choices is why developing a trusting, nonjudgmental approach is critical. There are 4 main approaches used in nutrition counseling—instructive counseling, guided counseling, CBT, and MI. These approaches are not mutually exclusive and can be used in combination.

Instructive Counseling

Instructive counseling[5] is when the athletic trainer provides instruction to the client about what to do. The benefit of instructive counseling is its brevity. This type of session can be short because the client is being told what they need to do. The disadvantage is that most clients typically do not respond well to the instructive counseling style because the client does not feel like they have a choice. In an instructive counseling session, the athletic trainer is telling the client what to do rather than partnering with the client to develop solutions.[5]

Athletic Trainer: I see on your food log that you use a lot of prepared shakes and eat a lot of fast food.

Betty: Yeah. My parents both work a lot. They just give me some money each week and let me eat whatever I want. I don't like vegetables. I don't know how to cook. I'm really busy with school and workouts, too. I need food that is fast and cheap. Those things fit the bill.

Athletic Trainer: You really need to start eating more vegetables. I want you to include at least one salad a day in your eating.

Betty is not likely to respond well to the athletic trainer's recommendations because she was not given a choice about the recommendation.

Guided Counseling

Guided counseling is a conversational session. The athletic trainer encourages the client to set goals and guides the client to find ways to reach them.[5] Many of the questions asked will be open-ended. The athletic trainer should also engage in active listening: summarizing what the client says, discussing pros and cons of changes with the client, and assessing the client's interest in making changes. During this stage, the athletic trainer should seek to ask for permission to make suggestions specific to recommending dietary changes.

Using the guided counseling approach can help the client feel more in charge and involved in the process.

Benefits of this approach include gaining insight from the client and gaining more buy-in with the changes since the client feels more in charge. Disadvantages of the guided counseling approach are that the client's motivations for making changes are not discussed and worked through and that ambivalence about making diet-specific changes is not addressed.

Athletic Trainer: What would you like to talk about today?

Sam: I'm feeling really stressed about my mom and having to do so much these days.

Athletic Trainer: You've got a lot to take care of right now.

Sam: Yeah. And, I'm frustrated about my eating and workouts. I just can't focus on eating the way we had planned. I have to cook for the whole family, and they don't like to eat the way I do. I can't fix 2 separate meals.

Athletic Trainer: Would you like some suggestions to help with your and your family's eating?

In this session, the athletic trainer is reflecting and summarizing Sam's concerns. Finally, the athletic trainer asks for permission to provide some suggestions to help Sam with the family's eating. By asking permission to offer suggestions, the athletic trainer is giving Sam the choice whether or not he wants suggestions at this point in the session. If Sam does

not want suggestions at this time, that is fine. The athletic trainer can continue listening, reflecting, and summarizing. At another point, the athletic trainer may want to ask again if Sam would like some suggestions.

Later in this chapter is a discussion on questions and responses that can be incorporated into the sessions.

Cognitive Behavioral Therapy

CBT "focuses on modifying dysfunctional emotions, behaviors, and thoughts by interrogating and uprooting negative or irrational beliefs."[6] CBT is based on the idea that thoughts and perceptions influence behaviors. When having a CBT-based session, the athletic trainer and client work to identify "harmful thoughts, assess whether they are an accurate depiction of reality, and, if they are not, employ strategies to challenge and overcome them."[6]

Benefits of CBT include client involvement in the process of identifying, evaluating, and modifying thoughts, and that it teaches strategies that can be used in other parts of the client's life even after they are no longer seeing the athletic trainer. A disadvantage with CBT is that if the athletic trainer finds that the client has complex mental health issues or the client is confronting anxiety and emotions, the athletic trainer would need to refer the client to an appropriate mental health counselor. It is recommended that an athletic trainer should seek additional information and training about CBT if this type of approach will be used in depth.

Betty: I'll never be able to eat better. There isn't enough time.

Athletic Trainer: Let's look at those thoughts and see if they are true. Is it true that there isn't enough time?

Betty: Yeah. I get up, get to school, have workouts, get home, eat, study, and spend time texting with my friends.

Athletic Trainer: You've said that you don't eat breakfast because you don't have time, right?

Betty: Yeah. There isn't time in the morning.

Athletic Trainer: Could we work together to find a few minutes, 5 or 10 minutes, at night when you could put together a breakfast you could grab in the morning?

Betty: Yeah. I think that would work.

Athletic Trainer: So, it looks like we can find time for breakfast.

In this interaction, Betty says there is no time. The athletic trainer calls that belief to her attention, questions whether it is accurate or not, then suggests they work together to find time to make a grab-and-go breakfast.

Motivational Interviewing

MI uses some aspects of guided counseling and adds more tools to be used in the counseling session. MI is a highly effective strategy, especially in combination with CBT.[5] MI can take more time than instructive or guided strategies and may require additional training.

Underlying MI are 4 key concepts: partnership, acceptance, compassion, and evocation.[7] The following definitions are adapted from those in *Motivational Interviewing in Nutrition and Fitness:*

1. **Partnership** is when the athletic trainer and client work together to find solutions to the issues the client is facing. The client is the expert of their body and experience.

2. **Acceptance** occurs when the athletic trainer communicates that the client has inherent value and potential, perceives and provides statements that reflect the client's meaning, that the client has the right to make choices, and the athletic trainer accentuates the client's strengths and efforts.

3. **Compassion** is when the athletic trainer acts with kindness and gives priority to the client's needs.

4. **Evocation** happens when the athletic trainer draws out the client's motivation for making a change.

The ambivalence that a client may feel and express during a session is also key in MI. If a client is expressing ambivalence about making a change, rather than listing all the reasons why a change should be made, the athletic trainer can work with the client to understand their motivation for wanting to change as well as the reasons for changing and not changing—all from the client's point of view.

> **Betty:** I don't know why coach wanted me to come talk to you. My eating and performance are OK.
>
> **Athletic Trainer:** Your eating and performance are fine and you don't understand why your coach wants you to improve your nutrition.
>
> **Betty:** Yeah. I mean there have been a few practices where I've been tired. Coach has said I could play in college if I can pick up my game.
>
> **Athletic Trainer:** You're interested in playing in college and having enough energy to have great practice sessions.
>
> **Betty:** I'd really like to play in college. And, play better for the team here. I'm just so busy. And, I don't know how to cook.
>
> **Athletic Trainer:** Playing better here and getting to play in college excites you. You have some challenges with cooking.
>
> **Betty:** Cooking scares me. I don't understand all the terms or even know what pan to use for what.
>
> **Athletic Trainer:** Cooking is scary. There seems like a lot to know about it.

> **Betty:** Exactly. No one ever taught me how. I just do shakes and buy food I can microwave. I wish the food tasted better.
>
> **Athletic Trainer:** You want food that tastes better than the microwave meals you've been buying. How could you get the food to taste better?

In this exchange, the athletic trainer reflects Betty's concerns and addresses her ambivalence about why she is even in the session. By listening and reflecting back Betty's thoughts, the athletic trainer is building rapport and practicing compassion, acceptance, and evocation. The athletic trainer becomes a partner when the client is asked about how she could work to make her food taste better. The athletic trainer is helping Betty find a solution to the issues she feels that she is facing.

Types of Questions and Responses—OARS

Open-ended questions, affirmations, reflection, and summary are abbreviated into the acronym OARS for MI. OARS are not specific to MI. They can be used in any type of nutrition counseling session.

Open-Ended Questions

Open-ended questions allow the client to think about their response and serve to spur discussion between the client and athletic trainer. Closed questions can be answered with just a few, or even one, words.

Open-ended questions frequently start with "how" or "what." If an athletic trainer wants to draw out more information about a particular topic, starting questions with "tell me about" can help the client provide more information about the topic.

Beginning a question with "why" can feel judgmental or condescending to the client. "Why" type questions should be used with care.

Following are some open-ended questions that can be used during counseling sessions. These questions go hand-in-hand with a nonjudgmental approach, guided counseling, and MI.

- "Tell me more about [fill in the blank]." This question is another way to gather more information about what the client has said. The "tell me more" question allows the athletic trainer and client to more deeply explore an area.

- "What do you think about [fill in the blank]?" This question is usually used after providing a suggestion for change. The client then has the opportunity to tell the athletic trainer what they think about the suggestion.

Affirmations

Affirmations help build self-efficacy in clients. When an athletic trainer affirms something a client has said, the athletic trainer builds rapport with their client. Affirmations can help point out something positive the client may not even be aware of.[9]

An athletic trainer provides an affirmation when they highlight the positive component of something a client says.[9]

> **Sam:** My mom will be finishing her treatment soon. It will still be a while after that until she gets her strength back. I'm planning on keeping up what I've been doing for the family until she is ready.
>
> **Athletic Trainer:** You care about your mom and your family. You can be counted on to help them, especially your mom.

Reflection

Reflective listening is when the athletic trainer "reflects what the client is thinking and feeling and expresses this understanding back to the client."[10] When the athletic trainer practices reflective listening, trust is built by making the client feel understood and validated.[10] Reflections are statements, not questions. Reflections should also be short.

Reflections can be provided a few times through the session to help the client clarify their motivation to change.

> **Betty:** Yeah. I mean there have been a few practices where I've been tired. Coach has said I could play in college if I can pick up my game.
>
> **Athletic Trainer:** You're interested in playing in college and having enough energy to have great practice sessions.

Summaries

Summaries are similar to reflections, except that they are longer and provide a few key pieces of information back to the client. This gives the client the opportunity to fully see the information that has been discussed during the session. Summaries can be particularly helpful in clarifying ambivalence, changing their talk, and changing the client's motivation to change.[11]

In the example here, the athletic trainer is summarizing part of the session with Sam.

> **Athletic Trainer:** Let's take a step back and look at the bigger picture. You haven't been able to work out as consistently as you had and keep to your eating plan. You've been picking up a lot of things your mom took care of, including cooking for the family. Your family doesn't like to eat the way you do, and you find it frustrating that you're eating the way they like, not the way that makes you feel good. How did I do?

When the athletic trainer asks at the end "How did I do?" the client is being asked to confirm, correct, or add to what the athletic trainer has summarized.

After a summary has been provided, ask the client if it is accurate or not. Then allow the client time to think through the summary and respond. The athletic trainer can be quiet for a few minutes to allow the client to process the information before answering.

Motivational Interviewing Phases

MI includes 2 main phases. The first phase is when the athletic trainer explores with the client their ideas and attitudes about where they are now and the changes they are considering making. Phase 2 is when suggestions and instruction are provided to the client.

Session Phase 1

Session Phase 1 is focused on listening to the client, understanding their perspective, and eliciting change talk. This time in the counseling session allows the athletic trainer to express empathy for the client.[8] The athletic trainer can use the 4 microskills (OARS) of MI discussed previously. Using OARS can help the athletic trainer draw out and emphasize the client's desire to change.

Once the client has expressed the desire to change and is ready to hear ideas for changing their behavior, the athletic trainer can move the session to Phase 2.

Session Phase 2

The first step in Phase 2 is to ask permission to offer suggestions to the client. Asking for permission allows the MI-based spirit of collaboration to continue through the session. The athletic trainer could ask, "May I offer a suggestion?" or "Would you like to hear a few ways you could make some changes?"[8]

The following exchange happens after the athletic trainer provided a summary to Betty.

> **Betty:** You've got it!
>
> **Athletic Trainer:** Would you like a few ideas on how to begin making these changes?

The athletic trainer is asking for permission from Betty. When Betty agrees to allow the athletic trainer to make suggestions, she is being a partner in the process rather than being told what to do by the athletic trainer.

When providing ideas on how the client can make changes, the athletic trainer should provide a few suggestions at a time, then ask for feedback from the client on the suggestions. The client should understand that if they do not like an idea that the athletic trainer has provided, it is indeed OK. The athletic trainer must remember that the client is the expert of their own body and life. They have the right to reject any ideas that they feel will not work for them. The athletic trainer can explain that their personal feelings will not be hurt and it will not damage the trust or relationship if the client does not like one of the suggestions provided by the athletic trainer.

Confidentiality

Nutrition counseling by athletic trainers falls under the confidentiality guidelines provided by National Athletic Trainers' Association and its *Code of Ethics*. If the client is a minor, the athletic trainer should understand who may or may not have access to the counseling session, either by attending the session with the client, a meeting before or after the client meeting, or through written communication or phone calls. If you have questions about confidentiality, contact the National Athletic Trainers' Association.

Notes

During the session the athletic trainer can make notes about the session to help them remember pertinent information or points to revisit later. Notes can also be made on the forms provided by the client. After the session, a summary of the session can be recorded either in paper format or electronically.

Summary notes should include:
- Client goals
- Summary of what was covered
- Summary of actions the client has agreed to work on
- Date and time of next session

All notes should be kept in a secure location and treated as any other confidential medical information. The athletic trainer should be aware whether or not they fall under the Health Insurance Portability and Accountability Act (HIPAA) and comply with the appropriate standards.

Terminology

As times change, so does the terminology used. Athletic trainers should be aware of and use appropriate terminology when interacting with clients to show respect, understanding, and to build rapport.

Gender

Gender terminology should be as inclusive as possible. Appropriate gender terminology should be used with the client to align with their gender expression. Gender terminology can be extensive. A few of the more frequently used terms are defined here.
- *Androgynous:* Identifying and/or presenting as neither distinguishably masculine nor feminine.
- *Cisgender:* A term used to describe a person whose gender identity aligns with those typically associated with the sex assigned to them at birth.

- *Gender expression:* External appearance of one's gender identity, usually expressed through behavior, clothing, haircut, or voice, and which may or may not conform to socially defined behaviors and characteristics typically associated with being either masculine or feminine.
- *Non-binary:* An adjective describing a person who does not identify exclusively as a man or a woman. Non-binary people may identify as being both a man and a woman, somewhere in between, or as falling completely outside these categories. While many also identify as transgender, not all non-binary people do.

The definitions here are quoted from Human Rights Campaign's *Glossary of Terms*.[12] Additional gender terms can be found at https://www.hrc.org/resources/glossary-of-terms.

Weight Bias

The terms "overweight" and "obese" "have a troubling history,"[13] and use of these terms is not encouraged in discussions with clients. These terms have been used to stigmatize those in larger bodies that has led many of them to avoid seeking medical treatment, including routine care. Athletic trainers can help their clients, and those they interact with, by not expressing terms that show weight bias. Appropriate terms that can be used to discuss larger body sizes include "people in larger bodies" or "higher-weight people."[13]

Conducting Counseling Sessions

Structuring the Initial Session

When meeting with the client for the first time, the following structure may be helpful. It encompasses the 2 phases of MI and includes additional information to set the stage for understanding the client's situation and goals.

Review Goals and Forms

Begin the session by reviewing the client's goals for the session. Understanding the client's goals for the session helps the athletic trainer structure the session after the forms are reviewed. As the athletic trainer reviews the client's goals and forms, they can identify what stage of change they are in, which can then guide the discussions.

As the nutrition and health history form is being reviewed, ask questions about the information provided. In particular, review the following items: food allergies/intolerances, injuries/surgeries, and illnesses. Asking about food dislikes and why the client may dislike a certain food, such as aversions due to taste, texture, or smell, is important so that those issues can be taken into consideration when making recommendations for other foods. The same can be done with foods that a client may like or prefer.

Review the medication and supplement history forms. The athletic trainer should understand why the client is taking the medication/supplement and any improvements or side effects they may be experiencing. If the client is subject to doping control, a discussion of supplement testing along with the risk associated with a positive doping test is appropriate if the client is using untested supplements. You may recommend that they only use supplements that have been tested or verified to ensure purity and contamination. Cost is a consideration that the athletic trainer can include in the discussion on supplements. Those that are tested/verified may be more expensive than those that have not gone through the testing/verification process. However, it is ultimately their decision what to put in their body. For more information on dietary supplements, refer to Chapter 6.

Session Phase 1

Ask the client which goal they would like to discuss first. Generally, the client should be doing most of the talking. The athletic trainer can use the OARS covered previously in this chapter to help the client clarify the goals, any ambivalence they are experiencing about making the changes necessary to achieve their goals, and elicit change talk.

Session Phase 2

When the client is ready to move on to talking about solutions, the athletic trainer can ask for permission to offer suggestions. This is discussed in more detail in the Session Phase 2 section under MI. The client should also clearly understand that it is OK if they do not like the suggestions offered. The athletic trainer is providing ideas to help the client achieve their goals. Toward the end of the session, the athletic trainer can briefly summarize what has been covered in the session, emphasize the changes the client has agreed to work on, and set a time for the next session if it is appropriate or warranted.

Structuring Follow-Up Sessions

Follow-up sessions are structured like initial sessions without the review of the forms. The session begins with the Session Phase 1 and asking the client what they would like to focus on for the session. The follow-up session then continues with the athletic trainer using OARS until the client is ready to move into Session Phase 2 to talk about suggestions and changes.

Timing for Sessions

At the beginning of the session, the athletic trainer can confirm with the client the amount of time available for the session. The athletic trainer could begin the session with, "Thanks for meeting with me today. We have 30 minutes together today." Then, the athletic trainer can move into the session.

Initial sessions can take anywhere from 45 to 60 minutes depending on the forms used and the amount of detail required by the forms. Follow-up sessions can take 15 to 30 minutes depending on the client and goals.

Conclusion

Athletic trainers are a trusted resource for their clients. Nutrition counseling can be incorporated into an athletic trainer's offerings as long as they are comfortable with providing nutrition information and it is not restricted by state licensure. Understanding the basics of nutrition counseling, the models of offering counseling, and how to structure and conduct nutrition counseling sessions will help the athletic trainer successfully offer nutrition counseling sessions. If at any time the athletic trainer is not comfortable providing nutrition counseling for any reason, the client should be referred to a registered dietitian.

Discussion Questions

1. You have a nutrition counseling session with a football player in his junior year. On his intake form, he states that his main goal is to "get control of his eating." As you review the information he has provided, you see that his eating is sporadic—some days he eats frequent, large meals and other days he eats only one small meal. Using each counseling approach discussed in the chapter, how would you approach his goals? Provide at least 3 questions you would ask him to help understand his eating and why he feels he needs to "get control of his eating."

2. A female soccer player has made an appointment with you for help in answering some nutrition questions she has. After reviewing the information she has provided prior to the session, you see her goal is to "lean out." Her forms show that she is at an appropriate weight and build for her position. Provide a question for each OARS that could help you understand her desire to "lean out."

3. One of your clients states in their session the following: "I'm so busy with school, workouts, practices, homework—just everything! I can't make eating a priority. I'm totally overwhelmed." Using the information from the discussion on MI and the OARS, provide 3 examples of how you would help this client.

4. Reflect on the counseling approaches provided in this chapter. Which are you most comfortable with and why? Which are you least comfortable with and why? How could you gain more experience with the one you are least comfortable with?

5. Reflect on the topics you are comfortable covering in a nutrition counseling session. Write down those topics and why you are comfortable with them. Reflect on the topics you are uncomfortable covering in a nutrition counseling session. Write down the topics and why you are uncomfortable with them. For each topic, find a registered dietitian to whom you can refer these clients.

Suggested Reading

Clifford D, Curtis L. *Motivational Interviewing in Nutrition and Fitness.* The Guilford Press; 2015.

Harrison C. *Anti-Diet: Reclaim Your Time, Money, Well-Being, and Happiness Through Intuitive Eating.* Little, Brown, Spark; 2019.

Tribole E, Resch E. *Intuitive Eating: A Revolutionary Program That Works.* St. Martin's Griffin; 2012.

References

1. Burns RD, Schiller MR, Merrick MA, Wolf KN. Intercollegiate student athlete use of nutritional supplements and the role of athletic trainers and dietitians in nutrition counseling. *J Am Diet Assoc.* 2004;104:246-249.

2. Institute of Medicine (US) Committee on Nutrition Services for Medicare Beneficiaries. *The Role of Nutrition in Maintaining Health in the Nation's Elderly: Evaluating Coverage of Nutrition Services for the Medicare Population.* National Academies Press; 2000:1-2.

3. Tribole E, Resch E. *Intuitive Eating: A Revolutionary Program That Works.* St. Martin's Griffin; 2012:62-63.

4. Prochaska JO, Velicer WF. The transtheoretical model of health behavior change. *Am J Health Promotion.* 1997;12(1):38-48.

5. Spahn JM, Reeves RS, Keim KS, et al. State of the evidence regarding behavior change theories and strategies in nutrition counseling to facilitate health and food behavior change. *J Am Diet Assoc.* 2010;110:879-891.

6. Psychology Today Staff. Cognitive behavior therapy. *Psychology Today.* Retrieved from https://www.psychologytoday.com/us/basics/cognitive-behavioral-therapy

7. Clifford D, Curtis L. *Motivational Interviewing in Nutrition and Fitness.* The Guilford Press; 2015:25-26.

8. Glovsky ER, Rose G. Motivational interviewing—a unique approach to behavior change counseling. *Today's Dietitian.* 2007;9(5):50-55.

9. Clifford D, Curtis L. *Motivational Interviewing in Nutrition and Fitness.* The Guilford Press; 2015:109-110.

10. Clifford D, Curtis L. *Motivational Interviewing in Nutrition and Fitness.* The Guilford Press; 2015:120-121.

11. Clifford D, Curtis L. *Motivational Interviewing in Nutrition and Fitness.* The Guilford Press; 2015:134-135.

12. HRC Foundation. *Human Rights Campaign Glossary of Terms.* Retrieved from https://www.hrc.org/resources/glossary-of-terms

13. Harrison C. *Anti-Diet: Reclaim Your Time, Money, Well-Being, and Happiness Through Intuitive Eating.* Little, Brown, Spark; 2019:11.

Financial Disclosures

Dr. Melissa Brown is the co-owner of Pro-Style Nutrition Consulting, LLC that developed and owns the intellectual property of study prep materials for the Board Certification Exam in Sports Dietetics.

Melanie Clark reported no financial or proprietary interest in the materials presented herein.

Kyla Cross reported no financial or proprietary interest in the materials presented herein.

Dr. Jon P. Gray reported no financial or proprietary interest in the materials presented herein.

Dr. Layci Harrison reported no financial or proprietary interest in the materials presented herein.

Christina Curry King was paid as an independent contractor to promote Enhanced Recovery Sports Drink and provide content for their website and social media platforms from April 2020 to April 2021.

Dr. Mark Knoblauch reported no financial or proprietary interest in the materials presented herein.

Dr. Tara LaRowe reported no financial or proprietary interest in the materials presented herein.

Dr. Tracey Ledoux reported no financial or proprietary interest in the materials presented herein.

Dr. Tabbetha D. Lopez reported no financial or proprietary interest in the materials presented herein.

Dr. Mindy A. Patterson reported no financial or proprietary interest in the materials presented herein.

Andrea Rudser-Rusin reported no financial or proprietary interest in the materials presented herein.

Brett Singer reported no financial or proprietary interest in the materials presented herein.

Sarah Snyder works for the NFL Baltimore Ravens, is on the Sports Nutrition Advisory Panel (American Dairy Association NE), and is president of the NFL Sports RD Society.

Dr. E. Joanna Soles reported no financial or proprietary interest in the materials presented herein.

Cathy Tillery reported no financial or proprietary interest in the materials presented herein.

Mandy Tyler reported no financial or proprietary interest in the materials presented herein.

Dr. Penny Wilson reported no financial or proprietary interest in the materials presented herein.

Index

Printed in the United States
by Baker & Taylor Publisher Services